Dedication

To the memory of my parents, who taught me the value of perseverance and hard work.

To my wife Hengameh, my daughters Mahkameh and Morvarid,
and also my precious granddaughters Laila and Anabelle,
thanks for your understanding and tremendous support.

Table of Contents

Part I Introduction

Chapter 1: Fundamentals of Math — 2
- Overview — 3
- Number Systems — 4
  - Arabic Numbers — 4
  - Roman Numerals — 4
- Conversion between Roman Numerals to Arabic Numbers — 6
- Metric System — 7
  - Units of Measure — 8
  - Terminology and Abbreviations — 9
  - Metric Notation — 10
- Apothecary System — 13
- Household System — 15
- Milliequivalents and Units — 16

Chapter 2: Celsius and Fahrenheit Temperature Conversions — 24
- Overview — 25
- Temperature — 25
  - Converting between the Celsius and Fahrenheit Scales — 25
  - Common Medication Temperatures in the Pharmacy — 27

Chapter 3: Fractions and Decimals — 31
- Overview — 32
- Fractions — 33
  - Distinguishing Types of Fractions — 33
  - Comparing Fractions — 35
  - Converting Improper Fractions to Mixed or Whole Numbers — 37
  - Converting Mixed or Whole Numbers to Improper Fractions — 37
  - Finding the Least Common Denominator — 39
  - Reducing Fractions to the Lowest Terms — 41
  - Adding Fractions — 42
  - Subtracting Fractions — 43
  - Multiplying Fractions — 44
  - Dividing Fractions — 45

Pharmaceutical Calculations

for Pharmacy Technicians

Third Edition

Pharmaceutical Calculations
for Pharmacy Technicians

Jahangir Moini, MD, MPH, CPhT

Professor and Former Director, Allied Health Sciences,
including the Pharmacy Technician Program,
Everest University, Melbourne, Florida
and Professor of Science and Health (retired),
Eastern Florida State College, Palm Bay, Florida

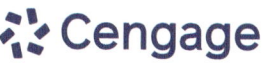

Australia • Brazil • Canada • Mexico • Singapore • United Kingdom • United States

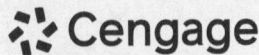

Pharmaceutical Calculations for Pharmacy Technicians, Third Edition
Jahangir Moini

SVP, Product: Cheryl Costantini

VP, Product: Thais Alencar

Portfolio Product Director: Jason Fremder

Associate Portfolio Product Director: Laura Stewart

Associate Portfolio Product Manager: Meryem Fqih

Product Assistant: Tennessee Sundermeyer

Learning Designer: Elinor Gregory

Content Manager: Ava O'Dea

Digital Project Manager: Andy Baker

Technical Editor: Obehi Enabulele

Developmental Editor: Peter McGahey

VP, Product Marketing: Jason Sakos

Director, Product Marketing: Neena Bali

Product Marketing Manager: Annie Gillingham

Content Acquisition Analyst: Erin McCullough

Production Service: Lumina Datamatics Ltd.

Senior Designer: Felicia Bennett

Cover Image Source: inxti/Shutterstock.com, paulista/Shutterstock.com

Interior Image Source: paulista/Shutterstock.com

Last three editions, as applicable: © 2013, © 2007

Copyright © 2024 Cengage Learning, Inc. ALL RIGHTS RESERVED.

No part of this work covered by the copyright herein may be reproduced or distributed in any form or by any means, except as permitted by U.S. copyright law, without the prior written permission of the copyright owner.

Unless otherwise noted, all content is Copyright © Cengage Learning, Inc.

The names of all products mentioned herein are used for identification purposes only and may be trademarks or registered trademarks of their respective owners. Cengage Learning disclaims any affiliation, association, connection with, sponsorship, or endorsement by such owners.

For product information and technology assistance, contact us at
**Cengage Customer & Sales Support, 1-800-354-9706
or support.cengage.com.**

For permission to use material from this text or product, submit all requests online at **www.copyright.com**.

Library of Congress Control Number: 2023904929

ISBN: 978-0-357-76597-5

Cengage
200 Pier 4 Boulevard
Boston, MA 02210
USA

Cengage is a leading provider of customized learning solutions. Our employees reside in nearly 40 different countries and serve digital learners in 165 countries around the world. Find your local representative at **www.cengage.com**.

To learn more about Cengage platforms and services, register or access your online learning solution, or purchase materials for your course, visit **www.cengage.com**.

Notice to the Reader
Publisher does not warrant or guarantee any of the products described herein or perform any independent analysis in connection with any of the product information contained herein. Publisher does not assume, and expressly disclaims, any obligation to obtain and include information other than that provided to it by the manufacturer. The reader is expressly warned to consider and adopt all safety precautions that might be indicated by the activities described herein and to avoid all potential hazards. By following the instructions contained herein, the reader willingly assumes all risks in connection with such instructions. The publisher makes no representations or warranties of any kind, including but not limited to, the warranties of fitness for particular purpose or merchantability, nor are any such representations implied with respect to the material set forth herein, and the publisher takes no responsibility with respect to such material. The publisher shall not be liable for any special, consequential, or exemplary damages resulting, in whole or part, from the readers' use of, or reliance upon, this material.

Printed at CLDPC, USA, 10-24

Decimals 51
    Converting Fractions to Decimals and Decimals to Fractions 52
    Adding Decimals 54
    Subtracting Decimals 54
    Multiplying Decimals 56
    Dividing Decimals 57
    Rounding Decimals 59

Chapter 4: Ratios, Proportions, and Percentages   64

Overview 65
Ratios 65
Proportions 67
Percentages 69
    Changing Percentages to Decimals 70
    Changing Decimals to Percentages 70
    Changing Percentages to Fractions 70
    Changing Fractions to Percentages 71
    Determining Percentages 71

Chapter 5: Percentage of Errors Due to Equipment   76

Overview 77
Measurement of Weight 77
Measurement of Volume 78
Percentage of Error 81
Calculating Percentage of Error When Weighing 81
Calculating Percentage of Error in Volumetric Measurement 82

Part II   Dosage Calculations

Chapter 6: Ratio and Proportion Method   88

Overview 89
Ratio and Proportion Expressed Using Common Fractions 89
    Dosage Calculations 91
Ratio and Proportion Expressed Using Colons 95
    Dosage Calculations 96
Calculations Using Different Units of Measure 97

Chapter 7: Dimensional Analysis — 109
- Overview 110
- Basic Dimensional Analysis 110
- Equations Requiring Metric Conversions 113
- Dosage Calculations Using Dimensional Analysis ... 116

Chapter 8: Formula Method — 128
- Overview 129
- Basic Formula 129
- Use with Metric Conversions 131
- Use with Units and Milliequivalent Calculations ... 132

Part III Concentrations and Dilutions

Chapter 9: Concentrations — 138
- Overview 139
  - Concentrations and Volumes of Solutions ... 140
- Weight/Weight 142
- Volume/Volume 143
- Weight/Volume 145
- Ratio Strength 148

Chapter 10: Dilutions and Solutions — 154
- Overview 155
- Dilutions 155
- Stock Solutions for Solids 155
  - Stock Vials and Ampules 156
- Liquid Dilutions 156
- Alligation 158

Part IV Medication Preparation

Chapter 11: Oral Medication Labels and Dosage Calculation — 170
- Overview 171
- Tablet and Capsule Labels and Calculations ... 171
- Oral Solution Labels 183
- Measurement of Oral Solutions 184

Chapter 12: Reconstitution of Powdered Drugs — 195

    Overview 196
    Reconstitution of a Single-Strength Solution 196
    Reconstitution of Multiple-Strength Solutions 205

Chapter 13: Parenteral Medication Labels and Dosage Calculation — 209

    Overview 210
    Reading Metric Solution Labels 210
    Percent and Ratio Solution Labels 211
    Solutions Measured in International Units 212
        Insulin Injections 212
        Types of Insulin 212
        Insulin Labels 213
        Mixing Insulins 214
        Measuring Insulin in an Insulin Syringe 215
        Combination Insulin Dosage 216
    Solutions Measured as Milliequivalents 223
    Calculating Parenteral Drug Dosages 225

Chapter 14: Intravenous Flow Rate Calculations — 238

    Overview 239
    IV Push 240
    Continuous Intravenous Infusions 243
        Solution Additives 246
        Percentage in IV Fluids 248
        Parenteral Nutrition 249
    Calculating IV Components as Percentages 249
        Calculating IV Flow Rates 251
        Calculating Flow Rates Using Ratio and Proportion 255
        Calculating Flow Rates Using Dimensional Analysis 258
        Calculating Flow Rates Using the Formula Method 259
        Calculating Flow Rates Using the Shortcut Method 262
        Adjusting IV Flow Rates 263
        Flow Rates for Electronic Regulation 268

Heparin Intravenous Calculations..271
    Calculating IV Flow Rate from Units Per Hour Ordered 273
    Calculating Units Per Hour Infusing from IV Flow Rate......................274
Intermittent Intravenous Injections 276
    IV Piggybacks (IVPB) 276

Chapter 15: Pediatric Drug Administration — 285

Overview 286
Calculating Pediatric Dosages 286
    Body Weight Dosage Calculations...287
    Body Surface Area (BSA) Dosage Calculations 295
    Clark's Rule 300
    Young's Rule 300
    Fried's Rule 300
Intramuscular Drugs...301
Intravenous Drugs 302
    Intermittent IV Drug Infusion Using a Volume
    Control Set 303
Daily Maintenance Fluid Needs 307

Chapter 16: Business Math for Pharmacy Technicians — 314

Overview 315
Markup..315
    Percent Markup 316
    Percent Markup Plus a Professional Fee 317
Gross Profit...317
Net Profit...318
Discounts..319
Depreciation 320
Inventory Turnover 321
    Average Wholesale Price 322
Wholesale Acquisition Cost..322
Insurance Reimbursements 323

Appendices

Appendix A: Answers to Stop and Review Exercises 327
Appendix B: Answer Key to Test Your Knowledge Questions 337
Appendix C: Case Studies with Answers 350
Glossary 353
Index 357

Preface

Pharmaceutical Calculations for Pharmacy Technicians, Third Edition, is developed for the pharmaceutical calculations course, a first course primarily for undergraduate and postgraduate pharmacy technician students. It features a great amount of expansion on the original edition, including three new chapters, plus a thorough reworking of the book's organization. However, other health science students whose roles involve drug therapy (such as medical assistants and nurses) should also find much of the material relevant to their studies. Some pharmaceutical calculation texts have been strong on pharmacy technician considerations, yet relatively weak in the organization of content and practice problems, or have lacked instructor resources and learning resources for students.

My goal in this book is to empower pharmacy technicians through an understanding of the fundamental skills of calculating drug dosages and converting them within the metric, apothecary, and household systems. Additional calculations in the book focus on pediatric dosages.

I believe that developing an understanding of basic math and becoming proficient in drug dosage calculation and conversion are critical skills for pharmacy technicians, in that they play an important role in preventing medication errors that occur all too frequently in the United States.

Organization of the Text

The book is organized in a natural progression of information, allowing users to master the information in order, ranging from simple to more complex. It is divided into 4 parts and 16 chapters, followed by 3 appendices. Chapters 1 through 5 focus on basic math skills such as number systems, conversions, terminology, abbreviations, fractions, decimals, ratios, proportions, percents, and errors due to equipment. Chapters 6 through 8 focus on dosage calculation methods, including ratio and proportion, dimensional analysis, and the formula method. Chapters 9 through 16 focus on topics concerning medication preparation. These topics include oral and parenteral medication labels, dosage calculations, reconstitution of powdered drugs, intravenous flow rate calculations, pediatric drug administration, and business math for pharmacy technicians.

The first two appendices feature answers to the Stop and Review exercises and the Test Your Knowledge questions. The third appendix features case studies with answers. There is also a glossary and index. This text is published in full color, which helps to illustrate key points and concepts. It highlights unique learning tools that will reinforce skills and competencies.

New to the Third Edition

- New online homework—textbook problems are now available in *WebAssign*, allowing instructors to assign autograded online homework, quizzes, and tests.
- New content—new sections on common medication temperatures in the pharmacy in Chapter 2 and depreciation in Chapter 16.
- Updated table of contents—the table of contents has been reorganized to provide an even better flow of information.
- Updated learning objectives—chapter learning objectives more precisely define the key concepts and skills students should understand.
- Updated Critical Thinking exercises—more Critical Thinking exercises have been added to several chapters.

Features of This Text

- **Learning objectives** outline the skills students should be able to perform upon completion of each chapter.
- **Worked examples** illustrate how to perform calculations.
- **Remember boxes** highlight important tips to help students be successful.
- **Stop and Review exercises** provide opportunities to practice calculations presented in each section.
- **Test Your Knowledge questions** are summative assessments that cover all the skills and concepts presented throughout the chapter.
- **Critical Thinking exercises** are scenario-based activities that ask students to apply what they've learned to real-world situations.
- **Case studies** at the back of the book are more comprehensive real-world scenarios in which students must think critically to determine the best course of action and apply what they've learned.

WebAssign

Built by educators, *WebAssign* offers flexible settings at every step to customize your course with online activities and secure testing. Students get everything in one place, including quality content and study resources designed to deepen understanding and an interactive eTextbook. Proven to support problem-solving skills, *WebAssign* fosters learning in any course delivery model.

Instructor Resources

Additional instructor resources are available online. Instructor assets include an Instructor's Manual, Complete Solution Manual, PowerPoint® slides, Educator's Guide, a test bank powered by Cognero®, and more. Sign up or sign in at **www.cengage.com** to search for and access this product and its online resources.

- Instructor's Manual—available for each chapter; describes the purpose and perspective of each chapter and incorporates suggested activities into the chapter outline
- Complete Solutions Manual—provides solutions and answers to textbook questions
- PowerPoint® slides—support lectures with definitions, examples, and activities
- Educator's Guide—offers suggested content for *WebAssign* to help you personalize your course
- Cengage Testing, powered by Cognero®—a flexible, online system that allows you to access, customize, and deliver a test bank from your chosen text to your students through your LMS or another channel outside of *WebAssign*
- Transition Guide—outlines changes between the second and third editions of the textbook

Acknowledgments

It is my pleasure to acknowledge the reviewers, past and present, who have helped with the development of this textbook over the years.

Christy Bevins, BS
Pharmacy Technology Professor and
Licensed Pharmacist
North Georgia Technical College
Clarkesville, Georgia

Brenda A. Ghigliotto
Pharmacy Technician Instructor
San Pablo, California

Christie E. Martin, ABD, MSM, CPhT
Pharmacy Program Coordinator
Northwest Vista College
San Antonio, Texas

Michelle Miller
Pharmacy Technician Instructor
Kirkwood Community College
Cedar Rapids, Iowa

Mary G. Nelson
Pharmacy Technician Specialty
Pharmacy Services, Inc.
Melbourne, Florida

Douglas Scribner, MEd, CPhT
Director of Pharmacy Technology
Central New Mexico Community College
Albuquerque, New Mexico

Bobbi Jane Steelman, CPT, BSEd, MAEd
Pharmacy Technician Program Director
Daymar Colleges Group
Bowling Green, Kentucky

Mohamad Tlass, BS, CPhT, PhTR
Pharmacy Technician Professor
Houston Community College
Houston, Texas

About the Author

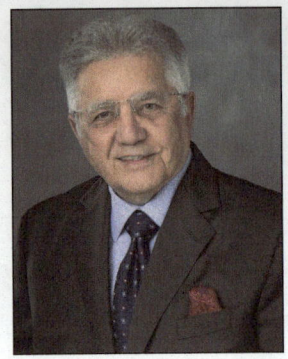

Dr. Moini was an assistant professor at Tehran University School of Medicine for nine years, teaching medical and allied health students. He was a professor and former director (for 15 years) of allied health programs at Everest University. Dr. Moini established the associate degree program for pharmacy technicians in 2000 at Everest's Melbourne, Florida, campus. For five years, he was also the director of the pharmacy technician program. Then he went to Eastern Florida State College, where he served as a professor of science and health for six years. He is now retired.

Dr. Moini was actively involved in teaching and helping students to prepare for service in various health professions, including the role of pharmacy technicians. He is an internationally published author of 51 allied health books (since 1999), including nine books related to pharmacy technology for Cengage Learning. His "Anatomy and Physiology for Health Professionals" was translated and released in South Korea and Japan. Also, his "Complications of Diabetes Mellitus" was translated and released in Spain.

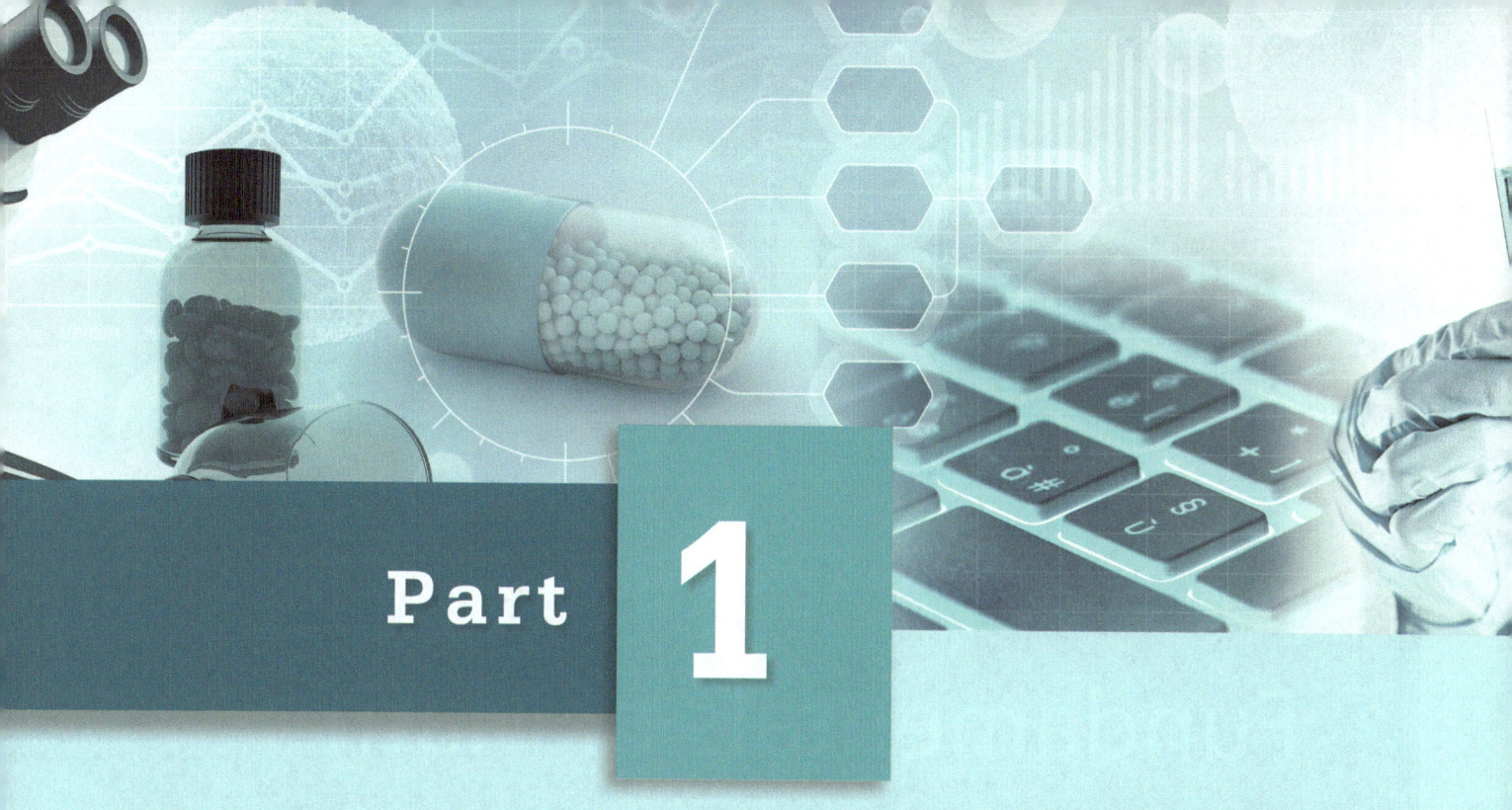

Part 1

Introduction

Chapter 1 Fundamentals of Math

Chapter 2 Celsius and Fahrenheit Temperature Conversions

Chapter 3 Fractions and Decimals

Chapter 4 Ratios, Proportions, and Percentages

Chapter 5 Percentage of Errors Due to Equipment

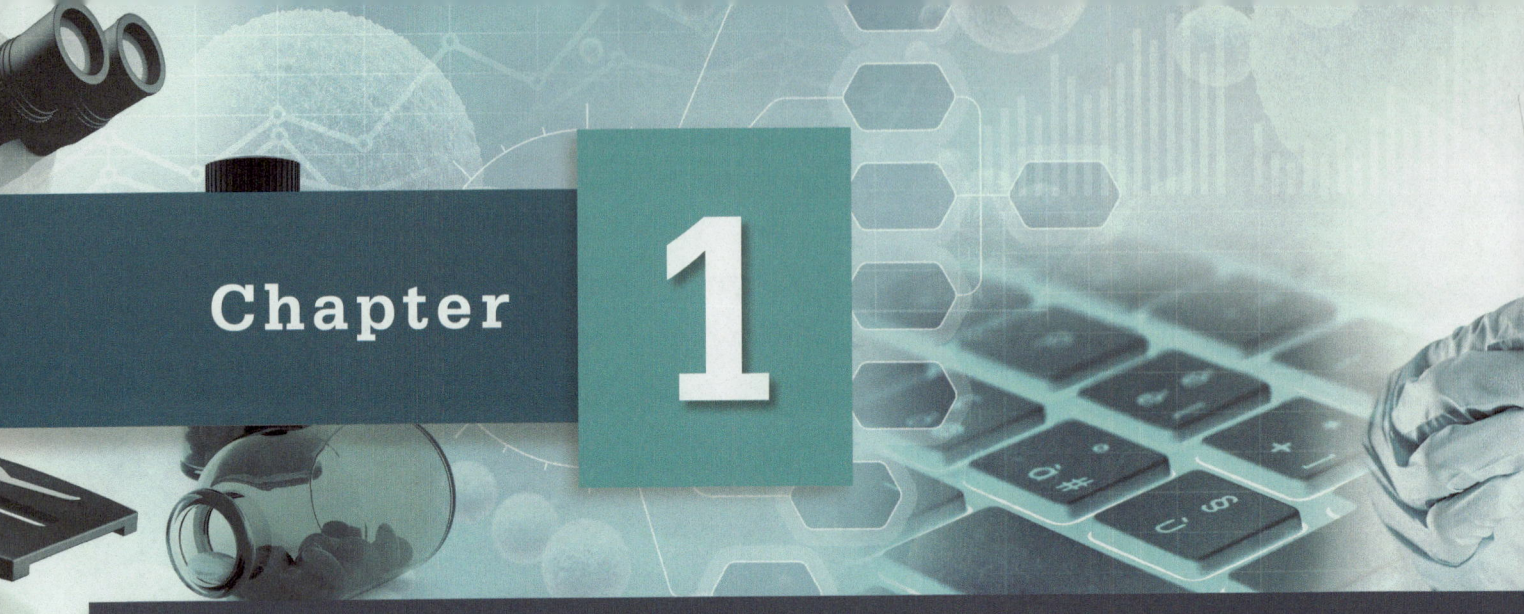

Chapter 1

Fundamentals of Math

Outline

Overview

Number Systems
- Arabic Numbers
- Roman Numerals

Conversion between Roman Numerals to Arabic numbers

Metric System
- Units of Measure
- Terminology and Abbreviations
- Metric Notation

Apothecary System

Household System

Milliequivalents and Units

Objectives

Upon completion of this chapter, you should be able to:

1. Convert Arabic numbers into Roman numerals, and Roman numerals into Arabic numbers.
2. Perform basic computations including addition, subtraction, multiplication, and division using Roman numerals and Arabic numbers.
3. List the basic units of weight, volume, and length.

Objectives continued

4. Demonstrate how to write abbreviations and use notation rules for metric, apothecary, and household units.
5. Calculate equivalent measurements within the metric system.
6. Compare apothecary and household equivalents.
7. Write measurements using apothecary symbols.
8. Interpret symbols from different systems that are used in pharmacy.
9. Convert equivalent household measurements.
10. Convert between household and metric measurements.
11. Calculate measurements in milliequivalents and units

Key Terms

apothecary system
Arabic numbers
exponent
gram
household system

international unit
liter
meter
metric system
milliequivalent

milliunit
Roman numerals
scientific notation
Système International (SI)
unit

Overview

To prevent medication errors, the pharmacy technician must be able to add, subtract, multiply, and divide whole numbers, fractions, and decimals. These are basic math skills/competencies that will contribute to a technician's success in preparing accurate dosages. Pharmacy technicians must be able to use basic mathematics to calculate the dosage of drugs by weight and measures of volume. The technician must be able to solve various types of mathematical problems. Therefore, it is essential for the pharmacy technician to have a sound knowledge of basic mathematical skills.

It also is necessary for pharmacy technicians to understand the systems of measurement and how to convert from one system to another in order to reduce the risk of medication errors. Three systems are used for measuring drugs and solutions: the metric, apothecary, and household systems. The weight of the patient and correct amount of the medication prescribed to the patient are essential factors in performing calculations in the various systems of measurement. Dosage calculations are most concerned with the measurement of weight and volume.

Number Systems

The two systems of numbers currently used in pharmacy are Arabic and Roman. Both systems are used in drug administration. The most common types of numbers used throughout the world today are Arabic. However, the pharmacy technician must also be able to interpret Roman numerals because they are still in use.

Arabic Numbers

Arabic numbers make up a system that is based on the digits 0, 1, 2, 3, 4, 5, 6, 7, 8, and 9. Any number can be represented by combining these digits. Arabic numbers can be written as whole numbers, fractions (for example, $\frac{1}{3}$), and decimals (for example, 0.6). The Arabic system is commonly used for counting.

Roman Numerals

Roman numerals consist of letters used to represent number values. The building blocks of the Roman system include the uppercase letters I, V, X, L, C, D, and M (**Table 1-1**).

Roman numerals are written as either uppercase or lowercase letters. For example, iv represents the number 4, and it is generally written in lowercase to distinguish it from the uppercase letters IV, which is the abbreviation for "intravenous." Sometimes a horizontal line is written above lowercase letters. When the letter "i" is written with this line, the dot of the i appears above the line.

Table 1-1   Roman Numerals

Roman Numeral	Arabic Equivalent
$\overline{SS}$ or $\overline{ss}$	$\frac{1}{2}$
I or i	1
V or v	5
X or x	10
L or l	50
C or c	100
D or d	500
M or m	1000

Reading Roman Numerals

Roman numerals are read by adding or subtracting the value of the letters. When a letter appears twice in a row, the value of the letter is counted twice (Example 1a). When it appears three times in a row, the value is counted three times (Example 1g). Letters are never used more than three times in a row. If a lower-valued letter follows a larger-valued letter, the letter values should be added (Example 1b). The letter with the largest number equivalent possible should be used to represent a value. If a lower-valued letter is placed before a higher-valued letter, the lower-valued letter is subtracted from the higher-valued letter (Example 2a).

■ Example 1:

a. ii = 1 + 1 = 2
b. vi = 5 + 1 = 6
c. vii = 5 + 1 + 1 = 7
d. xii = 10 + 1 + 1 = 12
e. xxv = 10 + 10 + 5 = 25
f. xxvii = 10 + 10 + 5 + 1 + 1 = 27
g. xxx = 10 + 10 + 10 = 30

■ Example 2:

a. iv = 5 − 1 = 4
b. ix = 10 − 1 = 9
c. XL = 50 − 10 = 40

When a Roman numeral of smaller value comes between two other Roman numerals with larger values, subtract the smaller numeral from the one to its right. Then, add the remaining values.

■ Example 3:

Calculate the Arabic number for xiv. In xiv, the letter i is located between two letters with larger values. Subtract i from v first, and then add.

$$xiv = x + iv = x + (v - i) = 10 + (5 - 1)$$
$$= 10 + 4 = 14$$

■ Example 4:

Calculate the Arabic for LXIX.

First, subtract I from X, and then add the remaining values.

$$LXIX = L + X + IX = L + X + (X - 1)$$
$$= 50 + 10 + (10 - 1) = 50 + 10 + 9 = 69$$

■ Example 5:

a. vi + xiii = 6 + 13 = 19
b. XII + VI = 12 + 6 = 18
c. XXIV − IX = 24 − 9 = 15
d. XLIX − XXXI = 49 − 31 = 18

> **》》》 Remember**
>
> - If a letter with a smaller value immediately follows a letter with a larger value, add their values.
> - If a letter with a smaller value appears immediately before a letter with a larger value, subtract the smaller value from the larger one. The uppercase letters V, L, and D cannot be subtracted from another number.
> - When a smaller-valued letter falls between two larger-valued letters, subtract the smaller value from the letter on the right, and then add that value to the letter on the left.

Use of Roman Numerals

Unlike the Arabic system used in everyday counting, the Roman system has no symbol for zero. Roman numerals are used less frequently in dosage calculations. In pharmacy practice, Roman numerals may be used to denote quantities on prescriptions (**Figure 1-1**). The use of this system is restricted because mathematical procedures would become extremely complicated if one were to attempt using these numerals in calculations. The technician needs to understand Roman numerals to interpret prescriptions and drug dosages correctly.

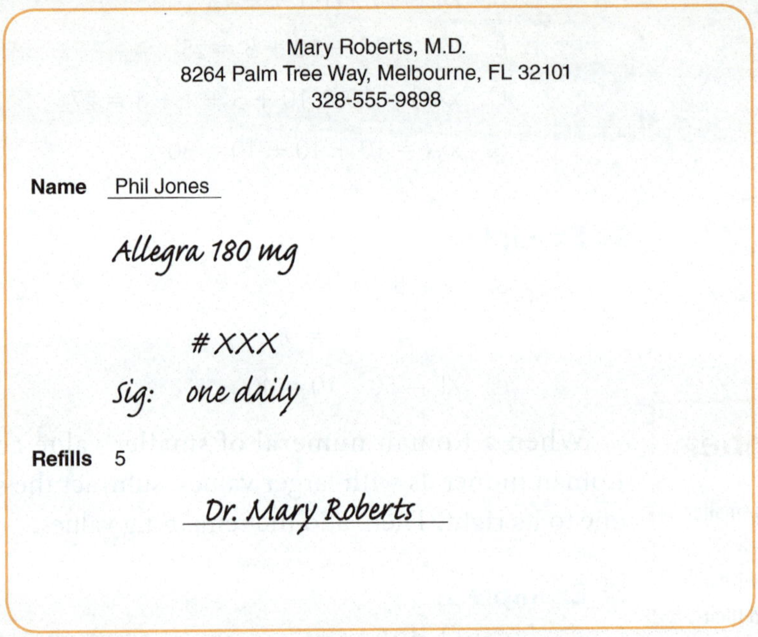

Mary Roberts, M.D.
8264 Palm Tree Way, Melbourne, FL 32101
328-555-9898

Name   Phil Jones

Allegra 180 mg

XXX

Sig: one daily

Refills   5

Dr. Mary Roberts

Figure 1-1 Roman numerals may be used on prescriptions.
© Cengage Learning 2013

Conversion between Roman Numerals to Arabic Numbers

To convert Roman numerals to Arabic numbers, convert the Roman symbols to Arabic symbols and add or subtract as described previously. See **Table 1-2** for a list of Roman numerals and their Arabic equivalents.

■ **Example 1:**

a. xv = 10 + 5 = 15

b. xxviii = 10 + 10 + 5 + 1 + 1 + 1 = 28

c. xix = 10 + (10 − 1) = 10 + 9 = 19

d. xxx = 10 + 10 + 10 = 30

Table 1-2 Converting the Roman System to Arabic

Roman Numeral	Arabic Number
I, i	1
II, ii	2
III, iii	3
IV, iv	4
V, v	5
VI, vi	6
VII, vii	7
VIII, viii	8
IX, ix	9
X, x	10
XI, xi	11
XII, xii	12
XIII, xiii	13
XIV, xiv	14
XV, xv	15
XVI, xvi	16
XVII, xvii	17
XVIII, xviii	18
XIX, xix	19
XX, xx	20
XXI, xxi	21
XXII, xxii	22
XXIII, xxiii	23
XXIV, xxiv	24
XXV, xxv	25
XXVI, xxvi	26
XXVII, xxvii	27
XXVIII, xxviii	28
XXIX, xxix	29
XXX, xxx	30

Metric System

The **metric system** was developed in France in the eighteenth century for scientific studies and calculations. In the United States, most people use the English system, which utilizes inches, feet, miles, pounds, and tons to describe length and weight. These units are hard to calculate because of how the units relate to each other. For example, 16 ounces equal 1 pound.

Today, the metric system is the official system of weight and measures used for weighing and calculating pharmaceutical preparations. The metric system is becoming the accepted system throughout the world. This system is sometimes referred to as the *International System of Units* (derived from the French, **Système International [SI]**). The SI metric system is the most widely accepted system. The basic units that make up the metric system are summarized in **Table 1-3**. Pharmacy technicians need to be concerned primarily with the divisions of weight, volume, and linear measurement of the metric system. Each of these divisions has a primary or basic unit.

Table 1-3   SI Metric System

System	Unit	Symbol	Equivalents
Weight	**gram (base unit)**	g	1 g = 1000 mg
	milligram	mg	1 mg = 1000 mcg = 0.001 g
	microgram	mcg	1 mcg = 0.001 mg = 0.00001 g
	kilogram	kg	1 kg = 1000 g
Volume	**liter (base unit)**	L (or l)	1 L = 1000 mL
	milliliter	mL	1 mL = 1 cc = 0.001 L
	cubic centimeter	cc	1 cc = 1 mL = 0.001 L
Length	**meter (base unit)**	m	1 m = 100 cm = 1000 mm
	centimeter	cm	1 cm = 0.01 m = 10 mm
	millimeter	mm	1 mm = 0.001 m = 0.1 cm

Units of Measure

The metric system has three basic units of measurements. Each of these divisions has a primary or basic unit as follows:

- Basic unit of weight is the **gram**, abbreviated as the lowercase letter g
- Basic unit of volume is the **liter**, abbreviated as the lowercase letter l or as an uppercase "L"
- Basic unit of length is the **meter**, abbreviated as the lowercase letter m

Terminology and Abbreviations

The metric system is a decimal system based on multiples of 10 and fractions of 10. It is important to learn the most commonly used prefixes and abbreviations of the metric system. The metric system uses prefixes with all measures. These prefixes indicate the size of the unit (root) being measured in multiples of 10. **Figure 1-2** details the use of prefixes as applied to the appropriate basic unit of measure. It shows that 10 g equals 1 dekagram, 100 g equals 1 hectogram, and 1000 g is referred to as 1 kilogram. Conversely, going down the scale, 0.1 g is referred to as 1 decigram, 0.01 g is called 1 centigram, and 0.001 g is known as a milligram.

1000	100	10	1	0.1	0.01	0.001
Kilo	Hecto	Deka	One	Deci	Centi	Milli
				$\frac{1}{10}$	$\frac{1}{100}$	$\frac{1}{1000}$

Figure 1-2 Metric systems prefixes and their decimal and fractional equivalents.
© Cengage Learning 2013

The basic structure of the metric system's prefixes is shown in **Table 1-4**. **Table 1-5** illustrates examples of common metric abbreviations.

Table 1-4 Prefixes

Prefixes for Larger Units	Prefixes for Smaller Units
giga (G) 1,000,000,000 (one billion) m = 1 Gm	deci (d) 0.1 (one-tenth) m = 1 dm
mega (M) 1,000,000 (one million) m = 1 Mm	centi (c) 0.01 (one-hundredth) m = 1 cm
kilo (k) 1000 (one thousand) m = 1 km	milli (m) 0.001 (one-thousandth) m = 1 mm
hecto (h) 100 (one hundred) m = 1 hm	micro (μ) 0.000001 (one-millionth) m = 1 μm
deka (D) 10 (ten) m = 1 Dm	nano 0.000000001 (one billionth) m = 1 nm

Table 1-5 Common Metric Abbreviations

Measure	Abbreviations
nanogram	ng
microgram	mcg
milligram	mg
gram	g
kilogram	kg
milliliter	mL
deciliter	dL

(Continues)

Table 1-5 (Continued)

Measure	Abbreviations
liter	L
millimeter	mm
centimeter	cm
meter	m
kilometer	km
kiloliter	kl

Metric Notation

The metric system uses decimals to express units of weight, volume, and length. From these units, temperature, speed, force, and other properties of the physical universe can be measured.

Recall that in the metric system, weight is described in grams, length is described in meters, and volume is described in liters. Each unit can increase or decrease by factors of 10, making calculations easier than in the English system. Note that prefixes like *kilo-* (thousand), *mega-* (million), *centi-* (hundredth), and *milli-* (thousandth) can be used to modify the units. For example, a kilometer is 1000 meters, and a centimeter is 0.01 meter.

For writing and interpreting metric notation accurately, remember the following rules:

- Do not guess about the true meaning. When in doubt, ask the writer for clarification.

- The abbreviation always follows the amount (for example, 25 g, not g 25).

- Decimals are used to designate fractional metric units (for example, 7.5 mL, not $7\frac{1}{2}$ mL).

- Use a leading zero to emphasize the decimal point for fractional metric units of less than 1 (for example, 0.75 mg, not .75 mg).

- Omit trailing zeros (for example, 6.5 g, not 6.50 g).

- Write the prefix before the basic unit of measure (such as putting "centi-" before the basic unit of measure "meter" = "centimeter").

■ **Example 1:**

To represent micrograms, write mcg, not gmc or microg.
- Use lowercase letters for metric abbreviations. However, use an uppercase "L" to represent liters.

■ **Example 2:**

Write mg in lowercase letters, not as the uppercase letters MG. Write mL with a lowercase m and an uppercase L, not ml written only in lowercase

> **Remember**
>
> - The basic unit of weight is the gram (a lowercase g).
> - The basic unit of volume is the liter (an uppercase L).
> - The basic unit of length is the meter (a lowercase m).
> - Prefixes accompany the basic units to denote the unit in multiples of 10.
> - Numbers in the metric system can be presented in scientific notation as a number × 10 to a particular power. To determine the power of 10, count the places from the decimal point in the number.

letters. Although the lowercase ml is technically correct, errors can be avoided by using an uppercase L.

- Insert a space between the quantity and the unit.

■ **Example 3:**

Write 15 L by using an uppercase L and include a space between the 15 and the uppercase L. The 15 and the uppercase L should not be written without a space between because it could cause an error if the reader mistakes the letter L for a number. Another example is when writing 75 kg, in which a space must be between the 75 and the lowercase kg, not written together without a space.

Exponents and Scientific Notation

An **exponent** is a way of expressing a number that is multiplied by itself (for example, $5 \times 5 \times 5 \times 5 = 5^4$; this is expressed as 5 to the 4th power). **Scientific notation** is a shorthand method for expressing large numbers that are a product of a number between 1 and 10 and a power of 10 (for example, 7,000,000 can be expressed as 7×10^6; 7 is multiplied by 1,000,000). Because the metric system uses factors of 10, the use of exponents and scientific notation is an easy way to express large metric units. An easy way to determine the power of 10 is to count the number of zeros in the number or the number of places after the decimal point (for example, 10^5 means "10 to the 5th power," which is expressed as $10 \times 10 \times 10 \times 10 \times 10$, equating to 100,000).

■ **Example 4:**

If you are given a value of 5.5×10^5, the number is equivalent to 550,000; 5.5 is multiplied by 100,000.

Stop and Review

Convert the following metric measures.

1. 2500 mL = _____ L
2. 630 mg = _____ g
3. 1600 mcg = _____ mg
4. 1300 mg = _____ g
5. 500 mL = _____ L
6. 150 mg = _____ g
7. 850 cc = _____ L
8. 250 mcg = _____ mg
9. 5500 mcg = _____ mg
10. 100 mg = _____ g

Stop and Review

Write the following measures by using official abbreviations and notation rules.

1. five grams = _____
2. two hundred milliliters = _____
3. five-tenths of a liter = _____
4. three-hundredths of a gram = _____
5. four hundred micrograms = _____
6. two-tenths of a milligram = _____
7. four-tenths of a milligram = _____
8. nine hundred micrograms = _____
9. ten and three-tenths micrograms = _____
10. two and seven-tenths kilograms = _____
11. five-hundredths of a gram = _____
12. six and four-tenths kilograms = _____

 Stop and Review

Abbreviate the following metric units.

1. milligram = _____
2. millimeter = _____
3. gram = _____
4. microgram = _____
5. kilogram = _____
6. meter = _____
7. milliliter = _____
8. liter = _____
9. centimeter = _____
10. kiloliter = _____

Apothecary System

The **apothecary system** is an old system of measurement. This system is not widely used today because it has been replaced by the metric system. The measures used in the apothecary system are approximate instead of exact. Pharmacy technicians must still be familiar with the apothecary system. Certain medications, especially older ones such as aspirin, quinine, and nitroglycerin, are still measured in apothecary units (**Figure 1-3**).

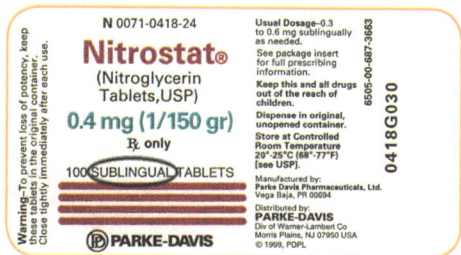

Figure 1-3 Some medications, such as nitroglycerin, still use apothecary systems of measurement.
Label reproduced with permission of Pfizer, Inc.

The basic unit of weight in the apothecary system is the grain (abbreviated as a lowercase gr). The apothecary system utilizes Roman numerals. The uppercase letters I, V, and X are the basic symbols of this system that pharmacy technicians use in dosage calculations. In medical notation, lowercase letters are typically used to designate Roman numerals such as i, v, and x.

Besides Roman numerals, apothecary notation also uses common fractions, special symbols, and units of measure that precede numeric values. The common units are the grain (abbreviated as a lowercase gr) and ounce (a lowercase oz or the ounce symbol, ʒ). **Table 1-6** lists commonly used apothecary system units of measure.

Table 1-6 Apothecary System Units of Measure

Solid Weight	Liquid Volume
60 grains = 1 dram	60 minims = 1 fluidram (fl dr)
8 drams = 1 ounce	8 fluidrams = 1 fluid ounce (fl oz)
12 ounces = 1 pound	

In the apothecary system, the symbol or abbreviation comes first, followed by the quantity, which is expressed in lowercase Roman numerals, for example, gr vi, which means 6 grains. Usually only the digits 1 through 10, 20, and 30 are expressed in Roman numerals. Most other quantities are expressed in Arabic numbers. However, numerals from 1 through 10, 20,

> > > **Remember**

- Apothecary measures are approximate, not exact.
- The basic unit of apothecary weight is the grain (lowercase gr).
- The apothecary system uses Roman numerals and fractions.
- The symbol or abbreviation comes first, followed by the quantity expressed in Roman numerals.

and 30 are written in Arabic if the entire unit measurement is written in full. For example, 18 grains would not be written xviii grains because the word *grains* is written out; it is either 18 grains or gr xviii.

Another difference between the metric system and the apothecary system is that fractions are used in the apothecary system when necessary. (Remember that metric quantities are expressed in decimals.) For example, the fraction three-quarters is notated as $\frac{3}{4}$ in the apothecary system but as 0.75 in the metric system. The exception to this rule is the fraction $\frac{1}{2}$. In apothecary notation, $\frac{1}{2}$ is expressed by the Roman numeral ss written below a straight line ($\overline{ss}$). **Table 1-7** shows the notations used in the apothecary system.

Table 1-7 Apothecary System Abbreviations

Term	Abbreviation	Symbol
Minim	min	♏
Dram	dr	ʒ
Ounce	oz	℥
Grain	gr	(none)
Pound	lb	(none)

Stop and Review

Write the following measurements using apothecary symbols.

1. 3 grains _____
2. $\frac{2}{3}$ dram _____
3. 8 ounces _____
4. 4 pounds _____
5. $\frac{1}{200}$ of a grain _____
6. $\frac{1}{2}$ dram _____
7. 3 ounces _____
8. 2 pounds _____
9. 2 pounds and 11 ounces _____
10. $\frac{1}{2}$ grain _____

Household System

The **household system** of measurement is still commonly used today. It was developed so that patients could measure out dosages at home using ordinary containers found in the kitchen. For example, cups and spoons are simple containers that anyone can use to administer or take medicine. Many over-the-counter medications provide guidelines for patients who depend on household measures. Pharmacy technicians should be familiar with the household system of measurement so that they can explain take-home prescriptions to their patients at the time of discharge. As **Table 1-8** shows, when dispensing medications, the four smallest measures are most frequently used. Household notation places the quantity in Arabic numerals (numbers and common fractions) before the abbreviation for the unit. This system has no standardized system of notation.

Table 1-8 Household Abbreviations

Unit	Abbreviation	Equivalents
Drop	gtt	60 drops = 1 tsp
Teaspoon	t (or tsp)	6 tsp = 1 oz
Tablespoon	T (or tbsp)	1 T = 3 t
Ounce (fluid)	oz (℥)	2 T = 1 oz
Ounce (weight)	oz	1 pound (lb) = 16 oz
Cup	C (or c)	1 c = 8 oz
Pint	pt	1 pt = 2 cups
Quart	qt	1 qt = 4 cups = 2 pt
Gallon	gal	4 qt = 1 gal

Household measurements are inaccurate, with wide variations in the size of teaspoons, tablespoons, and so forth. The generally accepted household measures are the following:

- 60 drops (lowercase gtt) = 1 teaspoon (lowercase tsp or t)
- 3 tsp = 1 tablespoon (lowercase tbsp or uppercase T)
- 16 tbsp = 1 glass (or a standard measuring cup)

Household measurements can be equated to apothecary units using the following:

- 1 drop = 1 minim
- 1 tsp = 1 dr
- 1 tbsp = $\frac{1}{2}$ oz

> **》》》 Remember**
>
> - The household system is a common system of measurement used by regular people in their homes.
> - It is very inaccurate due to variations in sizes of household measuring devices.
> - It is written in Arabic numbers, with abbreviations used for units of measure following the numbers.

- 2 tbsp = 1 oz
- 1 cup = 8 oz
- 1 glass = 8 oz
- 2 measuring cups = 1 pt

Stop and Review

Convert the following to the equivalent unit indicated using the household system.

1. 75 drops = _____ tsp

2. 24 oz = _____ cups

3. 3 tbsp = _____ oz

4. 4 cups = _____ oz

5. 8 tsp = _____ tbsp

Milliequivalents and Units

Some other measurements can be used for the quantity of medicine ordered. They include units (formerly abbreviated as an uppercase U), milliunits (formerly abbreviated as mU, with the m being lowercase and the U being uppercase), international units (no longer abbreviated as an uppercase IU to avoid confusion with the abbreviation IV that means "intravenous"), and milliequivalents (mEq, with the m being lowercase, the E being uppercase, and the q being lowercase). The quantity is shown in Arabic numbers with the symbol following. The **unit** is a standardized amount required to provide a desired effect. Medications such as insulin, heparin, and penicillin have their own meaning and numeric value related to the type of unit. One-thousandth of a unit is a **milliunit**. The equivalent of one unit is 1000 milliunits. Pitocin is one example of a medication measured in milliunits. The **international unit** is a unit of potency used to calculate vitamins and chemicals. The **milliequivalent** (mEq) is one-thousandth of an equivalent weight of a chemical substance. The mEq is the unit used to describe the concentration of serum electrolytes such as sodium, potassium, and calcium.

Medications that are measured in units, international units, and milliequivalents are prepared and administered in the same system. Therefore, there is no need to learn conversions for these systems.

■ Example 1:

What volume of a 1000 units/1 mL heparin stock drug is needed to prepare an order for Heparin 800 units?

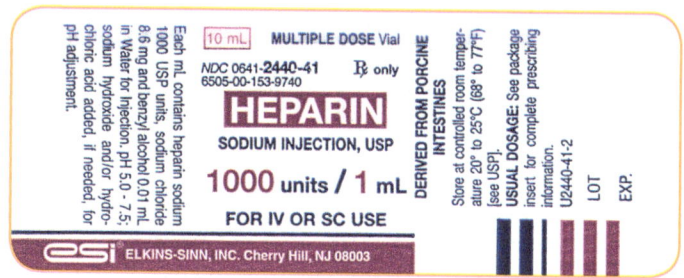

Heparin.
Courtesy of ESI Lederle, a Business Unit of Wyeth Pharmaceuticals, Philadelphia, PA

■ Example 2:

What volume of a 20 mEq per 15 mL potassium chloride stock drug is needed to prepare an order for potassium 5 mEq?

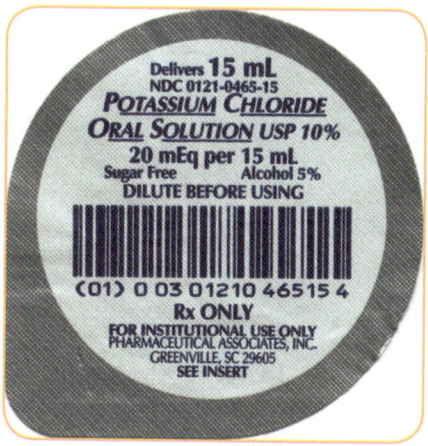

Potassium Chloride.
Courtesy of Pharmaceutical Associates, Inc.

■ Example 3:

What volume of an oxytocin 10 international units/1 mL stock drug, to be added to 1000 mL intravenous solution, is needed to prepare an order for oxytocin 2 milliunits (0.002 international unit) intravenous per minute?

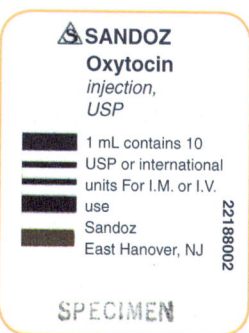

Oxytocin injection, USP 1 mL contains 10 USP or international units for I.M. or I.V. use.
© Cengage Learning 2013

> **Remember**
>
> - A unit is a standard of measurement based on the biological activity of a drug.
> - A milliunit is one-thousandth of a unit.
> - A milliequivalent is one-thousandth of a comparable substance whose chemical mass will combine with 1 gram of hydrogen or 8 grams of oxygen.
> - An international unit is a measurement of the potency of a vitamin or chemical.

Test Your Knowledge

Convert the following Arabic numbers to Roman numerals.

1. 5 _____
2. 18 _____
3. 9 _____
4. 16 _____
5. 19 _____
6. 22 _____
7. 24 _____
8. 27 _____
9. 29 _____
10. 30 _____
11. 45 _____
12. 89 _____
13. 112 _____
14. 155 _____
15. 198 _____
16. 202 _____
17. 506 _____
18. 534 _____
19. 1000 _____
20. 1025 _____

Convert the following Roman numerals to Arabic numbers.

21. IV _____
22. VII _____
23. IX _____
24. XIII _____

25. XIV _____

26. XVIII _____

27. XIX _____

28. XXIV _____

29. XXVII _____

30. XXIX _____

Convert the following Roman numerals to Arabic numbers.

31. VII + XI _____

32. VIII + IV _____

33. V + VI _____

34. xiv + xvii _____

35. xvi + v _____

36. XIX − xiii _____

37. xxvi − viii _____

38. XV − V _____

39. xiii − iv _____

40. ix − vi _____

Abbreviate the following units of measure.

41. minim _____

42. pint _____

43. grain _____

44. fluid ounce _____

45. dram _____

46. drop _____

47. fluid dram _____

48. quart _____

49. kilogram _____

50. liter _____

51. milligram _____

52. gram _____

53. milliliter _____

54. microgram _____

55. meter _____

56. centimeter _____

57. tablespoon _____

58. cup _____

59. teaspoon _____

60. gallon _____

61. ounce _____

Write the following metric measures using abbreviations and notation rules.

62. four-hundredths of a gram = _____

63. seventeen and five-tenths kilograms = _____

64. three and five-tenths kilograms = _____

65. five and three-tenths milliliters = _____

66. ten and four-tenths micrograms = _____

67. two hundred micrograms = _____

68. fifteen and two-tenths micrograms = _____

69. six-tenths of a liter = _____

70. eight grams = _____

71. four-tenths of a milliliter = _____

72. nine-hundredths of a milligram = _____

Write the amounts using either apothecary or household notation when appropriate.

73. five grains _____

74. one-half teaspoon _____

75. nine ounces _____

76. seven and one-half ounces _____

77. sixteen grains _____

78. one-half grain _____

79. four drams _____

80. twenty-five milliequivalents _____

81. ten thousand units _____

82. one-half tablespoon _____

83. three and one-half ounces _____

84. one-half ounce _____

Give the equivalents to each measurement.

85. 5 tablespoons = _____ t

86. 3 ounces = _____ T

87. 4 cups = _____ oz

88. 5 cups = _____ oz

89. 1 teaspoon = _____ gtt

90. 24 ounces = _____ cups

91. 90 drops = _____ t

92. 6 teaspoons = _____ T

Interpret the following symbols.

93. m = _____

94. ʒ = _____

95. ɱ = _____

96. gr = _____

97. qt = _____

98. oz = _____

99. ℥ = _____

100. (s̄s̄) = _____

101. mm = _____

102. g = _____

Write the symbols or abbreviations for the following measurements.

103. drop _____

104. grain _____

105. teaspoon _____

106. minim _____

107. tablespoon _____

108. dram _____

109. milliequivalent _____

110. pint _____

111. ounce _____

Complete the following statements with the correct words.

112. Meters and millimeters are metric units that measure _____.

113. Liters and milliliters are metric units that measure _____.

114. Grams and milligrams are metric units that measure _____.

Fill in the blanks with the correct equivalents to each measurement.

115. 1 kg = _____ g

116. 1000 mcg = _____ mg

117. 1 cm = _____ mm

118. 1 liter = _____ cc

119. 10 mL = _____ cc

120. 1 km = _____ m

121. 1 mm = _____ cm

Circle the correct metric notation.

122. mg10, 10 mG, 10.0 mg, 10 mg, 10 MG

123. 4.5 mL, 4.50 mL, 4.50 ML, $4\frac{1}{2}$ ML, 4.500 mL

124. 7 kg, 7.0 kg, 7-kg, 7 KG, kg 07

125. 2.5 mm, $2\frac{1}{2}$ mm, 2.5 Mm, 2.50 MM, $2\frac{1}{2}$ MM

126. 8.5 mcg, 8.50 mcg, $8\frac{1}{2}$ Mcg, 8.5 MCG, 8.5 MCG

Critical Thinking

1. A pharmacy technician is dispensing a prescription that reads: 15 mL of cough suppressant three times per day (tid) for 10 days. The technician must answer the following questions:

    a. Which household equipment should the patient use?

    b. How much medication should the patient take, given the device he was recommended to use?

    c. If the medication is supplied in half-pint bottles, how many bottles will the patient need during the 10 days?

2. A pharmacy technician is reading a prescription:

    tetracycline 250 mg Capsule
    # LXIV

    The technician cannot remember the numeric equivalent for the Roman numeral L. He needs to know it in order to dispense the physician's request. What is the next step that he should take?

3. How many tablets of a 0.625 mg tablet are required to fill a prescription for conjugated estrogen, 1.25 mg?

4. What is the equivalent Arabic number for the Roman numeral CCXL?

5. To convert kilograms to pounds, you must multiply by 2.2. For example, 4 kilograms (kg) multiplied by 2.2 is equal to 8.8 lb. How many kilograms equals a weight of 16.4 lb?

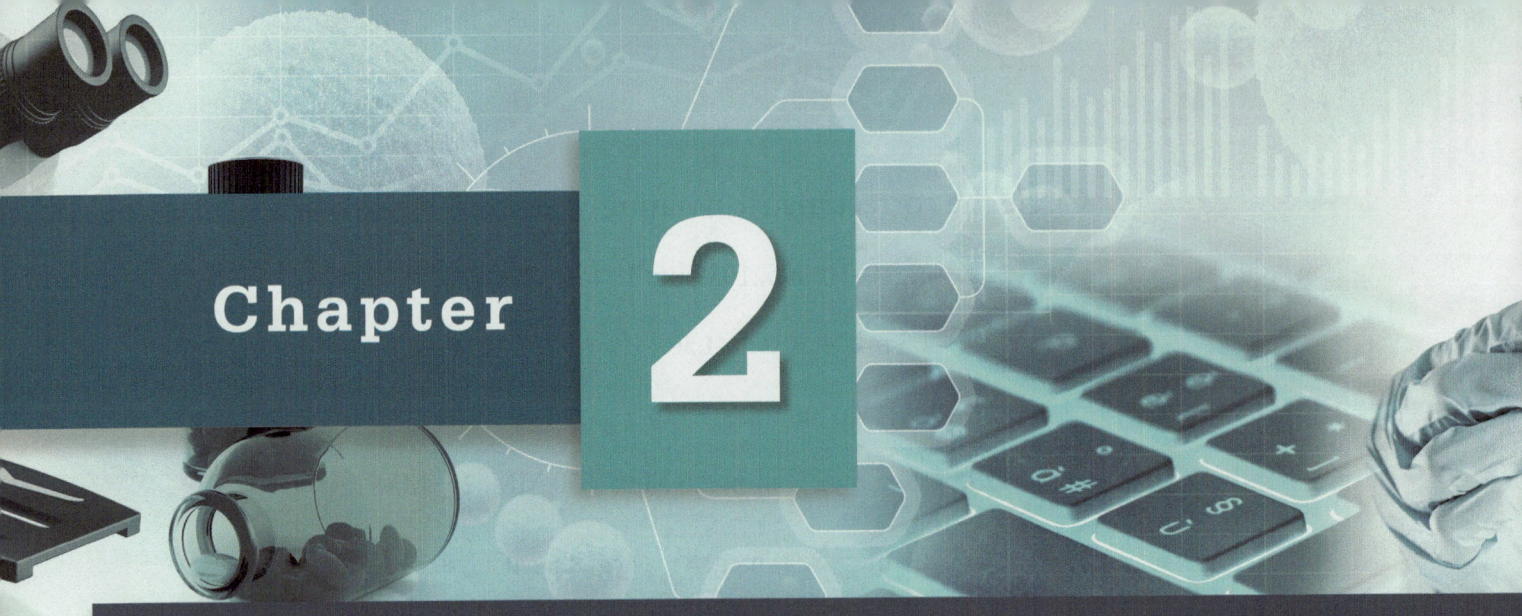

Chapter 2

Celsius and Fahrenheit Temperature Conversions

Outline

Overview

Temperature

    Converting between the Celsius and Fahrenheit Scales

    Common Medication Temperatures in the Pharmacy

Objectives

Upon completion of this chapter, you should be able to:

1. Convert between Celsius and Fahrenheit temperatures.
2. List common medication temperatures in the pharmacy.
3. Explain what the pharmacy technician is required to do concerning incorrect refrigerator and freezer temperatures.
4. Identify which vaccines must be frozen, not refrigerated.

Key Terms

Celsius scale
centigrade

Fahrenheit scale
temperature

Overview

Pharmacy technicians should be familiar with measurements of temperature and also be able to convert them. Correct temperatures are essential for the proper storage of drugs and vaccines. Many different medications and substances must be kept refrigerated until use. The temperature of the pharmacy refrigerator must be kept constant and requires regular monitoring by the pharmacy technician. Many medications list storage temperatures in either Celsius or Fahrenheit. Also, because body temperature is measured as part of diagnosing medical conditions, the ability to convert between Celsius and Fahrenheit temperatures is essential for pharmacy technicians.

Temperature

Temperature is defined as a relative measure of sensible heat or cold. Normally, the human body is maintained at a constant level of 98.6° Fahrenheit (F) (or 37° Celsius [C]) by the body's Thermotaxis nerve mechanism that balances heat gains and heat losses.

Temperature scales have two basic points: from when water starts to freeze and when it starts to boil. Between these two temperatures, a scale is made. The most popular scales are the Celsius (created by Anders Celsius) and Fahrenheit (made by Gabriel Fahrenheit) scales. The **Fahrenheit scale** is defined so that the freezing point of water occurs at 32 degrees Fahrenheit and the boiling point occurs at 212 degrees Fahrenheit. This means that there are 180 divisions between the freezing point and boiling point.

The **Celsius scale** differs in that the freezing point of water occurs at 0 degrees Celsius and the boiling point occurs at 100 degrees Celsius. This scale (also referred to as "**centigrade**") exists on 100-unit divisions and is also known as a "centiscale." In 1948, the "centidegrees" (centigrade scale) was replaced by "degrees Celsius" (°C).

Converting between the Celsius and Fahrenheit Scales

Temperatures are most often reported in Fahrenheit and, occasionally, also in Celsius. A formula has been developed to compute conversions between the two scales based on the differences between the freezing and boiling points of each scale (**Figure 2-1**). Recall that there are 100 degrees between the boiling and freezing points on the Celsius thermometer, and 180 degrees between the boiling and freezing points on the Fahrenheit thermometer. The ratio of the difference between the Fahrenheit and Celsius scales can be expressed as 180:100, or:

$$\frac{180}{100}$$

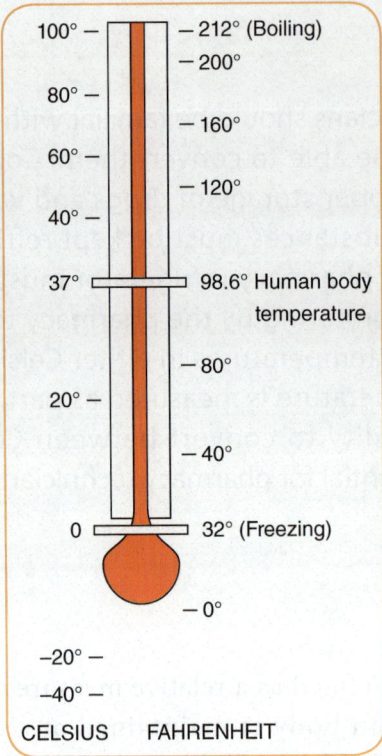

Figure 2-1 Comparison of Celsius and Fahrenheit scales.
© Cengage Learning 2013

When reduced, this ratio is equivalent to 1.8.

This equivalent of 1.8 is constantly used in temperature conversions between Fahrenheit and Celsius via the following formulas:

$$°C = \frac{°F - 32}{1.8} \text{ and } °F = (1.8 \times °C) + 32$$

■ Example 1:

Convert: 99.4°F to °C.

Substituting 99.4 for °F in the conversion formula, 99.4°F = °C:

$$\frac{99.4 - 32}{1.8} = \frac{67.4}{1.8} = 37.4°C$$

Use the following formula to convert a temperature from Celsius to Fahrenheit:

$$°F = (1.8 \times °C) + 32$$

■ Example 2:

Convert: 20°C to °F.

Substituting 20 for °C in the conversion formula:

$$(1.8 \times 20) + 32 = 36 + 32 = 68$$

Thus, 20°C = 68°F.

》》》 Remember

- To convert Fahrenheit to Celsius, use the following formula:

$$°C = \frac{°F - 32}{1.8}$$

- To convert Celsius to Fahrenheit, use the following formula:

$$°F = (1.8 \times °C) + 32$$

Common Medication Temperatures in the Pharmacy

Most over-the-counter and prescription medications can be stored at room temperature, and will remain stable. The active ingredient(s) in any medication may change in molecular form when exposed to different temperatures. This can result in decomposition of the medication, making it less potent or resulting in new or different effects on the body. Many medications can be maintained at temperatures as low as 52°F (11°C), such as the liquid forms of amoxicillin and interferon beta. A few medications maintain their composition even if they are frozen. No medications can be stored at temperatures above 86°F (30°C) because they will become degraded. Examples of medication storage recommendations include the following:

- Lipitor (atorvastatin calcium) and Norvasc (amlodipine besylate)—room temperature
- Toprol (metoprolol succinate) and Synthroid (levothyroxine)—room temperature, but can be temporarily transported at temperatures between 59°F (15°C) and 86°F (30°C)
- Veletri (epoprostenol)—must be kept between 35.6°F (2°C) and 46.4°F (8°C)

Factors that can expose medications to dangerously high temperatures include hot weather, storing medications in a car for an extended period of time, putting medications into luggage while traveling on a plane, loss of power in pharmacies, and non-temperature-regulated delivery trucks for mail-order medications.

> **Remember**
>
> - The pharmacy technician must be aware of the proper temperatures for all vaccines stored in the pharmacy. The majority of vaccines must be refrigerated at between 35.6°F (2°C) and 46.4°F (8°C), with a preferred average of 41°F (5°C). Some live vaccines must be frozen at between 5°F (−15°C) and −58°F (−50°C), including varicella (chickenpox), and zoster (shingles) vaccines. Of the COVID-19 vaccines, the Pfizer vaccine must be frozen while it is being transported at −94°F (−70°C), and the Moderna vaccine requires a less cold temperature, but is still frozen during transport, at −4°F (−20°C). These vaccines can be refrigerated once they arrive at a storage facility. The Pfizer vaccine can be refrigerated for up to 31 days, and the Moderna vaccine can be refrigerated for up to 30 days. If a pharmacy technician discovers that any refrigerator or freezer in the pharmacy is not at the required temperature, they must document the findings and alert the pharmacist.

Stop and Review

Convert the following temperatures.

1. 37°C = _____ °F
2. 93°F = _____ °C
3. 62°F = _____ °C
4. 104°F = _____ °C
5. 42.7°C = _____ °F
6. 188°F = _____ °C
7. 100°C = _____ °F
8. 87°C = _____ °F
9. 109°F = _____ °C
10. 22°C = _____ °F

Convert the following statements of temperature to Celsius or Fahrenheit.

11. Normal body temperature is 98.6°F. _____

12. Medication must not be exposed to a temperature >88°F. _____

13. A patient has a fever of 102.8°F. _____

14. You need to keep a vaccine at a temperature of 6°C. _____

15. A physician orders antipyretic medication and adds a note that the patient should stop taking it if his body temperature lowers to 38.5°C. _____

Another method can be used to convert Fahrenheit to Celsius: subtract 32 and then multiply the result by $\frac{5}{9}$.

1. To begin, subtract 32 from the Fahrenheit number.

2. Divide the answer by 9.

3. Multiply the answer by 5.

■ **Example 3:**

Convert: 95°F to Celsius.

$$95 - 32 = 63 \quad 63 \div 9 = 7 \quad 7 \times 5 = 35°C$$

Table 2-1 lists a few common temperatures with approximate descriptions.

Table 2-1 Common Temperatures

°F	°C	Description
212	100	Boiling point of water
98.6	37	Normal body temperature
86	30	Very hot summer day
72	22	Room temperature
68	20	Mild spring day
50	10	Warm winter day
32	0	Freezing point of water
20	−7	Very cold winter day

Chapter 2 • Celsius and Fahrenheit Temperature Conversions

 Test Your Knowledge

Give the following temperature equivalents as indicated. Those temperatures given in °F should be converted to °C and vice versa.

1. 63.4°F _____
2. 99.5°F _____
3. 87.2°F _____
4. 178°F _____
5. 132°F _____
6. 32°F _____
7. 112°F _____
8. 212°F _____
9. 44°F _____
10. 97.8°F _____
11. 164°F _____
12. 48°F _____
13. 0°C _____
14. 6.8°C _____
15. 2.4°C _____
16. 37.4°C _____
17. 100°C _____
18. 43.6°C _____
19. 32°C _____
20. 8.4°C _____
21. 55°C _____
22. 17°C _____
23. 0.12°C _____
24. 27°C _____

Critical Thinking

1. A prescription is written for a child who has a fever of more than 101°F. She is to be given acetaminophen every 4 hours. Her mother asks a pharmacy technician to tell her the Celsius temperature equivalent of 101°F.

2. A vaccine must be kept in the pharmacy refrigerator at 8°C. What is the equivalent Fahrenheit temperature?

3. Most medications must be kept at home at average room temperature, which is 20°C. What is the equivalent Fahrenheit temperature?

4. A hospital pharmacy technician routinely checked refrigerator and freezer temperatures for accuracy. One day, he discovered the temperatures to be higher than required, and the freezer containing live vaccines had a temperature of 10°F. What must the pharmacy technician do?

5. COVID-19 vaccinations were scheduled to be given in a health clinic, and the frozen vaccines were brought there by a pharmacist. Which COVID-19 vaccines must be frozen during transport?

6. What is the lowest temperature that amoxicillin should be refrigerated at?

7. At which temperature should Lipitor and Toprol be stored?

8. At what temperature will all medications become degraded?

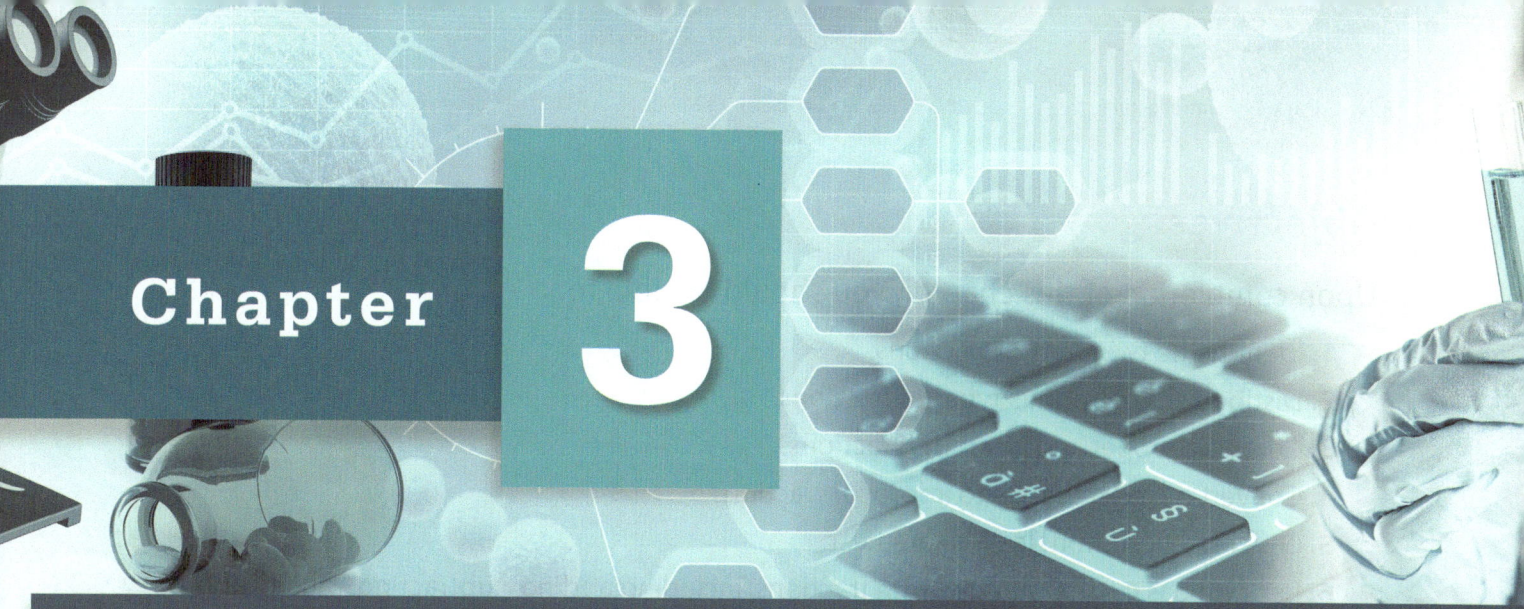

Chapter 3

Fractions and Decimals

Outline

Overview

Fractions
- Distinguishing Types of Fractions
- Comparing Fractions
- Converting Improper Fractions to Mixed or Whole Numbers
- Converting Mixed or Whole Numbers to Improper Fractions
- Finding the Least Common Denominator
- Reducing Fractions to the Lowest Terms
- Adding Fractions
- Subtracting Fractions
- Multiplying Fractions
- Dividing Fractions

Decimals
- Converting Fractions to Decimals and Decimals to Fractions
- Adding Decimals
- Subtracting Decimals
- Multiplying Decimals
- Dividing Decimals
- Rounding Decimals

Objectives

Upon completion of this chapter, you should be able to:

1. Identify the two parts of fractions.
2. Distinguish the various types of fractions.
3. Compare proper and improper fractions.
4. Convert mixed numbers to improper fractions.
5. Order fractions from least to greatest.
6. Perform basic computations with fractions, including adding, subtracting, multiplying, dividing, finding the lowest common denominator, and reducing.
7. Convert fractions to mixed numbers and decimals.
8. Convert decimals to fractions.
9. Perform basic computations with decimals, including adding, subtracting, multiplying, and dividing.
10. Round decimals to the nearest whole number, tenth, hundredth, and thousandth.
11. Order decimal numbers from least to greatest.

Key Terms

common fraction
complex fraction
decimal fraction
denominator
dividend

divisor
fraction
improper fraction
mixed fraction
multiplicand

multiplier
numerator
proper fraction
quotient

Overview

Correct dosage calculations play a large role in ensuring that medications are administered accurately and safely. Pharmacy technicians must learn fractions and decimals to be able to calculate the dosage of drugs by weight and measures of volume. The pharmacy technician must also be able to convert from fractions to decimals as well as from decimals to fractions. Fractions and decimals provide a way to express the relationship of parts to a whole. Fractions measure a portion or part of a whole amount. The decimal system provides another way to represent whole numbers and their fractional parts. Pharmacy technicians use fractions and decimals in their daily work and must be able to work with decimals and fractions proficiently.

Fractions

Fractions can help pharmacy technicians interpret and act on physicians' orders, read prescriptions, and understand patient records and information in the pharmacy literature. Fractions are used in household and apothecary measures for dosage calculations. A **fraction** is a portion of a whole number and represents parts of the whole. The top number is called the **numerator**. The bottom number is called the **denominator**, which represents the whole. Therefore, a fraction has two parts. It can never equal zero. The diagram in **Figure 3-1** represents fractions of a whole.

$$\frac{\text{Numerator (3 parts)}}{\text{Denominator (4 parts)}} = \frac{3}{4}$$

The fraction $\frac{3}{4}$ is used to represent "three-fourths." It means three parts out of a total four parts that make up the whole. The fraction bar also means "divided by." Thus, $\frac{3}{4}$ can be read as "three divided by four," or $3 \div 4$. This definition is important when one changes fractions into decimals.

Distinguishing Types of Fractions

The two types of fractions are common and decimal. A **common fraction** usually is represented as equal parts of a whole. A **decimal fraction** is commonly referred to simply as a decimal. Decimals are covered later in this chapter. The four types of common fractions are proper, improper, mixed, and complex.

Proper Fractions

A **proper fraction** has a numerator that is smaller than the denominator. When the numerator is smaller than the denominator, the value of the fraction is always less than 1 (**Figure 3-2**).

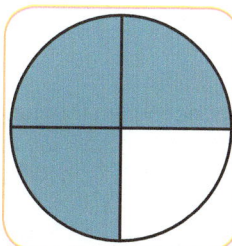

Figure 3-1 The fraction 3/4 means three parts out of a total of four parts that make up the whole.
© Cengage Learning 2013

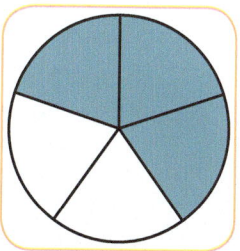

Figure 3-2 The value of a proper fraction is always less than 1.
© Cengage Learning 2013

■ **Example 1:**

$$\frac{3}{5} = \frac{\text{numerator}}{\text{denominator}} = < 1$$

Other examples of proper fractions are $\frac{2}{5}, \frac{1}{10}, \frac{26}{47},$ and $\frac{125}{1000}$.

Improper Fractions

An **improper fraction** has a numerator that is equal to or greater than the denominator. The symbol < means "is less than," and > means "is greater than." When the numerator is larger than the denominator, the value of the fraction is always greater than 1 (**Figure 3-3**).

$$\frac{\text{numerator}}{\text{denominator}} > 1 \text{ or } \frac{6}{4} = > 1$$

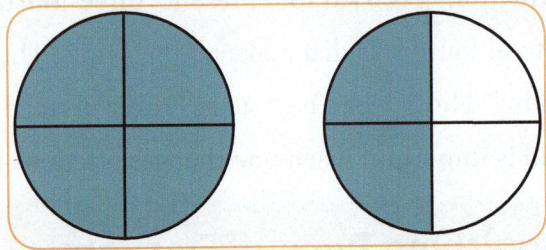

Figure 3-3 The value of an improper fraction is always greater than 1.
© Cengage Learning 2013

When the numerator is equal to the denominator, the value of the fraction is always exactly 1 (**Figure 3-4**). If the numerator = the denominator, then:

$$\frac{\text{numerator}}{\text{denominator}} = 1 \text{ or } \frac{6}{6} = 1$$

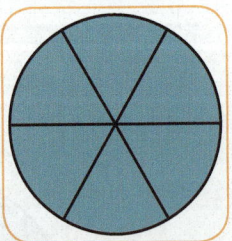

Figure 3-4 The value of an improper fraction when the numerator and the denominator are equal is always 1.
© Cengage Learning 2013

■ **Example 2:**

Examples of improper fractions include:

$$\frac{7}{5}, \frac{19}{13}, \frac{153}{18}, \text{ and } \frac{1200}{100}$$

Example 3:

Examples of improper fractions that equal 1 include:

$$\frac{7}{7}, \frac{16}{16}, \frac{111}{111}, \text{ and } \frac{1333}{1333}$$

Mixed Fractions

A **mixed fraction** has a whole number and a proper fraction that are combined. The value of the mixed fraction is always greater than 1 (**Figure 3-5**).

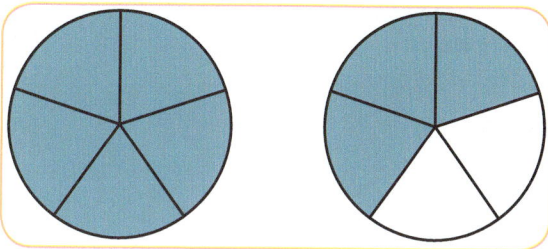

Figure 3-5 The value of a mixed fraction is always greater than 1.
© Cengage Learning 2013

Example 4:

$$1\frac{3}{5} = 1 + \frac{3}{5} \text{ or } 1\frac{3}{5} > 1$$

Complex Fractions

A **complex fraction** is a fraction in which the numerator or the denominator, or both, may be a whole number, proper fraction, or mixed fraction. The value may be less than, greater than, or equal to 1.

Example 5:

$$\frac{\frac{4}{9}}{\frac{1}{3}} > 1, \frac{\frac{4}{9}}{2} < 1, \frac{1\frac{4}{9}}{\frac{1}{3}} > 1, \frac{\frac{1}{2}}{\frac{2}{4}} = 1$$

Comparing Fractions

When calculating some drug dosages, it is helpful for the pharmacy technician to know whether the value of one fraction is greater than or less than the value of another fraction. The size of fractions can be determined by comparing the numerators when the denominators are the same, or comparing the denominators when the numerators are the same. If the numerators are the same, the fraction with the smaller denominator has the greater value (**Figure 3-6**).

> ### Remember
>
> - A proper fraction has a numerator that is smaller than the denominator.
>
> - An improper fraction has a numerator that is equal to or greater than the denominator.
>
> - A mixed fraction has a whole number and a proper fraction that are combined.
>
> - A complex fraction is a fraction in which the numerator or the denominator, or both, may be a whole number, proper fraction, or mixed fraction.

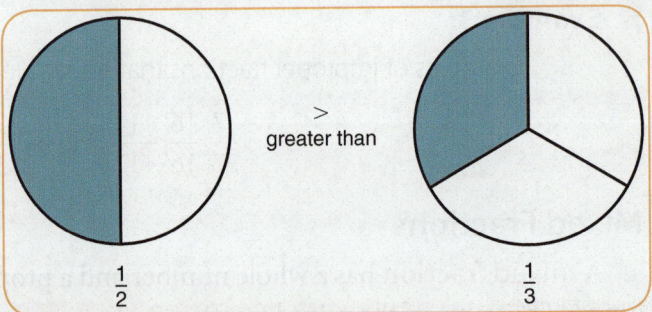

Figure 3-6 If the numerators are the same, the fraction with the smaller denominator has the greater value.
© Cengage Learning 2013

■ Example 6:

Compare $\frac{1}{2}$ and $\frac{1}{3}$.

Numerators are both 1.

Denominator 2 is less than 3.

Therefore, $\frac{1}{2}$ has the greater value.

On the contrary, if both the denominators are the same, the fraction with the smaller numerator has the lesser value (**Figure 3-7**).

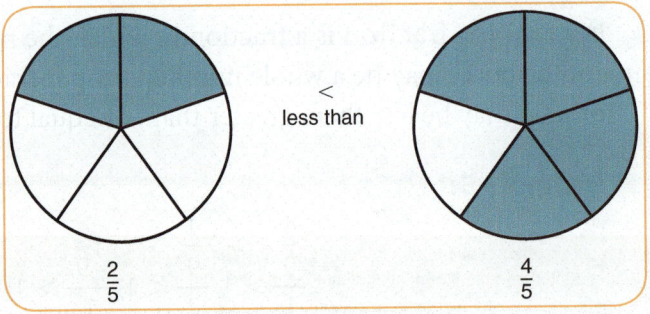

Figure 3-7 If the denominators are the same, the fraction with the smaller numerator has the lesser value.
© Cengage Learning 2013

> **》》》 Remember**
>
> - If the numerators are the same, the fraction with the smaller denominator has the greater value.
>
> - If the denominators are the same, the fraction with the smaller numerator has the lesser value.

■ Example 7:

Compare $\frac{2}{5}$ and $\frac{4}{5}$.

Denominators are both 5.

Numerator 2 is less than 4.

Therefore, $\frac{2}{5}$ has a lesser value.

Converting Improper Fractions to Mixed or Whole Numbers

To convert an improper fraction to an equivalent mixed number or whole number, divide the numerator by the denominator.

■ **Example 8:**

$$\frac{6}{3} = 6 \div 3 = 2 \text{ (whole number)}$$

However, in some cases, the numbers do not divide equally. Therefore, a mixed number is the result.

■ **Example 9:**

$$\frac{15}{4} = 15 \div 4 = 3\frac{3}{4} \text{ (mixed number)}$$

Because the closest whole number less than 15 that 4 will divide into is 12, 3 is the whole number (4 multiplied by 3 equals 12). Now 15 minus 12 is the remainder, which equals 3. Therefore, 3 out of 4 is the remainder. This fraction is already expressed in the lowest terms, which means that a number can be reduced no further.

■ **Example 10:**

$$\frac{9}{4} = 9 \div 4 = 2\frac{1}{4}$$

$$\frac{11}{4} = 11 \div 4 = 2\frac{3}{4}$$

Converting Mixed or Whole Numbers to Improper Fractions

To convert a mixed number to an improper fraction with the same denominator, multiply the whole number by the denominator and add the numerator. Place that value in the numerator, and use the denominator of the fraction part of the mixed number.

■ **Example 11:**

Convert $1\frac{3}{7}$ to an improper fraction.

The whole number is 1. The denominator of the fraction is 7. The numerator of the fraction is 3.

Step 1: Multiply the whole number by the denominator of the fraction.

$$1 \times 7 = 7$$

Step 2: Add the product from step 1 to the numerator of the fraction.

$$7 + 3 = 10$$

Step 3: Write the sum from step 2 over the original denominator.

Therefore, the answer is $\frac{10}{7}$.

Thus,

$$1\frac{3}{7} = \frac{10}{7}$$

 Stop and Review

Answer the following questions relating to common fractions.

1. What is the denominator in $\frac{15}{80}$? _____

2. What is the denominator in $\frac{75}{5}$? _____

3. What is the denominator in $\frac{60}{60}$? _____

4. What is the numerator in $\frac{25}{100}$? _____

5. What is the numerator in $\frac{9}{6}$? _____

6. What is the numerator in $\frac{82}{82}$? _____

7. Which of the following fractions is a proper fraction? _____

   a. $\frac{27}{26}$ c. $\frac{43}{63}$

   b. $\frac{7}{7}$ d. $\frac{95}{90}$

8. Which of the following fractions is an improper fraction? _____

   a. $\frac{39}{38}$ c. $\frac{19}{92}$

   b. $\frac{39}{48}$ d. $\frac{45}{102}$

Convert the following improper fractions to mixed or whole numbers.

9. $\frac{60}{20}$ _____

10. $\frac{72}{72}$ _____

11. $\frac{26}{4}$ _____

12. $\frac{9}{5}$ _____

>>> **Remember**

- To convert an improper fraction to an equivalent mixed number or whole number, divide the numerator by the denominator.

- To convert a mixed number to an improper fraction with the same denominator, multiply the whole number by the denominator and add the numerator. Place that value in the numerator, and use the denominator of the fraction part of the mixed number.

13. $\dfrac{146}{30}$ _____

14. $\dfrac{200}{8}$ _____

15. $\dfrac{160}{80}$ _____

16. $\dfrac{93}{9}$ _____

Convert the following mixed numbers to improper fractions.

17. $6\dfrac{12}{18}$ _____

18. $19\dfrac{9}{19}$ _____

19. $5\dfrac{1}{10}$ _____

20. $2\dfrac{1}{4}$ _____

21. $3\dfrac{8}{9}$ _____

22. $56\dfrac{4}{8}$ _____

23. $150\dfrac{2}{3}$ _____

24. $192\dfrac{4}{6}$ _____

Finding the Least Common Denominator

>>> **Remember**

- The least common denominator is the smallest number into which all of the denominators will divide equally.

It is frequently necessary to find a least common denominator (LCD) for a group of fractions. The least common denominator is the smallest number into which each of the denominators of each of the fractions in the group will divide exactly.

For example, 12 is the least common denominator for the fractions $\dfrac{1}{4}$ and $\dfrac{1}{3}$ because it is the smallest number that both 4 and 3 divide into exactly. For the fractions $\dfrac{1}{4}, \dfrac{1}{6}$, and $\dfrac{1}{8}$, the least common denominator is 24.

The number 48 could have been selected because 4, 6, and 8 also divide exactly into this number, but the least common denominator is the smallest number that all the denominators divide into exactly.

If the least common denominator for a group of fractions cannot be determined by looking, use the following procedure.

■ Example 12:

Find the least common denominator of $\frac{1}{5}, \frac{1}{6}, \frac{2}{9}, \frac{5}{12}$, and $\frac{3}{24}$.

Solution:

Write all the denominators in a horizontal row:

5 6 9 12 24

Starting with the number 2, find the smallest whole number that divides exactly into two or more of the denominators. (If two or more of the denominators cannot be exactly divided by the number 2, try the number 3, and so on.)

Write the results of the division directly under the denominators, and bring down all the denominators that cannot be divided, thus completing a totally new row of numbers.

2	5	6	9	12	24
	5	3	9	6	12

Repeat the process until the final row of numbers contains no numbers that can be exactly divided by any whole number other than 1.

2	5	6	9	12	24
2	5	3	9	6	12
3	5	3	9	3	6
	5	1	3	1	2

The least common denominator can then be determined by multiplying each divisor (vertical numbers) and each number in the last row (horizontal numbers).

LCD = 2 × 2 × 3 × 5 × 1 × 3 × 1 × 2

LCD = 2 × 2 × 3 × 5 × 3 × 2 (the 1s can be dropped)

LCD = 360

When the least common denominator is obvious, this procedure is unnecessary.

■ Example 13:

Find the least common denominator of $\frac{1}{4}, \frac{3}{12}, \frac{3}{20}$, and $\frac{7}{40}$.

Solution:

Write the row of denominators:

	4	12	20	40	divide this row by 2
2	2	6	10	20	divide this row by 2
2	1	3	5	10	divide this row by 5
5	1	3	1	2	which is only divisible
	1	3	1	2	by 1

Therefore, the least common denominator is determined by multiplying $2 \times 2 \times 5 \times 1 \times 3 \times 1 \times 2 = 120$.

Reducing Fractions to the Lowest Terms

When calculating dosages, it is usually easier to work with fractions using the smallest numbers possible. Finding these equivalent fractions is called *reducing the fraction to the lowest terms* or *simplifying the fraction*. To reduce a fraction to the lowest terms, *divide* both the numerator and denominator by the *largest nonzero whole number* that will go evenly into both the numerator and the denominator.

■ Example 14:

Reduce $\dfrac{6}{12}$ to the lowest terms.

The largest number that will divide evenly into both 6 (numerator) and 12 (denominator) is 6.

$$\frac{6}{12} = \frac{6 \div 6}{12 \div 6} = \frac{1}{2} \text{ in lowest terms}$$

Stop and Review

Find the lowest common denominator for these fractions.

1. $\dfrac{1}{4}, \dfrac{1}{3}, \dfrac{1}{6}$ _____

2. $\dfrac{2}{3}, \dfrac{5}{6}$ _____

3. $\dfrac{2}{3}, \dfrac{3}{4}, \dfrac{4}{5}$ _____

4. $\dfrac{8}{10}, \dfrac{12}{20}$ _____

5. $\dfrac{7}{8}, \dfrac{7}{16}$ _____

6. $\dfrac{3}{4}, \dfrac{1}{3}$ _____

7. $\dfrac{7}{8}, \dfrac{1}{4}, \dfrac{2}{3}$ _____

8. $\dfrac{1}{2}, \dfrac{1}{16}$ _____

9. $\dfrac{17}{4}, \dfrac{18}{8}$ _____

10. $\dfrac{1}{2}, \dfrac{3}{4}$ _____

Reduce these fractions.

11. $\dfrac{6}{12}$ _____

12. $\dfrac{4}{6}$ _____

13. $\dfrac{6}{8}$ _____

14. $\dfrac{9}{81}$ _____

15. $\dfrac{3}{6}$ _____

16. $\dfrac{10}{20}$ _____

17. $\dfrac{3}{9}$ _____

18. $\dfrac{56}{64}$ _____

19. $\dfrac{18}{24}$ _____

20. $\dfrac{105}{135}$ _____

Adding Fractions

If fractions have the same denominator, simply add the numerators and keep the value of the common denominator the same. Then reduce to the lowest terms. In Example 12, the result is 4/10. The largest number that the numerator and denominator can be divided by is 2. Therefore, 4 divided by 2 equals 2, and 10 divided by 2 equals five. The lowest terms of this fraction is therefore 2/5.

■ **Example 15:**

$$\dfrac{1}{10} + \dfrac{3}{10} = \dfrac{4}{10}$$

■ **Example 16:**

$$\dfrac{4}{18} + \dfrac{3}{18} + \dfrac{6}{18} = \dfrac{13}{18}$$

The preceding final fraction is already expressed in the lowest terms.

If you gave an infant $\dfrac{1}{2}$ tablespoon of medication before breakfast, $\dfrac{3}{8}$ tablespoon before lunch, $\dfrac{3}{4}$ tablespoon with dinner, and $\dfrac{3}{8}$ tablespoon at bedtime, you must add the fractions to determine the total amount of medication you have given the infant.

To add the fractions, you must first find the common denominator in all the fractions. A common denominator means the same number on the bottom of two or more fractions. Next add the numerators together and keep the value of the common denominator the same. At the end, reduce the numerator and denominator to the lowest terms.

■ Example 17:

Add $\frac{1}{6}$ and $\frac{4}{12}$. To obtain a common denominator of 12, it is necessary to multiply the numerator and denominator of $\frac{1}{6}$ by 2. (*Note:* Both the numerator and denominator must be multiplied so that the value of the fraction remains constant.)

$$\frac{1}{6} \times 2 = \frac{2}{12}$$

Now we have a common denominator and are able to simply add the numerators.

$$\frac{2}{12} + \frac{4}{12} = \frac{6}{12}$$

Be sure to reduce the final answer.

$$\frac{2}{12} + \frac{4}{12} = \frac{6}{12} = \frac{1}{2}$$

When reduced to the lowest terms, $\frac{6}{12}$ is $\frac{1}{2}$. (The largest number that may be divided into both the numerator and denominator is 6.) So $\frac{6}{12}$ (after both the numerator and denominator are divided by 6) becomes $\frac{1}{2}$.

> **》》》 Remember**
>
> - To add fractions:
>
>   Step 1: Find the least common denominator.
>
>   Step 2: Add the numerators together; keep the denominators the same.
>
>   Step 3: Reduce the answer to the lowest terms.

Subtracting Fractions

If fractions have the same denominator, subtract the smaller numerator from the larger numerator. Keep the denominator the same, and then reduce to the lowest terms to obtain the final answer.

■ Example 18:

$$\frac{6}{8} - \frac{2}{8} = \frac{4}{8} = \frac{1}{2}$$

If fractions do not have the same denominator, you must change the fractions so that they have the smallest common denominator. Then they can be subtracted as in the preceding example.

■ Example 19:

$$\frac{13}{24} - \frac{2}{12} =$$

The first fraction cannot be reduced to lowest terms because the numerator, 13, and the denominator, have no common number that can be divided into them. Therefore, the second fraction must be converted. This

> **Remember**
>
> - To subtract fractions:
>
>   Step 1: Find the least common denominator.
>
>   Step 2: Subtract the numerators; keep the denominators the same.
>
>   Step 3: Reduce the answer to the lowest terms.

is done by multiplying its numerator and denominator by the number 2, which converts it into the fraction 4/24. This can then easily be subtracted from the first fraction.

■ **Example 20:**

$$\frac{2}{12} \times \frac{2}{2} = \frac{4}{24}$$

Now that the second fraction has been converted, you may continue with the subtraction as follows.

■ **Example 21:**

$$\frac{13}{24} - \frac{4}{24} = \frac{9}{24}$$

■ **Example 22:**

$$\frac{9}{24} = \frac{3}{8}$$

Subtracting fractions is similar to adding fractions. To subtract fractions, you must write equivalent fractions with a common denominator. Then subtract the numerators (the difference is the new numerator). Keep the common denominator and reduce your answer to its lowest terms.

■ **Example 23:**

Subtract: $\frac{2}{6} - \frac{3}{12}$

Find a common denominator.

Multiplying the numerator and denominator by 2 produces 12 as the lowest common denominator.

$$\frac{2}{6} - \frac{3}{12} = \frac{4}{12} - \frac{3}{12}$$

Subtract the numerators: $4 - 3 = 1$

Keep the common denominator: $\frac{1}{12}$

Multiplying Fractions

To multiply fractions, first multiply the numerators. Second, multiply the denominators, then place the product of the numerators over the product of the denominators, and, finally, reduce to the lowest terms.

■ **Example 24:**

$$\frac{3}{5} \times \frac{2}{4} = \frac{6}{20} = \frac{3}{10}$$

In the case of having two fractions that you need to multiply, which could be reduced before multiplying, you may do so as follows.

> **Remember**

- To multiply fractions:

  Step 1: Reduce all fractions to the lowest terms.

  Step 2: Multiply the numerators.

  Step 3: Multiply the denominators.

  Step 4: Reduce to the lowest terms.

■ **Example 25:**

$$\frac{3}{6} \times \frac{4}{6}$$

Reduce $\frac{3}{6}$ to $\frac{1}{2}$, then reduce $\frac{4}{6}$ to $\frac{2}{3}$, and then multiply.

$$\frac{1}{2} \times \frac{2}{3} = \frac{2}{6} = \frac{1}{3}$$

■ **Example 26:**

Multiply $\frac{2}{6} \times \frac{3}{4}$.

The product of the numerators is $2 \times 3 = 6$. The product of the denominators is $6 \times 4 = 24$. Thus, $\frac{2}{6} \times \frac{3}{4} = \frac{6}{24}$. If $\frac{6}{624}$ is reduced, the result is $\frac{1}{4}$.

$$\frac{2}{6} \times \frac{3}{4} = \frac{6}{24} = \frac{1}{4}$$

■ **Example 27:**

Multiply $4 \times \frac{2}{4}$.

First, convert 4 to the improper fraction $\frac{4}{1}$.

Now solve.

$$4 \times \frac{2}{4} = \frac{4}{1} \times \frac{2}{4} =$$

$$\frac{4 \times 2}{1 \times 4} = \frac{8}{4} = 2$$

■ **Example 28:**

Multiply: $1\frac{4}{7} \times 2\frac{3}{5}$

First, convert the mixed fractions to improper fractions.

$$1\frac{4}{7} = \frac{11}{7} \text{ and } 2\frac{3}{5} = \frac{13}{5}$$

Now multiply the numerators and denominators.

$$1\frac{4}{7} \times 2\frac{3}{5} = \frac{11}{7} \times \frac{13}{5} =$$

$$\frac{11 \times 13}{7 \times 5} = \frac{143}{35}$$

$\frac{143}{35}$ converts to $4\frac{3}{35}$

Dividing Fractions

To divide fractions, first invert (or turn upside down) the divisor, and then multiply. The divisor is the number (or in this case, fraction) by which another number (or fraction) is to be divided. In this example, 2/8 is the divisor.

> **Remember**

- To divide fractions:

  Step 1: Reduce all fractions to the lowest terms.

  Step 2: Invert the divisor.

  Step 3: Multiply the fractions.

  Step 4: Reduce to the lowest terms.

■ **Example 29:**

$$\frac{4}{8} \div \frac{2}{8} = ?$$

Invert the divisor. Note that 2/8 has now become 8/2.

$$\frac{4}{8} \times \frac{8}{2} = \frac{32}{16}$$

Reduce, and then multiply the numerators and then the denominators.

$$\frac{32}{16} = \frac{2}{1} = 2$$

■ **Example 30:**

$$\frac{32}{12} \div \frac{2}{3} = ?$$

Invert the divisor.

$$\frac{32}{12} \times \frac{3}{2} = \frac{96}{24}$$

Simplify.

$$\frac{16}{4} \times \frac{1}{1} = 4$$

■ **Example 31:**

$$3\frac{2}{5} = \frac{5 \times 3 + 2}{5} = \frac{17}{5}$$

■ **Example 32:**

$$6\frac{3}{7} = \frac{7 \times 6 + 3}{7} = \frac{45}{7}$$

To divide fractions, multiply the **dividend** (the fraction being divided) by the reciprocal of the **divisor** (the fraction performing the division). First, reduce all fractions to the lowest terms. Next invert (turn upside down) the divisor. Then multiply the two fractions and reduce to the lowest terms.

■ **Example 33:**

Suppose you have $\frac{3}{4}$ bottle of liquid medication available. The usual dose you would give a patient is $\frac{1}{16}$ bottle, and you want to know how many doses remain in the bottle. You solve this problem by dividing fractions. To solve $\frac{3}{4} \div \frac{1}{16}$, $\frac{3}{4}$ is the dividend and $\frac{1}{16}$ is the divisor. Therefore, multiply the dividend $\frac{3}{4}$ by the reciprocal of the divisor $\frac{1}{16}$. To determine the reciprocal, the divisor is inverted (or turned upside down).

$$\frac{3}{4} \div \frac{1}{16} = \frac{3}{4} \times \frac{16}{1}$$

You now solve this as a multiplication problem.

$$\frac{3}{4} \times \frac{16}{1} = \frac{48}{4} = \frac{12}{1} = 12$$

The bottle has 12 doses remaining.

Example 34:

Divide $\frac{1}{2}$ by $\frac{1}{4}$.

The problem has no mixed or whole numbers. Invert (flip) the divisor of $\frac{1}{4}$ to find its reciprocal, $\frac{4}{1}$. Then multiply the dividend by the reciprocal of the divisor.

$$\frac{1}{2} \div \frac{1}{4} = \frac{1}{2} \times \frac{4}{1} = \frac{4}{2} = \frac{2}{1} = 2$$

Example 35:

Divide $\frac{1}{75}$ by $\frac{1}{150}$.

The problem has no mixed or whole numbers. Invert the divisor of $\frac{1}{150}$ to find its reciprocal, $\frac{150}{1}$.

Then multiply the dividend by the reciprocal of the divisor.

$$\frac{1}{75} \div \frac{1}{150} = \frac{1}{75} \times \frac{150}{1} = \frac{150}{75} = 2$$

Example 36:

Simplify the following:

$$\frac{\frac{3}{4}}{\frac{1}{16}}$$

The numerator is $\frac{3}{4}$ and the denominator is $\frac{1}{16}$. Rewrite the complex fraction as a regular division problem and then solve it.

$$\frac{3}{4} \div \frac{1}{16} = \frac{3}{4} \times \frac{16}{1}$$

Now solve it as a multiplication problem.

$$\frac{3}{4} \div \frac{1}{16} = \frac{3}{4} \times \frac{16}{1} = \frac{48}{4} = 12$$

Stop and Review

Add the following fractions.

1. $\dfrac{1}{6} + \dfrac{3}{8} =$ _____

2. $\dfrac{1}{9} + \dfrac{7}{8} =$ _____

3. $4 + \dfrac{3}{5} =$ _____

4. $\dfrac{3}{8} + \dfrac{3}{4} + \dfrac{7}{12} =$ _____

5. $\dfrac{1}{6} + \dfrac{3}{6} =$ _____

6. $\dfrac{2}{10} + \dfrac{4}{20} =$ _____

7. $3 + \dfrac{8}{11} =$ _____

8. $\dfrac{1}{7} + \dfrac{2}{12} =$ _____

9. $\dfrac{1}{3} + \dfrac{1}{5} + \dfrac{1}{7} =$ _____

10. $\dfrac{2}{5} + \dfrac{4}{15} =$ _____

11. $\dfrac{1}{5} + \dfrac{1}{4} + \dfrac{1}{3} =$ _____

12. $\dfrac{5}{6} + \dfrac{7}{9} =$ _____

13. $2\dfrac{3}{6} + \dfrac{1}{5} =$ _____

14. $\dfrac{3}{5} + \dfrac{4}{15} =$ _____

15. $3\dfrac{1}{2} + 2\dfrac{1}{2} =$ _____

Subtract the following fractions.

16. $7\dfrac{7}{15} - 4\dfrac{4}{15} =$ _____

17. $\dfrac{7}{25} - \dfrac{2}{25} =$ _____

18. $\dfrac{11}{3} - \dfrac{2}{6} =$ _____

19. $6\dfrac{1}{3} - \dfrac{5}{6} =$ _____

20. $6\dfrac{7}{7} - 2\dfrac{21}{5} =$ _____

Chapter 3 • Fractions and Decimals   49

21. $7 - \dfrac{3}{7} =$ _____

22. $\dfrac{4}{7} - \dfrac{3}{21} =$ _____

23. $\dfrac{3}{4} - \dfrac{1}{6} =$ _____

24. $1\dfrac{7}{8} - \dfrac{1}{4} =$ _____

25. $2\dfrac{5}{8} - \dfrac{1}{2} =$ _____

26. $14\dfrac{9}{10} - 3\dfrac{1}{2} =$ _____

27. $14 - \dfrac{3}{7} =$ _____

28. $8\dfrac{1}{12} - 3\dfrac{1}{4} =$ _____

29. $25 - 17\dfrac{7}{9} =$ _____

30. $1\dfrac{2}{3} - 1\dfrac{1}{12} =$ _____

Stop and Review
Multiply these fractions.

1. $\dfrac{1}{3} \times \dfrac{1}{5} =$ _____

2. $\dfrac{2}{7} \times \dfrac{4}{5} =$ _____

3. $\dfrac{2}{5} \times \dfrac{6}{8} =$ _____

4. $\dfrac{5}{3} \times \dfrac{8}{10} =$ _____

5. $\dfrac{6}{9} \times \dfrac{2}{6} =$ _____

6. $\dfrac{9}{7} \times \dfrac{7}{2} =$ _____

7. $\dfrac{10}{16} \times \dfrac{5}{9} =$ _____

8. $\dfrac{3}{8} \times \dfrac{4}{9} =$ _____

9. $\dfrac{12}{9} \times \dfrac{2}{2} =$ _____

10. $\dfrac{14}{12} \times \dfrac{4}{5} =$ _____

11. $3\dfrac{1}{3} \times \dfrac{9}{15} =$ _____

12. $1\dfrac{5}{6} \times 7\dfrac{4}{5} =$ _____

13. $3\dfrac{6}{8} \times 7\dfrac{2}{9} =$ _____

14. $1\dfrac{7}{8} \times \dfrac{4}{5} =$ _____

15. $\dfrac{3}{6} \times \dfrac{7}{16} \times \dfrac{3}{4} =$ _____

16. $\dfrac{8}{5} \times \dfrac{3}{10} \times \dfrac{4}{5} =$ _____

17. $\dfrac{14}{36} \times \dfrac{2}{24} \times 14 =$ _____

18. $7 \times \dfrac{5}{15} \times \dfrac{5}{14} =$ _____

19. $\dfrac{45}{22} \times \dfrac{14}{7} \times \dfrac{7}{24} =$ _____

20. $\dfrac{12}{24} \times \dfrac{7}{8} \times \dfrac{15}{18} =$ _____

Stop and Review
Divide these fractions.

1. $\dfrac{4}{8} \div \dfrac{6}{9} =$ _____

2. $\dfrac{5}{11} \div \dfrac{3}{4} =$ _____

3. $\dfrac{4}{9} \div \dfrac{1}{2} =$ _____

4. $\dfrac{1}{5} \div \dfrac{3}{4} =$ _____

5. $\dfrac{5}{7} \div \dfrac{2}{6} =$ _____

6. $\dfrac{6}{9} \div \dfrac{3}{7} =$ _____

7. $\dfrac{9}{10} \div \dfrac{3}{5} =$ _____

8. $\dfrac{5}{14} \div \dfrac{23}{36} =$ _____

9. $1\dfrac{5}{7} \div \dfrac{4}{5} =$ _____

10. $\dfrac{5}{8} \div 1\dfrac{3}{4} =$ _____

11. $6\dfrac{2}{9} \div 2\dfrac{3}{8} =$ _____

12. $5\dfrac{1}{2} \div 1\dfrac{1}{6} =$ _____

13. $1\dfrac{5}{6} \div 7 =$ _____

14. $8 \div \dfrac{3}{6} =$ _____

15. $\dfrac{\frac{9}{12}}{\frac{4}{6}} =$ _____

16. $\dfrac{\frac{2}{7}}{\frac{3}{8}} =$ _____

Decimals

Generally, decimal fractions or decimal numbers are referred to simply as *decimals*. Decimal fractions are used with the metric system, which is the system most often used in the calculation of drug dosages. The pharmacy technician must be able to manipulate decimals easily and accurately. Each decimal fraction consists of a numerator that is expressed in numerals, a decimal point placed so that it designates the value of the denominator, and the denominator that is understood to be 10, or some power of 10. In writing a decimal fraction, always place a zero to the left of the decimal point so that the decimal point can readily be seen. This also ensures that the decimal will not be mistaken for the whole number 1. **Table 3-1** shows some examples.

》》》 Remember

- Whole numbers are to the left of the decimal point.
- Fractions are to the right of the decimal point.
- Always write a zero to the left of the decimal point when the decimal number has no whole number part. Using the zero makes the decimal point more noticeable. It also helps prevent errors caused by illegible handwriting.

Table 3-1 Equivalent Mixed Fractions and Decimals

Mixed Fraction	Decimal	Description
$15\dfrac{3}{10}$	15.3	Fifteen and three-tenths
$85\dfrac{7}{10}$	85.7	Eighty-five and seven-tenths
$172\dfrac{25}{100}$	172.25	One hundred seventy-two and twenty-five hundredths
$\dfrac{42}{100}$	0.42	Forty-two hundredths
$2\dfrac{355}{1000}$	2.355	Two and three hundred fifty-five thousandths

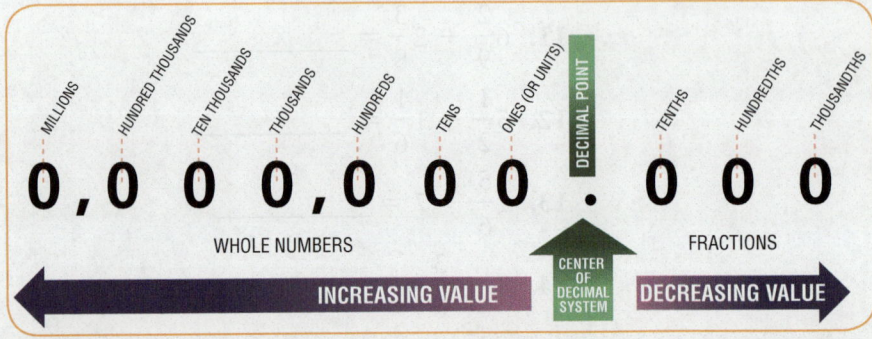

Figure 3-8
© Cengage Learning 2013

To understand how to read and write decimals, examine **Figure 3-8**, which shows that all whole numbers are to the left of the decimal point and all fractions are to the right.

Converting Fractions to Decimals and Decimals to Fractions

Recognizing that there is a relationship between fractions and decimals is useful when it becomes necessary to convert a fraction to its decimal equivalent. To accomplish this task, simply divide the numerator of the fraction (the top of the fraction) by the denominator of the fraction (the bottom number of the fraction).

■ Example 1:

Convert $\frac{3}{4}$ to a decimal.

Solution:

Divide the numerator of the fraction by the denominator.

$$\begin{array}{r} 0.75 \\ 4\overline{)3.00} \\ \underline{2.8} \\ 20 \\ \underline{20} \end{array}$$

Therefore, $\frac{3}{4} = 0.75$

■ Example 2:

Convert $\frac{1}{100}$ to a decimal.

Solution:

Divide the numerator of the fraction by the denominator.

$$\begin{array}{r} 0.01 \\ 100\overline{)1.00} \\ \underline{1.00} \end{array}$$

Therefore, $\frac{1}{100} = 0.01$

>>> **Remember**

- All decimal fractions and decimal numbers are referred to simply as *decimals*.

- To convert fractions to decimals, divide the numerator by the denominator.

- To convert decimals to fractions, make the number without the decimal point the numerator. The number 1 followed by as many zeros as decimal places becomes the denominator. Then reduce to the lowest terms.

Example 3:

Convert 0.75 to a fraction.

Solution:

Make the decimal number without the decimal point the numerator of the fraction. The number 1 followed by as many zeros as there are digits to the right of the decimal point is the denominator.

$$\frac{75}{100} = \frac{3}{4}$$

Therefore, $0.75 = \frac{3}{4}$

Stop and Review

Change the following fractions into decimals.

1. $\frac{1}{2}$ _____
2. $\frac{2}{5}$ _____
3. $\frac{1}{6}$ _____
4. $\frac{5}{8}$ _____
5. $\frac{2}{15}$ _____
6. $\frac{1}{158}$ _____
7. $\frac{3}{200}$ _____
8. $\frac{1}{12}$ _____
9. $\frac{1}{500}$ _____
10. $\frac{1}{3000}$ _____

Change the following decimals to fractions.

11. 0.005 _____
12. 0.009 _____
13. 0.0033 _____
14. 0.05 _____
15. 0.25 _____

16. 0.0002 _____

17. 0.075 _____

18. 0.15 _____

19. 0.84 _____

20. 2.75 _____

Adding Decimals

To add decimals, write the decimals in a column, with the decimal points placed directly under each other. Then add the numbers, as in the addition of whole numbers, and place the decimal point in the sum directly under the decimal points in the column.

■ Example 4:

Add 4.27 and 0.51.

To perform the operation, write it as follows.

```
  4.27
+ 0.51
```

Then add vertically to keep the decimal points aligned.

```
  4.27
+ 0.51
  4.78
```

■ Example 5:

Add 18.4 + 7.52 + 8 + 0.631.

To perform the operation, write it as follows.

```
   18.4
    7.52
    8
+   0.631
```

Then add.

```
   18.4
    7.52
    8.0
+   0.631
   34.551
```

Subtracting Decimals

To subtract decimals, write the decimals in columns, keeping the decimal points under each other. Then subtract the decimals, as with whole

>>> **Remember**

- To add decimals:

  Step 1: Write the decimals in a column, aligning the decimal points.

  Step 2: Add the columns vertically right to left, carrying numbers over as necessary.

  Step 3: Place the decimal point in the answer directly under the decimal point in the column.

numbers. A zero may be added after the decimal without changing the value. Then place the decimal point in the remainder, directly under the decimal point in the column. Remember to carry numbers over as necessary when subtracting.

■ Example 6:

Subtract 68.07 − 17.44.

To perform the operation, write it as follows.

```
 68.07
−17.44
 50.63
```

■ Example 7:

Subtract 9.5 − 3.008.

To perform the operation, write it as follows.

```
 9.5
−3.008
```

Or

```
 9.500
−3.008
 6.492
```

Stop and Review

Add or subtract the following numbers.

1. 9.32 + 4.92 = _____
2. 155.07 + 31.02 = _____
3. 17.435 + 0.034 = _____
4. 72.308 + 4.916 = _____
5. 4.06 + 0.8 = _____
6. 5.45 + 0.009 = _____
7. 0.025 + 0.68 = _____
8. 8 + 0.033 = _____
9. 53.62 − 0.07 = _____
10. 18.36 − 1.225 = _____
11. 7.88 − 0.08 = _____

))) Remember

- To subtract decimals:

  Step 1: Write the decimals in a column, aligning the decimal points.

  Step 2: Subtract the columns vertically right to left, borrowing numbers as necessary.

  Step 3: Place the decimal point in the answer directly under the decimal point in the column.

12. 16.5 − 0.9 = _____

13. 5.22 − 0.6 = _____

14. 12.8 − 0.777 = _____

15. 9 − 0.023 = _____

16. 17 − 0.07 = _____

Multiplying Decimals

To multiply decimals, first find the product as usual. Second, count the number of decimal places in both the **multiplicand** (the number being multiplied) and the **multiplier** (the number doing the multiplying). Finally, mark the total number of decimal places in the product and insert a decimal point.

■ **Example 8:**

Step 1: Multiply 3.07 × 0.8.

3.07 (multiplicand)

× 0.8 (multiplier)
_____

2456 (product)

Step 2:

Count the number of decimal places in the multiplicand and multiplier.

3.07

× 0.8 =   Total of three decimal places

Step 3:

By counting decimal places from right to left, mark off three decimal places in the product.

New decimal = 2.456

■ **Example 9:**

Step 1: Multiply 3.85 × 2.2.

3.85 (multiplicand)

× 2.2 (multiplier)
_____

8470 (product)

Step 2:

Count the number of decimal places in the multiplicand and multiplier.

3.85

× 2.2 =   Total of three decimal places

Step 3:

Mark off three decimal places in the product.

New decimal = 8.47

>>> **Remember**

- To multiply decimals:

Step 1: Multiply the whole numbers.

Step 2: Add the number of decimal places in the numbers being multiplied.

Step 3: Place the decimal point in the answer the number of spaces to the left equal to the number of decimal places in the numbers being multiplied.

Stop and Review
Multiply the following numbers.

1. 9.7 × 8.6 = _____
2. 4.9 × 0.7 = _____
3. 6.28 × 3.3 = _____
4. 7.06 × 0.08 = _____
5. 0.77 × 0.7 = _____
6. 0.082 × 0.6 = _____
7. 0.009 × 0.03 = _____
8. 0.25 × 0.85 = _____
9. 5.04 × 18 = _____
10. 17 × 0.08 = _____
11. 0.003 × 19.7 = _____
12. 0.007 × 55.05 = _____

Dividing Decimals

To divide a decimal by a whole number, first write the problem as usual. Second, place a decimal point in the quotient line directly above the decimal in the dividend, and then find the **quotient** (the answer). Division is written using several symbols, such as 1 ÷ 2, or $\frac{1}{2}$. The divisor (the number performing the division) is on the right of the symbol in the first example and on the bottom of the symbol in the second example. The divisor must be a whole number (a number with no decimal point), and the decimal point must be correctly placed in the answer. When a decimal number is being divided by a whole number, the decimal point is placed directly above the decimal point in the dividend (number being divided). When a number is being divided by a decimal number, the decimal point in the divisor must be moved to the right as many places as needed to make the divisor a whole number. The decimal point in the dividend must be moved the same number of places to the right. The decimal point in the quotient is placed directly above the new position of the decimal point in the dividend.

■ **Example 10:**

Divide 0.6 ÷ 0.02.

First, write the problem as a fraction.

$$\frac{0.6}{0.02}$$

Second, move the decimal point two places to the right in both the numerator and the denominator. The denominator is now a whole number.

$$\frac{0.6}{0.02} = \frac{60}{2}$$

This step is equivalent to multiplying.

$$\frac{0.6}{0.02} \times \frac{100}{100}$$

Third, complete the division

$$\frac{0.6}{0.02} = \frac{60}{2} = 30$$

so that 0.6 ÷ 0.02 = 30.

■ **Example 11:**

Divide 0.088 ÷ 0.11.

First:

$$\frac{0.088}{0.11}$$

Second:

$$\frac{0.088}{0.11} = \frac{8.8}{11} = 0.8$$

Move the decimal point two places to the right, in both the numerator and denominator, so that the denominator (divisor) is a whole number.

Third, complete the division:

$$0.088 \div 0.11 = 0.8$$

>>> **Remember**

- To divide decimals:

    Step 1: Write the division problem as a fraction.

    Step 2: Move the decimal point so that the denominator is a whole number.

    Step 3: Move the decimal point in the numerator the same number of places to the right.

    Step 4: Complete the division.

 Stop and Review

Divide the following numbers.

1. 6.2 ÷ 1.4 = _____

2. 36.8 ÷ 0.6 = _____

3. 84.6 ÷ 1.8 = _____

4. 0.004 ÷ 0.002 = _____

5. 1.5 ÷ 0.5 = _____

6. 0.62 ÷ 0.4 = _____

7. 0.08 ÷ 0.02 = _____

8. 14.6 ÷ 2 = _____

9. 60 ÷ 0.6 = _____

10. 0.88 ÷ 8.8 = _____

11. 39.06 ÷ 100 = _____

12. 4.44 ÷ 1000 = _____

13. 66.666 ÷ 0.03 = _____

14. 82.82 ÷ 0.004 = _____

15. 126.26 ÷ 2000 = _____

16. 38.42 ÷ 2.1 = _____

17. 6.6 ÷ 0.11 = _____

18. 77.7 ÷ 3.3 = _____

19. 0.888 ÷ 1000 = _____

20. 8.875 ÷ 3.25 = _____

Rounding Decimals

To round a decimal, it is necessary to obtain an answer one decimal place after the desired place. Therefore, if the last digit is less than 5, the last digit is simply dropped. However, if the last digit is 5 or greater, the prior digit must increase by one number.

■ Example 12:

Round 3.3 to the nearest whole number.

Consider the tenths column. Because 3 is less than 5, the answer is 3, and 0.3 is discarded. Round 3.57 to the nearest tenth. Because the hundredths column is 7, and this number is greater than 5, the answer is 3.6 and the 7 is dropped.

Round 2.896 to the nearest hundredth. Because the last digit is 6, and this number is greater than 5, the answer is 2.90 and the 6 is dropped.

> **Remember**
>
> - To round decimals:
>
>   Step 1: If the last digit is less than 5, the last digit is simply dropped.
>
>   Step 2: If the last digit is 5 or greater, the number is increased by one, and the last digit is dropped. This is also described as "if the last digit is 5 or greater, round up."

Test Your Knowledge

Calculate the following numbers and give the answer in the lowest terms.

1. $\dfrac{8}{4} + \dfrac{2}{6} = $ _____

2. $\dfrac{3}{5} + 1\dfrac{2}{5} = $ _____

3. $\dfrac{4}{10} + \dfrac{2}{20} + \dfrac{1}{50} = $ _____

4. $8 + \dfrac{5}{8} + \dfrac{1}{4} + \dfrac{6}{12} = $ _____

5. $\dfrac{18}{9} - \dfrac{4}{6} = $ _____

6. $\dfrac{4}{5} - \dfrac{3}{4} = $ _____

7. $6\dfrac{1}{2} - 2\dfrac{7}{8} = $ _____

8. $3 - \dfrac{2}{7} = $ _____

9. $\dfrac{8}{6} \times \dfrac{2}{4} = $ _____

10. $\dfrac{7}{7} \times \dfrac{3}{14} = $ _____

11. $4\dfrac{6}{3} \times \dfrac{10}{5} = $ _____

12. $\dfrac{6}{8} \times 11 = $ _____

13. $\dfrac{2}{8} \div \dfrac{4}{6} = $ _____

14. $\dfrac{17}{13} \div \dfrac{3}{56} = $ _____

15. $2\dfrac{7}{8} \div \dfrac{2}{6} = $ _____

16. $\dfrac{1}{4} \div 1\dfrac{1}{4} = $ _____

Chapter 3 • Fractions and Decimals

Convert the following mixed numbers to improper fractions.

17. $1\frac{2}{7} =$ _____

18. $21\frac{3}{8} =$ _____

19. $8\frac{6}{10} =$ _____

20. $6\frac{4}{8} =$ _____

21. $4\frac{3}{6} =$ _____

22. $11\frac{2}{6} =$ _____

Reduce the following fractions to their lowest terms.

23. $\frac{12}{48} =$ _____

24. $\frac{66}{92} =$ _____

25. $\frac{48}{8} =$ _____

26. $\frac{92}{8} =$ _____

27. $\frac{112}{62} =$ _____

28. $\frac{186}{93} =$ _____

Find the least common denominator, and then write an equivalent fraction for each.

29. $\frac{5}{10}$ and $\frac{3}{5} =$ _____

30. $\frac{6}{3}$ and $\frac{4}{9} =$ _____

31. $\frac{7}{10}, \frac{1}{4},$ and $\frac{2}{3} =$ _____

32. $\frac{3}{5}, \frac{3}{2},$ and $\frac{1}{6} =$ _____

Round to the nearest tenth.

33. 4.62 = _____

34. 7.75 = _____

35. 8.991 = _____

36. 0.053 = _____

Round to the nearest hundredth.

37. 8.091 = _____

38. 0.444 = _____

39. 64.004 = _____

40. 9.882 = _____

Round to the nearest whole number.

41. 20.4 = _____

42. 6.86 = _____

43. 0.821 = _____

44. 12.668 = _____

Calculate the following numbers.

45. 0.021 + 0.88 = _____

46. 7.18 + 14.38 = _____

47. 4.69 + 0.7 = _____

48. 16 + 0.008 + 1.3 = _____

49. 5.47 − 0.39 = _____

50. 6.26 − 3.31 = _____

51. 0.684 − 0.89 (*Note:* The answer to this problem will be a negative decimal.)
_____

52. 19.02 − 0.647 = _____

53. 5.3 × 7.9 = _____

54. 0.67 × 0.004 = _____

55. 9 × 0.992 = _____

56. 12.09 × 1.009 = _____

57. 48.62 ÷ 2.1 = _____

58. 6.876 ÷ 3.36 = _____

59. 4.4 ÷ 0.11 = _____

60. 1.6 ÷ 0.08 = _____

Circle the correct answer.

61. Which is the largest number?   0.015   0.15   0.024

62. Which is the smallest number?   0.325   0.6   0.073

63. True or false? 0.465 = 0.0465

64. True or false? 4.6 grams = 4.06 grams

65. True or false? 8.8 ounces = 8.800 ounces

Critical Thinking

A pharmacy technician is opening a box of instruments in various sizes. The technician is asked to arrange a set of instruments on the shelf in order, from smallest to largest on the basis of the instruments' diameters. The diameters are marked $\frac{1}{4}, \frac{1}{16}, \frac{1}{2}, \frac{7}{16}, \frac{3}{16},$ and $\frac{5}{16}$.

1. How should the technician arrange the instruments?

   _____

2. Look at the pattern of increase in these measurements. Are any instruments missing in the sequence? If so, which ones?

   _____

A stock bottle of medication contains 500 mg. It is used for compounding medications. Three prescriptions were filled by using this medication. The first was for 125 mg, the second was for 62.5 mg, and the third was for 25.25 mg.

3. What was the total amount of this medication used to fill these three prescriptions?

   _____

4. How much of the medication was not used?

   _____

5. If the bottle had originally contained 1000 mg instead of 500 mg, how much of the medication would be left unused?

   _____

Chapter 4

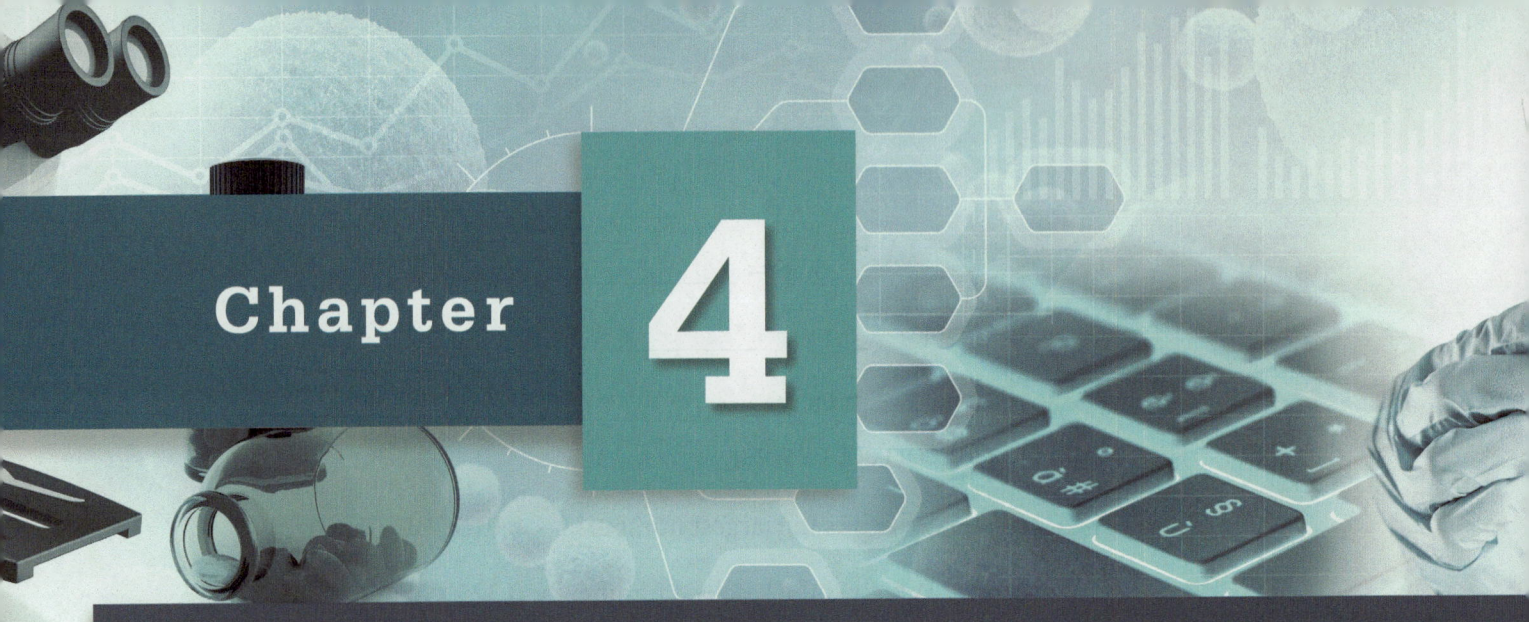

Ratios, Proportions, and Percentages

Outline

Overview
Ratios
Proportions
Percentages
  Changing Percentages to Decimals
  Changing Decimals to Percentages
  Changing Percentages to Fractions
  Changing Fractions to Percentages
  Determining Percentages

Objectives

Upon completion of this chapter, you should be able to:

1. Solve for *X* using proportions.
2. Convert percentages into ratios and fractions.
3. Convert ratios and fractions into percentages.
4. Convert percentages to decimals.
5. Convert decimals to percentages.
6. Convert percentages to fractions.
7. Convert fractions to percentages.
8. Convert fractions to ratios.
9. Determine percentages of various whole numbers.

Key Terms

extremes

means

percentages

proportion

Overview

Pharmacy technicians must understand percentages, ratios, and proportions to deal with a variety of medications and treatments and to ensure accuracy in preparing and calculating these medications. The ability to express percentages and ratios, and how they are related to fractions and decimals, is a skill that is essential to correctly measuring and calculating medications. The pharmacy technician needs to practice using percentages, ratios, and proportions to become skilled in this area of mathematics.

Ratios

A ratio is the relation between two numbers. Ratios may be used to relate a quantity of liquid medication to a quantity of intravenous solution. Pharmacy technicians can also use ratios to calculate dosages of dry medication such as caplets or tablets. Ratios are written either as fractions or linearly. The two numbers in a ratio (or "quantities") are separated by a colon (:). The use of the colon is a traditional way to write the division sign within a ratio, which is expressed as "4 is to 9" in the following example.

■ Example 1:

$\frac{4}{9}$ may be expressed as a ratio: 4:9.

A ratio also can be expressed as a fraction. The first number of the ratio becomes the numerator and the second number becomes the denominator. When expressed as a fraction, a ratio can be reduced to its lowest terms.

■ Example 2:

5:250 may be expressed as a fraction.

$$\frac{5}{250} = \frac{1}{50}$$

■ Example 3:

$$7:21 = \frac{7}{21} = \frac{1}{3}$$

> **Remember**
> - Ratios express a relationship.
> - The quantities in a ratio are separated by a colon.
> - To change a ratio into a fraction, the first number in the ratio becomes the numerator and the second number becomes the denominator.
> - Ratios should be expressed in lowest terms.

■ **Example 4:**

4:8 can be expressed as $\frac{4}{8}$ and can be reduced to $\frac{1}{2}$.

Ratios should generally be expressed in lowest terms, such as the following: $\frac{5}{25}$, which reduces to $\frac{1}{5}$. Therefore, the ratio 5:25 should be written as 1:5. Another example would be $\frac{25}{100}$, which can be reduced to $\frac{1}{4}$, or 1:4.

Stop and Review

Convert the following fractions into ratios.

1. $\frac{250}{1000} =$ _____
2. $\frac{20}{100} =$ _____
3. $\frac{40}{60} =$ _____
4. $\frac{6}{8} =$ _____
5. $\frac{300}{900} =$ _____
6. $\frac{25}{200} =$ _____
7. $\frac{60}{1200} =$ _____
8. $\frac{75}{1500} =$ _____
9. $\frac{3}{9} =$ _____
10. $\frac{25}{50} =$ _____
11. $\frac{40}{100} =$ _____
12. $\frac{17}{170} =$ _____
13. $\frac{50}{1000} =$ _____
14. $\frac{8}{100} =$ _____
15. $\frac{20}{4000} =$ _____

16. $\dfrac{150}{3000} =$ _____

17. $\dfrac{500}{2000} =$ _____

18. $\dfrac{32}{160} =$ _____

19. $\dfrac{10}{40} =$ _____

20. $\dfrac{12}{120} =$ _____

Proportions

A **proportion** is the relationship between two equal ratios. Because ratios are usually written as fractions, a proportion is also expressed as two equal fractions. The proportion (equation) uses an equal sign or double colon to demonstrate that the ratios on both sides of the equal sign (=) or double colon (::) are equal. Therefore, a proportion can be shown in two ways.

As two equal fractions:

$$\frac{A}{B} = \frac{C}{D}$$

or using a colon:

$$A:B = C:D$$

When two ratios are equal, the cross products of the ratios are equal. Using cross products tests whether the two ratios are equal. To find the cross products of a proportion, multiply the outer terms, called the **extremes**, and the middle terms, called the **means**. This relationship is shown in **Figure 4-1**. In a proportion, the product of means is equal to the product of extremes.

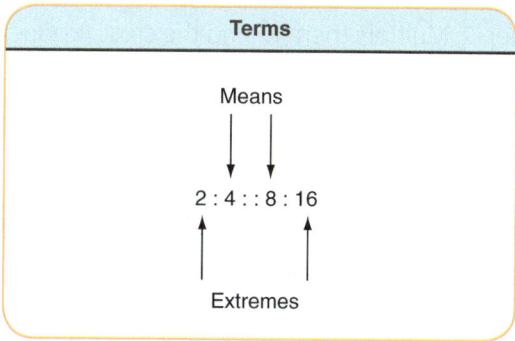

Figure 4-1 The means and the extremes.
© Cengage Learning 2013

> **Remember**
>
> - A proportion is the relationship between two equal ratios.
> - An equal sign or double colon represents the relationship between the two parts.
> - Both sides of the proportion must be the same. This can be verified by multiplying the means and the extremes.

Example 1:

$$A:B = C:D \text{ or } A \times D = B \times C$$

$$\frac{5}{10} = \frac{13}{26}$$

or, $5 \times 26 = 10 \times 13$, $130 = 130$

Example 2:

$$20:25 = 4:5$$

In this example, 20 and 5 are the extremes, and 25 and 4 are the means. Because the cross products are both equal to 100, these ratios are equal and this proportion is true ($20 \times 5 = 25 \times 4$ or $100 = 100$).

To write a ratio proportion as a fraction proportion, use the following rule.

1. Change the double colon to an equal sign.
2. Convert both ratios to fractions.

Example 3:

$$3:5 :: 9:15 \text{ or}$$
$$3:5 = 9:15 \text{ or}$$
$$\frac{3}{5} = \frac{9}{15}$$

Example 4:

$$5:100 :: 50:1000 \text{ or}$$
$$5:100 = 50:1000 \text{ or}$$
$$\frac{5}{100} = \frac{50}{1000}$$

In a case when one quantity is missing from the proportion, substitute the letter X for the missing term. You must take three steps:

Step 1: Write the proportion as a fraction.

$$\frac{5}{30} = \frac{10}{X}$$

Step 2: Multiply them to find the cross products.

$$\frac{5}{30} = \frac{10}{X} \quad \text{(cross multiply)}$$

$$5 \times X = 10 \times 30$$

$$5X = 300$$

Step 3: Divide them to solve for X.

$$X = \frac{300}{5} = 60$$

> **Remember**
>
> - To solve for X:
>   Write the proportion.
>   Cross multiply.
>   Divide to solve for X.

Stop and Review

Solve for X in the following proportions.

1. 6:30 = 15:X _____
2. 2:10 = 3:X _____
3. 5:20 = 3:X _____
4. 50:250 = 10:X _____
5. 21:63 = 45:X _____
6. 32:128 = 4:X _____
7. 8:72 :: 5:X _____
8. 0.4:0.8 = X:80 _____
9. 30:120 = X:12 _____
10. 128:1 = X:5 _____
11. X:625 = 1:5 _____
12. 20:40 = X:100 _____

Percentages

Percent (denoted by the symbol %) stands for "hundredths." A percent is a ratio of a number to 100, and is also referred to as a percentage. Note that **percentages** can be written in the form of "X" with the symbol %, or X%. Think of the symbol % to be a distortion of the 100 in a ratio of X:100. The ratio of 30 to 100 is 30 percent, or 30%; this is the same as 30 hundredths, or 0.30. A percent may be expressed as a fraction, a decimal, or a ratio, each of which provides a way to express the relationship of parts to a whole. The term *percentages* is preferred when referring to any lesser amount that is in relation to a whole amount.

■ **Example 1:**

Percent	Fraction	Decimal	Ratio
30%	= $\frac{30}{100}$	= 0.30	= 30:100

Percentages are frequently used to show the strength of intravenous (IV) solutions. They are also used to indicate the strength of medications such as ointments; for example, two percent (2%) of an ointment means 2 parts of 100, and 0.9% of a solution means 0.9 part (less than 1 part) of 100.

Changing Percentages to Decimals

To change a percentage to a decimal, move the decimal point two places to the left to signify hundredths, and add zeros as necessary. This also can be done by removing the percent sign and dividing by 100.

■ **Example 2:**

Convert 38% to a decimal.

$$38\% = 38.\% = .38. = 0.38$$

■ **Example 3:**

Convert 125% to a decimal.

$$125\% = 125.\% = 1.25. = 1.25$$

■ **Example 4:**

Convert $15\frac{1}{2}\%$ to a decimal.

$$15\frac{1}{2} = 15\frac{5}{10}\% = 15.5\% = 015.5\% = 0.15.5 = 0.155$$

Changing Decimals to Percentages

To change a decimal to a percentage, move the decimal point two places to the right to signify hundredths, and add zeros as necessary. This also can be done by multiplying by 100 and adding the percent sign.

■ **Example 5:**

Convert 0.22 to a percent.

$$0.22 \times 100 = 22\%$$
$$0.22 = 0.22. = 22\%$$

Changing Percentages to Fractions

To convert a percentage to a fraction, first convert it to a decimal, and then convert the decimal to a fraction. Another way is to put the percent over 100 and reduce.

■ **Example 6:**

Change 30% to a fraction.

$$30 \div 100 = 0.30$$
$$\frac{3}{10}$$

■ **Example 7:**

Change 0.1% to a fraction.

$$0.1 \div 100 = 0.001$$
$$\frac{1}{1000}$$

> **))) Remember**
>
> - Percentages stand for hundredths.
> - Percentages can be expressed as ratios, decimals, or fractions.
> - To change a percent to a decimal, move the decimal point two places to the left or divide by 100.
> - To change a decimal to a percent, move the decimal point two places to the right or multiply by 100.
> - To change a percent to a fraction, convert the percent to a decimal and then the decimal to the fraction.
> - To change a fraction to a percent, convert the fraction to a decimal and then the decimal to a percent.
> - To determine a specific percentage, change the percent to a decimal or fraction and then multiply by the number.

Changing Fractions to Percentages

To change a fraction to a percentage, convert the fraction to a decimal, and then convert the decimal to a percentage by multiplying by 100 and adding a percent sign.

■ **Example 8:**

Convert $\frac{3}{5}$ to a percent.

$$\frac{3}{5} = 0.6 = 60\%$$

■ **Example 9:**

Convert $\frac{1}{4}$ to a percent.

$$\frac{1}{4} = 0.25 = 25\%$$

Determining Percentages

To determine the percentage of a given number, first convert it to a decimal or fraction. Next multiply the decimal or fraction by the number.

■ **Example 10:**

What percent of 10 ounces is 3 ounces? You are looking for a percentage in this case.

Convert the percentage to a decimal or fraction.

$$10\% = 0.1 = \frac{1}{10}$$

Next multiply the decimal or fraction by the number.

$$0.1 \times 3 = 0.3 = 30\%$$

Another way to solve this is shown here.

$$\frac{1}{10} = \frac{X}{3}$$

$$3 = 10X \text{ or } 10X = 3$$

X divided by 10 = 3 divided by 10.

$$X = \frac{3}{10} \text{ or } X = 0.30 = 30\%$$

Stop and Review

Solve the following problems on determining percentages.

1. 60% of 20 = _____

2. 50% of 1000 = _____

3. 0.02% of 100 = _____

4. $\frac{1}{2}$% of 2000 = _____

5. 25% of 1000 = _____

6. 10% of 75 = _____

7. $\frac{8}{10}$% of 1000 = _____

8. 75% of 250 = _____

9. $\frac{1}{4}$% of 1200 = _____

10. 7% of 500 = _____

11. 0.9% of 1200 = _____

12. 5% of 5000 = _____

13. $\frac{1}{2}$% of 250 = _____

14. 15% of 400 = _____

15. 20% of 150 = _____

Test Your Knowledge

Express the following percentages as decimals.

1. 6% _____
2. 35% _____
3. 0.3% _____
4. 0.01% _____
5. 0.004% _____

Express the following decimals as percentages.

6. 0.16 _____
7. 0.09 _____
8. 1.4 _____
9. 12.8 _____
10. 2.6 _____

Express the following percentages as fractions and reduce the answers to the lowest terms.

11. 5%   _____

12. 20%   _____

13. 0.3%   _____

14. 25%   _____

15. 0.05%   _____

Express the following fractions as percentages.

16. 3/25   _____

17. 4/5   _____

18. 3/4   _____

19. 3/10   _____

20. 7/20   _____

Express the following as ratios.

21. $\dfrac{1}{3}$ _____

22. $\dfrac{1}{500}$ _____

23. $\dfrac{\frac{2}{3}}{\frac{3}{4}}$ _____

24. $\dfrac{2}{150}$ _____

25. $\dfrac{\frac{1}{500}}{\frac{1}{1000}}$ _____

Express the following percentages as ratios.

26. 1%   _____

27. 50%   _____

28. 12.5%   _____

29. 0.25% _____

30. 0.33% _____

Solve for X in the following proportions.

31. 1:5 = X:20 _____

32. X:3 = 7:21 _____

33. $\frac{1}{2}$:X = 3:12 _____

34. $\frac{1}{3}$:$\frac{2}{3}$ = $\frac{1}{6}$:X _____

35. 25:X = 75:1500 _____

36. $\frac{1}{6}$:$\frac{1}{8}$ = X:3 _____

37. 0.3:0.4 = X:0.5 _____

38. 0.5:0.125 = 2:X _____

39. 0.25:3 = 0.75:X _____

40. $\frac{1}{150}$:$\frac{1}{100}$ = X:1 _____

Are the following statements true or false?   True   False

41. 3:5 and 12:20 are equal ratios.   ____   ____

42. If cross products are equal, the ratios are equal.   ____   ____

43. A proportion is the relationship between two equal quotients.   ____   ____

44. 7 miles in 10 minutes = 3.5 miles in 5 minutes.   ____   ____

45. If $\frac{x}{15} = \frac{2}{36}$, then x = 3.   ____   ____

46. If $\frac{3}{5} = \frac{6}{10}$, then 3 × 6 = 5 × 10.   ____   ____

47. 6 for $0.85 is better than 8 for $1.00.   ____   ____

48. $\frac{4}{5} = \frac{16}{18}$ ____   ____

49. 18 for $0.56 is better than 9 for $1.50.   ____   ____

50. $\frac{25}{55} = \frac{4}{8}$ ____   ____

Critical Thinking

A pharmacy technician received a prescription for 125 mcg of a medication to be taken once daily. The pharmacy has 0.25 mg scored tablets on hand and the drug label from the manufacturer indicates that 0.25 mg is equivalent to 250 mcg. The technician calculated that the patient should take two tablets per dose.

1. Is the pharmacy technician performing the calculation correctly?

2. If not, how many tablets should the patient take?

A pharmacy technician is required to determine the ratio strength of a medication. She must convert 0.8% to the correct ratio strength. A ratio strength is written in the format 1:10 or 2:50 (these are just examples of how ratios appear).

3. What decimal is equivalent to 0.8%, in comparison to 100?

4. If 100 is divided by 0.8, what is the result?

5. What is the final ratio strength?

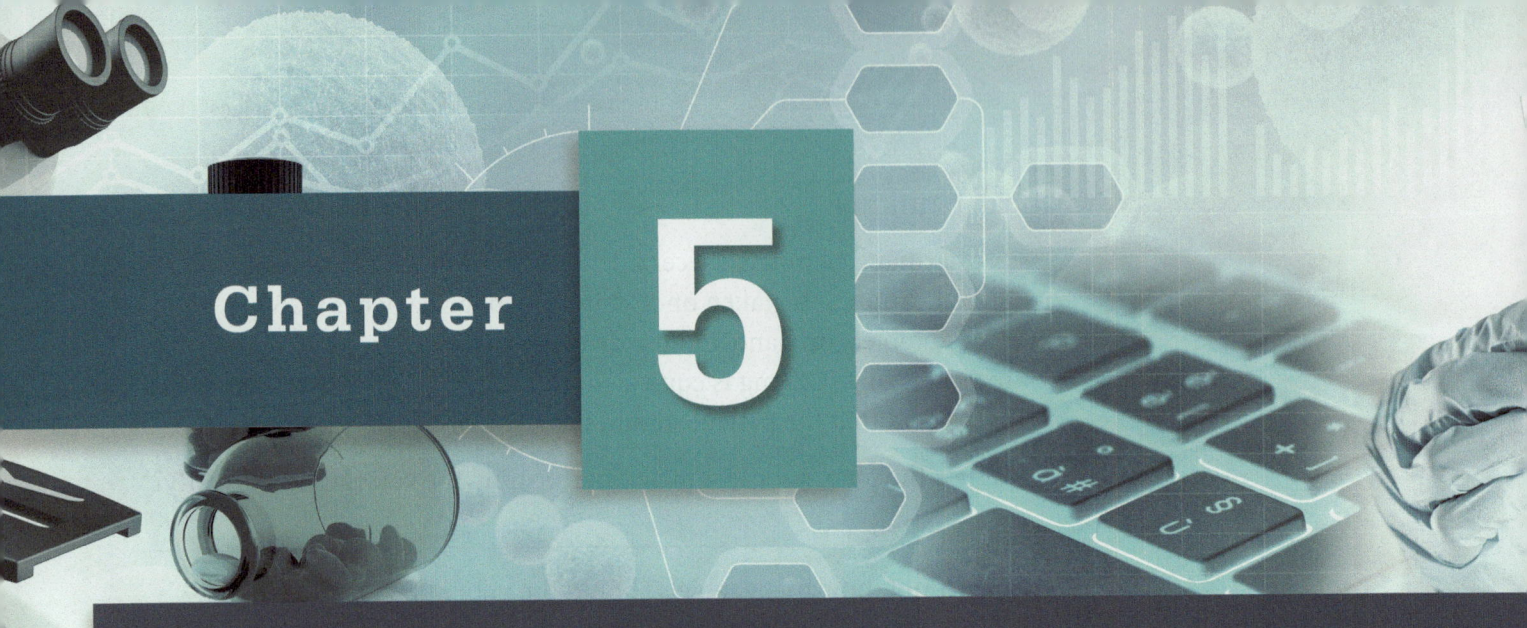

Chapter 5

Percentage of Errors Due to Equipment

Outline

Overview
Measurement of Weight
Measurement of Volume
Percentage of Error
Calculating Percentage of Error When Weighing
Calculating Percentage of Error in Volumetric Measurement

Objectives

Upon completion of this chapter, you should be able to:

1. Given a sensitivity requirement for a Class A prescription balance, calculate dosages within a certain percentage error.
2. Calculate the smallest amount of medication to be measured by a specific device.
3. Calculate the percentage of error for weight and volume measurements.
4. Describe equipment used to measure weight and volume.
5. Explain how errors in dosing can occur due to equipment.

Key Terms

class A prescription balances
conical graduates
cylindrical graduates
electronic balances
meniscus
pipets

Overview

The pharmacy technician must understand how to utilize the proper equipment to measure weight and volume for dosages. The ability to calculate percentage of error when weighing and conducting volumetric measurement is essential to the duties of the pharmacy technician. The demands of today's practice of pharmacy require skillful use of calculators when performing dosage calculations. State boards of pharmacy often require pharmacies to provide minimum lists of equipment for compounding prescriptions.

Measurement of Weight

Many types of equipment are available to measure weight in the pharmacy. Balances, scales, and metal weights are commonly utilized on a day-to-day basis. The correct equipment to use for each type of measurement is based on the task at hand. For example, prescription balances are commonly used in extemporaneous compounding, while **electronic balances** are used for assay tests. All weighing equipment must be calibrated and tested for accuracy and sensitivity.

Medicinal substances are usually weighed on **Class A prescription balances**. These balances are sensitive enough to weigh as little as 6 mg in each weighing pan and can weigh up to 120 grams in each weighing pan. They include torsion balances (see **Figure 5-1**) and electronic balances (see **Figure 5-2**).

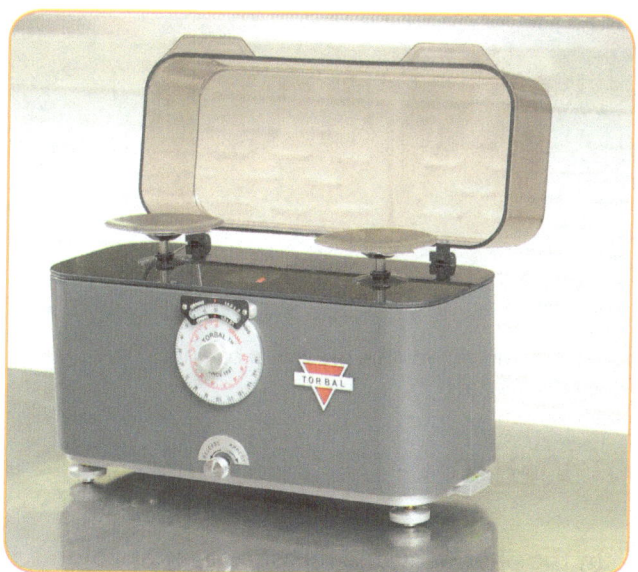

Figure 5-1 Class A prescription balance.
© Cengage Learning 2013

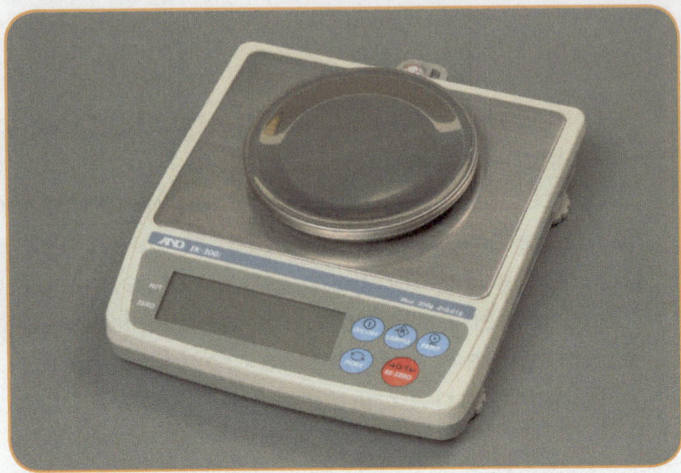

Figure 5-2 Electronic balance.
© Cengage Learning 2013

The *sensitivity requirement* of a balance is defined as the load that will cause a change of one division on its index plate. This is determined by first leveling the balance and then determining its rest point. Following this, the smallest weight that causes the rest point to shift one division on the index plate reveals the sensitivity requirement of the balance. High-precision electronic analytical balances are even more accurate for very small quantities. They are often able to weigh 0.1 mg of a substance, self-calibrate, and have easy-to-read digital displays. Metric weights used with balances are shown in **Figure 5-3**.

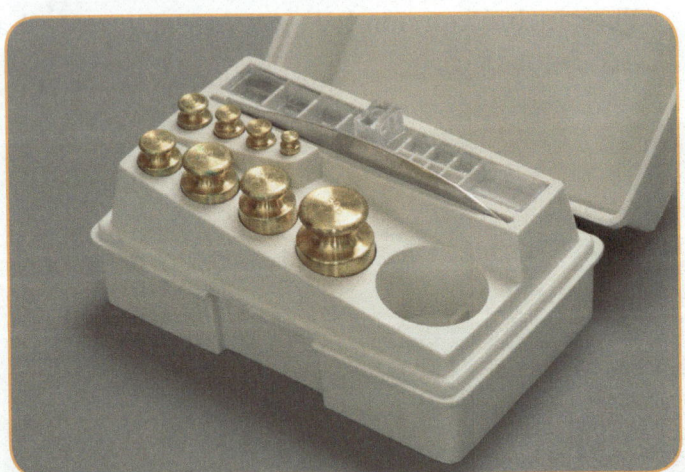

Figure 5-3 Metric weights used with balances.
© Cengage Learning 2013

Measurement of Volume

In the pharmacy, the measurement of volume involves the use of a variety of equipment, including burettes, graduates, calibrated syringes, **pipets**, micropipets, and others. The level of precision needed determines the choice of the correct measuring instrument. Cylindrical and conical (cone-shaped) graduates are the most commonly used types of equipment for volumetric measurements.

Cylindrical graduates (see **Figure 5-4**) are calibrated in metric units. **Conical graduates** (see **Figure 5-5**) are usually calibrated in both metric and apothecary units. Graduates are made of glass or plastic and *usually* range in capacity from 5 mL to 1000 mL. To decrease errors, the smallest size graduate should be used to measure a specific quantity. In general, the thinner the graduate, the less error in reading the **meniscus** of the liquid contained (see **Figure 5-6**). To accurately read the amount of a substance inside a graduate, it should be placed on a flat, level surface.

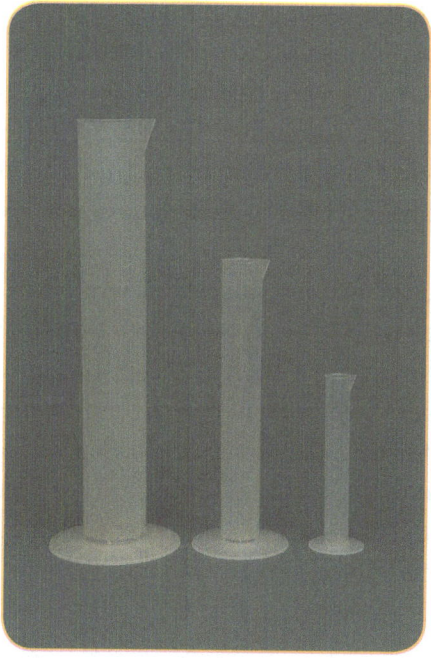

Figure 5-4 Cylindrical graduates.
© Cengage Learning 2013

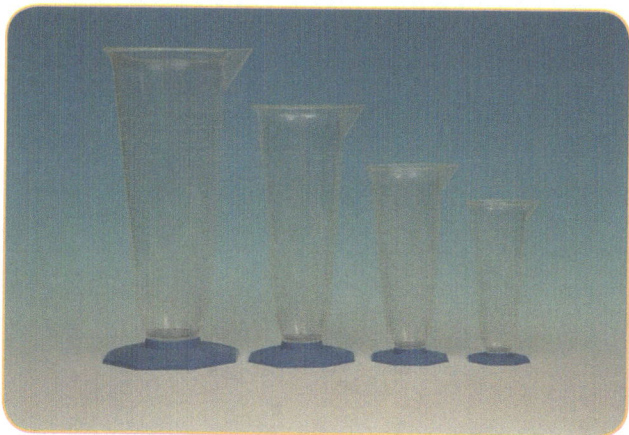

Figure 5-5 Conical graduates.
© Cengage Learning 2013

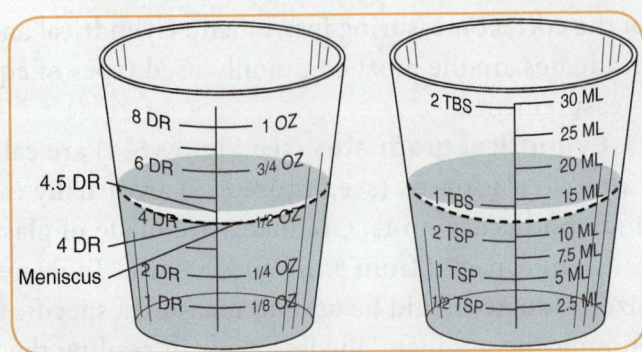

Figure 5-6 How to read the meniscus.
© Cengage Learning 2013

Both the *United States Pharmacopeia* and the *National Bureau of Standards Handbook* discuss how deviations affect errors in reading the meniscus when working with different sizes of graduates. It is essential for the pharmacy technician to select the proper type of graduate and also to ascertain that its size is the most correct for the amount being measured. They must carefully observe the meniscus at eye level to achieve the desired measurement.

The household measurement system, while still used in homes throughout the United States, is highly inaccurate due to the discrepancies in sizes of manufactured equipment such as teaspoons and tablespoons. While teaspoons are (in general) equivalent to 5 mL, and tablespoons are considered to be 15 mL, calibrated droppers that can contain these quantities are preferred because they are more accurate and precise (see **Figure 5-7**). Calibrated dosage spoons, hypodermic syringes, and medicine cups are also preferred over household equipment (see **Figures 5-8** and **5-9**).

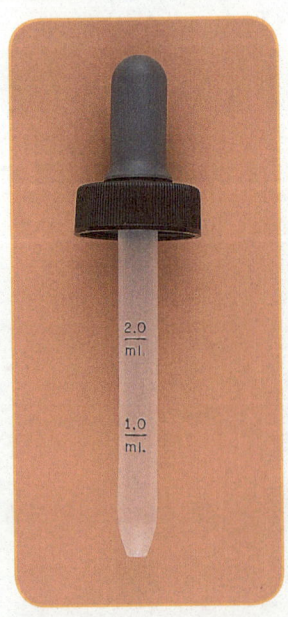

Figure 5-7 Calibrated dropper.
© Cengage Learning 2013

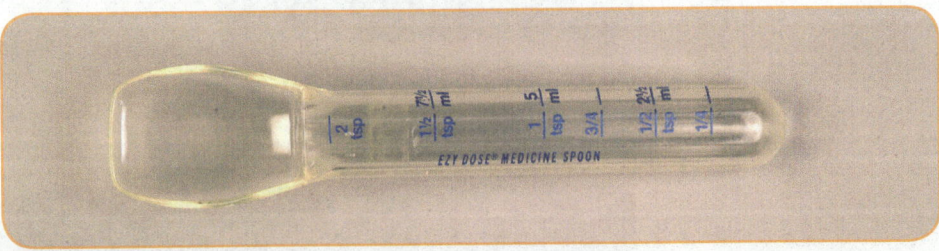

Figure 5-8 Calibrated spoon.
© Cengage Learning 2013

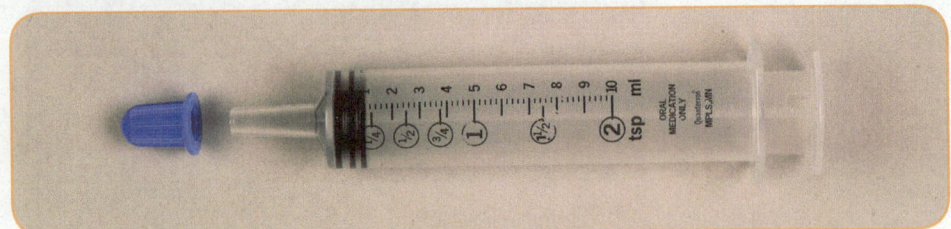

Figure 5-9 Oral syringe.
© Cengage Learning 2013

Chapter 5 • Percentage of Errors Due to Equipment

> **))) Remember**
>
> An oral syringe should never be confused with a syringe used for injections. Serious medication errors may occur as a result of such confusion.

Oral syringes are calibrated in both metric and household units. They are available in many different sizes to ensure accuracy for small dosages.

Medicine cups (see **Figure 5-10**) are preferred for larger dosages (usually from 2 teaspoons to 2 tablespoons).

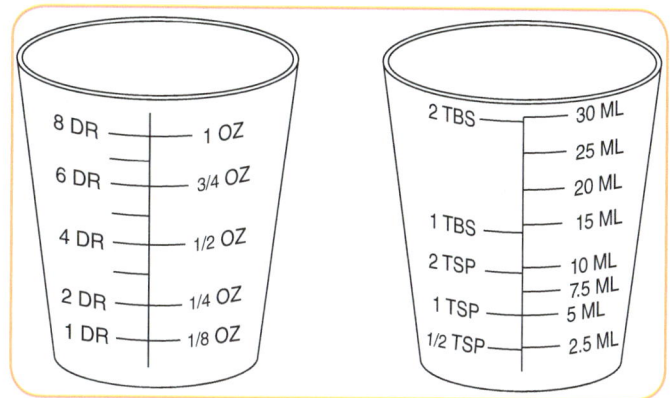

Figure 5-10 Medicine cup with approximate equivalent measures.
© Cengage Learning 2013

> **))) Remember**
>
> It is important to make sure that, no matter what type of equipment is used for measuring a medication, the calibrations on the device match the unit of measurement listed in the dosage instructions.

Because drops are often used for medications, official medicine droppers are preferred because they better control the size of each drop. Droppers with round openings that have an external diameter of approximately 3 millimeters deliver accurate drop sizes when held vertically. These droppers are calibrated to deliver approximately 20 drops of water per mm.

Percentage of Error

Pharmacy technicians as well as pharmacists must understand how inaccurate measurements may cause medication errors, and how these may vary in significance. Two quantities are important when measuring weight or volume:

- The *apparent* weight or volume that is measured
- The possible deficiency or excess of the actual quantity that is obtained

Percentage of error is the maximum potential error multiplied by 100 and then divided by the desired quantity.

$$\frac{\text{Error} \times 100\%}{\text{Desired quantity}} = \text{Percentage of error}$$

Calculating Percentage of Error When Weighing

The percentage of error when weighing is easily calculated using the preceding formula.

■ Example 1:

If the maximum potential error is ±5 mg in a total of 100 mg, what is the percentage of error?

$$\frac{5 \times 100\%}{100} = 5\%$$

Therefore, in this example, the percentage of error is 5%.

■ Example 2:

A prescription calls for 600 mg of a substance. The amount is weighed, and the pharmacy technician double-checks it by using a more sensitive balance to weigh it again. This reveals the amount to be 575 mg. The difference is 25 mg, so what is the percentage of error?

$$\frac{25 \times 100\%}{600} = 4\%$$

Therefore, in this example, the percentage of error is 4%.

If a certain percentage of error is not to be exceeded, and the maximum potential error of a measuring instrument is known, you can calculate the smallest quantity that can be measured within the desired accuracy.

$$\frac{100 \times \text{Maximum potential error}}{\text{Permissible percentage of error}} = \text{Smallest quantity}$$

■ Example 3:

On a balance that is sensitive to 6 mg, what is the smallest quantity that can be weighed with a potential error of no more than 5 percent?

$$\frac{100 \times 6 \text{ mg}}{5(\%)} = 120 \text{ mg}$$

Therefore, the smallest quantity that can be weighed with a potential error of no more than 5 percent is 120 mg.

Calculating Percentage of Error in Volumetric Measurement

The percentage of error in volumetric measurement can be calculated easily, by relating the volume in error to the desired volume.

■ Example 1:

A graduated cylinder is used to measure 30 mL of a medication. To double-check, the pharmacy technician uses a narrow-gauge burette and finds that 32 mL was actually measured. What is the percentage of error?

The volume of error is 32 mL − 30 mL = 2 mL.

Therefore,

$$\frac{2\ mL \times 100\%}{30\ mL} = 6.7\%$$

The percentage of error in this example is 6.7%.

Stop and Review
Answer the following questions.

1. What is the potential error (in terms of percentage) if 100 mg of a powdered medication is weighed on a balance with a sensitivity requirement of 6 mg?

2. If a 20-mL graduate weighs 85.49 grams, and 15 mL of distilled water is measured in it, the combined weight of the graduate and water is 100.28 grams. Because 15 mL of water should weigh 15 grams, calculate the weight of the measured water, and then express any deviation from 5 g as a percentage of error.

3. On a prescription balance with a sensitivity requirement of 0.06 g, what is the smallest amount that can be weighed with a maximum potential error of not more than 12%?

4. A pharmacy technician weighed 40 mg of menthol on a balance with a sensitivity requirement of 4 mg. Calculate the percentage of error that may have been incurred.

5. A pharmacy technician is directed to weigh 15 g of a substance in order to limit the percentage of error to 0.5%. What is the maximum potential error in milligrams the technician would not be allowed to exceed?

Test Your Knowledge

Answer the following questions.

1. A pharmacist weighed 0.075 g of a substance on a balance insensitive to quantities smaller than 0.005 g. What was the maximum potential error in terms of percentage?

2. A pharmacist weighed 500 mg of a substance on a balance of unknown accuracy. When checked on a more accurate balance, the weight was found to be 495 mg. Calculate the percentage of error in the first weighing.

3. A graduate weighs 42.85 g. When 10 mL of water is measured in it, the weight of the graduate and water is 45.95 g. Calculate the weight of the water and express any deviation from 10 g as the percentage of error.

4. A pharmacist prepared an ointment using 28.5 g of zinc oxide instead of the 30.5 grams required. Calculate the percentage of error on the basis of the desired quantity.

5. A pharmacist weighed 0.365 g of morphine sulfate on a balance of unknown accuracy. When checked on a better balance, the weight was found to be 0.385 g. Calculate the percentage of error in the first weighing.

6. A pharmacist measured 70 mL of a medication by difference, starting with 100 mL. He noted that the graduate used contained 35 mL of glycerin. Calculate the percentage of error incurred in the measurement.

7. A pharmacy technician did not calibrate a balance before weighing 225 mg of codeine sulfate. She later found that because of lack of calibration, a 10% error (over the desired amount) had occurred. If this error percentage is accurate, how much codeine sulfate was actually weighed?

8. A pharmacist measures 800 mL in a 1000 mL cylindrical graduate that is calibrated in 10 mL units. What is the percentage of error that might be incurred in the measurement?

9. How would you weigh 0.15 g of atropine sulfate and diluent of lactose with an error not greater than 5% if the prescription balance has a sensitivity requirement of 0.06 grams?

10. How would you weigh 0.006 g of a substance with an error not greater than 5% if the prescription balance has a sensitivity requirement of 0.004 gram?

Critical Thinking

A 4-year-old child has been on an oral antibiotic for 7 days. She still has all the same symptoms as when she started taking the antibiotic. Her mother called the pharmacy and spoke to a pharmacy technician. She tells him that though the antibiotic is supposed to continue for another 7 days, it is still almost $\frac{3}{4}$ full. The pharmacy technician asks the mother how she is administering the medication. She explains that she is administering one spoonful three times per day. The pharmacy technician asks what type of spoon she is using because the prescription was for "one teaspoonful three times per day." The mother says the child will only allow her to use a plastic spoon that was inside the packaging of her favorite doll.

1. What mistake has occurred in dosing?

2. Why is the child still exhibiting symptoms?

A pharmacy technician weighed 1 g of a substance on a balance of unknown accuracy. When he checked the substance's weight on a more accurate balance, the weight was found to be 995 mg.

3. What is the percentage of error in the first weight that was obtained?

4. What would the percentage of error be if the first weight of the substance was 500 mg and the second weight was 450 mg?

A pharmacy technician is required to measure a liquid medication's volume in apothecary units. Which type of equipment must be used?

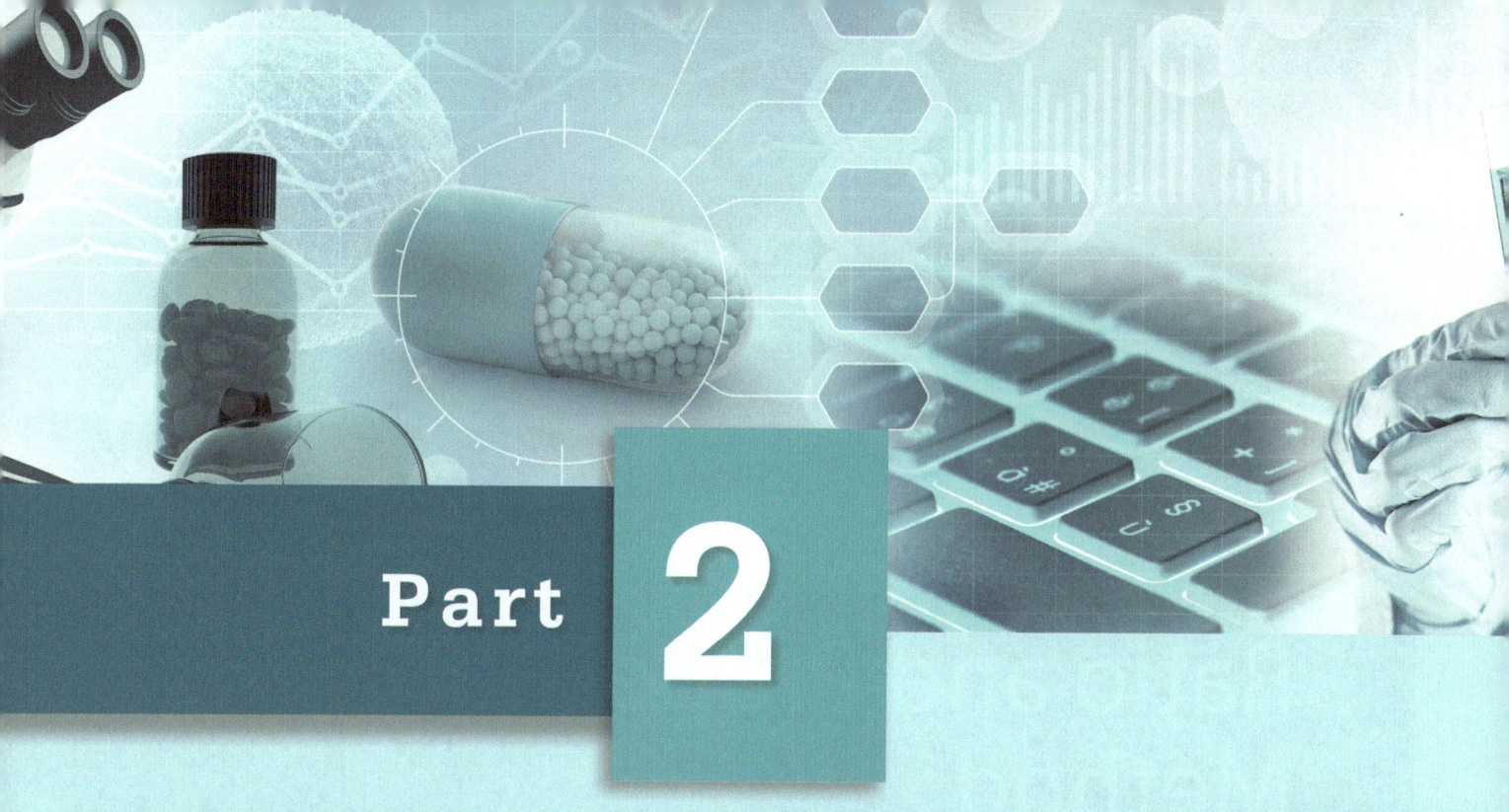

Part 2

Dosage Calculations

Chapter 6 Ratio and Proportion Method
Chapter 7 Dimensional Analysis
Chapter 8 Formula Method

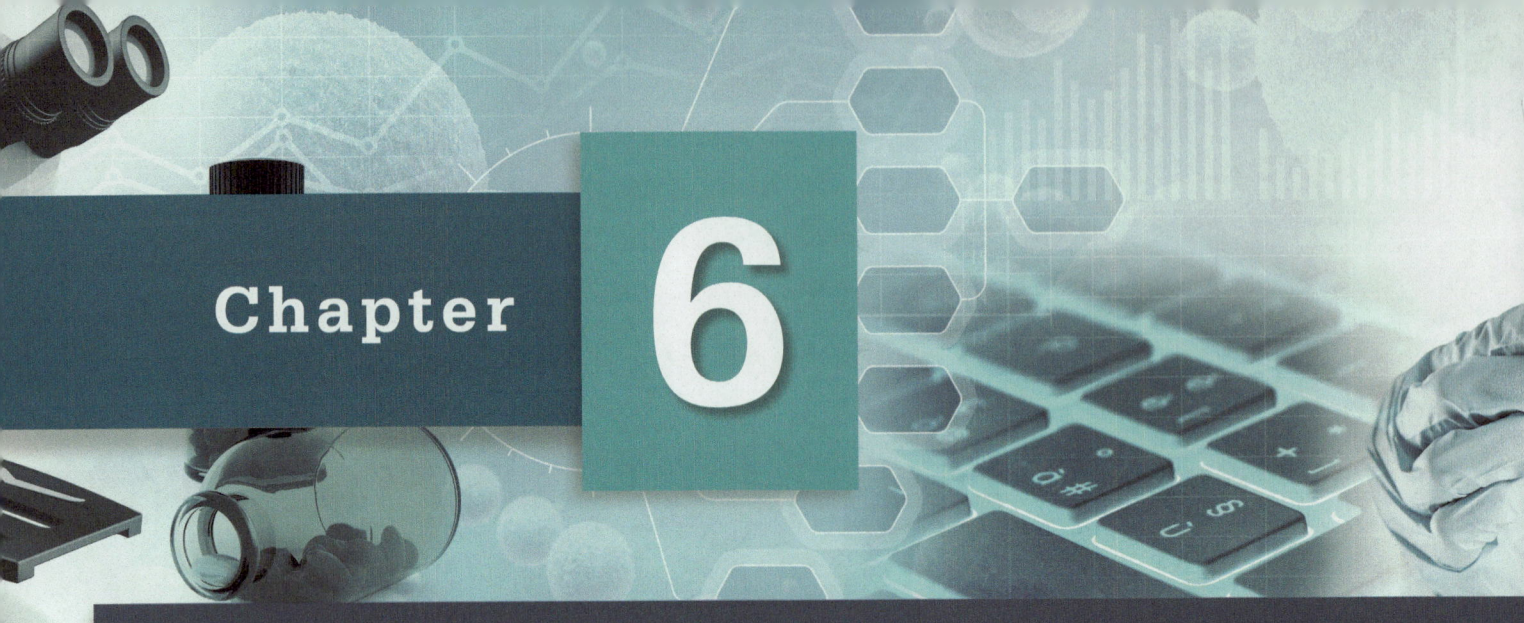

Chapter 6

Ratio and Proportion Method

Outline

Overview
Ratio and Proportion Expressed Using Common Fractions
    Dosage Calculations
Ratio and Proportion Expressed Using Colons
    Dosage Calculations
Calculations Using Different Units of Measure

Objectives

Upon completion of this chapter, you should be able to:

1. Cross-multiply proportions to determine if they are true.
2. Calculate dosages to the nearest tenth or hundredth using the ratio and proportion method.
3. Demonstrate the use of colons in the ratio and proportion method for dosage calculations.
4. Perform calculations using different units of measure.

Key Terms

common fractions
proportion
ratio
true proportion

Overview

Ratio and proportion form the basis for nearly all calculations. The ratio and proportion method is a concept that is widely understood and used. **It is important for pharmacy technicians to be able to interpret such calculations and identify where to start.** A ratio states the relation of one quantity to another. Ratios may be written as common fractions (implying division) or with a colon between the two numbers.

In previous chapters, this book discussed how to read the dosage strengths on drug labels. Each of these strengths was expressed as a ratio: a specific weight (strength of a drug in forms such as tablets, capsules, or certain volumes of solution). Liquid preparations are commonly measured in mL, and their strengths are called concentrations. Common dosage strengths are expressed as follows: 50 mg per mL, 100 mcg per tablet, and 1000 units per mL.

Ratio and Proportion Expressed Using Common Fractions

A **ratio** is made up of two numbers or quantities that have a significant relationship. They can be expressed (written) as **common fractions** or separated by a colon (:). A **proportion** is used to show the relationship between two ratios. The ratios in a proportion are separated by an equal (=) sign. Conversions may be made by setting up a proportion of two ratios expressed as fractions. A **true proportion** contains two ratios that are equal (for example, $\frac{1}{50} = \frac{2}{100}$). In a true proportion, the cross-multiplied products will be identical.

The pharmacy technician must make sure that the units in the numerators match and that the units in the denominators match. The units in each ratio must then be labeled.

> **》》》 Remember**
>
> In a proportion, the ratio for a known equivalent equals the ratio for an unknown equivalent. The following two steps are involved in this method:
>
> 1. Set up a proportion of two equivalent ratios.
> 2. Cross-multiply to solve for an unknown quantity (*X*).

■ **Example 1:**

Convert: 1.5 g to grains (gr)

Known approximate equivalent: 1 g = gr 15

This proportion in fractional form looks like this.

$$\frac{gr\ 15}{1\ g} = \frac{gr\ x}{1.5\ g} \quad \text{(Cross-multiply)} \quad 22.5 = 1x$$

Therefore, $x = 22.5$

In the preceding equation, the unknown *x* is the numerator. It is important that the sequence is the same (the numerator units match and the denominator units match). Remember, a proportion must compare "like things" to "like things."

■ Example 2:

Convert: 10 grains to milligrams

$$\frac{\text{gr i}}{60 \text{ mg}} = \frac{\text{gr } 10}{x \text{ mg}} \quad x = 60 \times 10 = 600 \text{ mg}$$

■ Example 3:

Convert: 75 mL to tsp

Known approximate equivalent: 1 tsp = 5 mL

$$\frac{1 \text{ t}}{5 \text{ mL}} = \frac{x \text{ t}}{75 \text{ mL}} \quad 5x = 75$$

$$\frac{5x}{5} = \frac{75}{5} \quad x = \frac{75}{5} \text{ t} = 15 \text{ t}$$

■ Example 4:

Convert: 176 lb to kg

Known approximate equivalent: 1 kg = 2.2 lb

$$\frac{1 \text{ kg}}{2.2 \text{ lb}} = \frac{x \text{ kg}}{176 \text{ lb}} \quad \text{(Cross-multiply)} \quad 2.2x = 176$$

$$\frac{2.2x}{2.2} = \frac{176}{2.2} \quad x = \frac{176}{2.2} = \text{kg} = 80 \text{ kg}$$

■ Example 5:

How many tablets are needed for a 100 mg dose if 1 tablet contains 50 mg?

$$\frac{1 \text{ tablet}}{50 \text{ mg}} = \frac{x \text{ tablets}}{100 \text{ mg}}$$

Therefore,

$$50X = 100 \text{ mg, so } X = 2 \text{ tablets}$$

■ Example 6:

Cross-multiply this proportion to determine if it is a true proportion.

$$\frac{1 \text{ mL}}{10 \text{ units}} = \frac{2 \text{ mL}}{20 \text{ units}}$$

Therefore,

$$1 \times 20 = 10 \times 2$$

$$20 = 20$$

Yes, this is a true proportion because the products of cross-multiplying—20—are equal.

Dosage Calculations

In dosage calculations, ratio and proportion are important because they can be used when only one ratio is known (or complete), and the second ratio is incomplete.

■ Example 1:

A solution strength of 8 mg per mL is needed to prepare a dosage of 10 mg. The solution strength available (8 mg per mL) provides the *known ratio*. The dosage to be given is the *incomplete ratio* (10 mg). The letter *X* is used to represent the mL that will contain 10 mg. Notice that both numerators are expressed as milligrams while both denominators are expressed as milliliters. The ratios in a proportion must be written in the same sequence of measurement units.

$$\frac{8 \text{ mg}}{1 \text{ mL}} = \frac{10 \text{ mg}}{X \text{ mL}}$$

The first fraction is a complete ratio that expresses the drug strength. The second fraction is an incomplete ratio that expresses the dosage to give. By cross-multiplying, it is easy to see that:

$$8X = 10; \text{ therefore, the answer is } 1.25 \text{ mL}$$

The ordered dosage of 10 mg is contained in 1.25 mL.

It is important to double-check your calculations and to assess that each answer is logical. In the preceding example, because 1 mL contains 8 mg, you need a larger volume than 1 mL to obtain 10 mg. The answer, 1.25 mL, is larger, so it is logical. While this does not verify that the calculation is correct, at least it shows you that you set up the proportion correctly and cross-multiplied sufficiently.

■ Example 2:

A dosage of 20 mg has been ordered. The strength available is 25 mg in 1.5 mL.

$$\frac{25 \text{ mg}}{1.5 \text{ mL}} = \frac{20 \text{ mg}}{X \text{ mL}}$$

When you cross-multiply:

$$25X = 1.5 \times 20$$

Therefore, $X = 1.2$ mL.

Because the dosage ordered (20 mg) is smaller than the strength available (25 mg in 1.5 mL), the answer should be smaller than 1.5 mL, and it is. Therefore, it is logical.

■ Example 3:

The solution strength on hand is 80 mg per mL. A dosage of 200 mg is ordered.

$$\frac{80 \text{ mg}}{1 \text{ mL}} = \frac{200 \text{ mg}}{X \text{ mL}}$$

Therefore,

$$80X = 200$$

$$\text{So, } X = 2.5 \text{ mL.}$$

This answer is logical because 2.5 mL is larger than the strength available, and the dosage ordered (200 mg) is larger than the solution on hand (80 mg per mL) and must be contained in more than 1 mL.

■ Example 4:

Shortcuts can be used to simplify the math in these problems. To do so, after cross-multiplying, immediately divide by the number in front of X. You can also reduce numbers to their lowest common terms whenever possible. For example, you have a 300 mg per 1.2 mL solution and need to prepare a dosage of 120 mg.

$$\frac{300 \text{ mg}}{1.2 \text{ mL}} = \frac{120 \text{ mg}}{X \text{ mL}}$$

Cross-multiply and immediately divide by the number in front of X:

$$X = \frac{1.2 \times 120}{300}$$

Reduce the 120 and 300 numbers by 60. Do the final division, and, depending on the medication you are using, round to the nearest tenth.

$$X = \frac{1.2 \times 2}{5} = \frac{2.4}{5} = 0.48 = 0.5 \text{ mL}$$

A dosage of 120 mg requires fewer mL than the 300 mg per 1.2 mL strength available. Therefore, the smaller 0.5 mL answer is logical.

■ Example 5:

You have on hand a 1.5 mg in 0.5 mL solution. You must prepare a 2 mg dosage.

$$\frac{1.5 \text{ mg}}{0.5 \text{ mL}} = \frac{2 \text{ mg}}{X \text{ mL}}$$

Therefore,

$$X = \frac{1 \times 2}{3} = \frac{2}{3} = 0.66 = 0.7 \text{ mL}$$

Because the 0.7 mL answer is a larger volume than the 1.5 mg in 0.5 mL dosage strength, it is logical for this 2 mg dosage.

■ Example 6:

The solution available is 80 mg per mL. A 120 mg dosage is ordered.

$$\frac{80 \text{ mg}}{1 \text{ mL}} = \frac{120 \text{ mg}}{X \text{ mL}}$$

Therefore,

$$X = \frac{120}{80} = \frac{3}{2} = 1.5 \text{ mL}$$

Because the 120 mg dosage ordered requires a volume larger than the 80 mg per mL available dosage strength, the answer, 1.5 mL, is larger and, therefore, logical.

Stop and Review
Using the Ratio and Proportion Method

1. Use the ratio and proportion method to convert each of the following amounts to the unit indicated. Indicate the approximate equivalent used in the conversion.

   a. 160 mL = _____ L

   b. 84 lb = _____ kg

   c. 30 mg = _____ gr

   d. 625 mcg = _____ mg

   e. 2 qt = _____ L

   f. 32 g = _____ mg

   g. 18.5 cm = _____ in.

   h. gr $\overline{ss}$ = _____ mg

   i. gr $\frac{1}{8}$ = _____ mg

   j. 250 mL = _____ L

2. Determine if these proportions are true by cross-multiplying.

   a. $\dfrac{34 \text{ mg}}{2 \text{ mL}} = \dfrac{51 \text{ mg}}{3 \text{ mL}}$ _____

   b. $\dfrac{15 \text{ mg}}{4 \text{ mL}} = \dfrac{45 \text{ mg}}{12 \text{ mL}}$ _____

   c. $\dfrac{1.3 \text{ mL}}{46 \text{ mg}} = \dfrac{0.65 \text{ mL}}{23 \text{ mg}}$ _____

   d. $\dfrac{2.3 \text{ mL}}{150 \text{ units}} = \dfrac{1.9 \text{ mL}}{130 \text{ units}}$ _____

   e. $\dfrac{40 \text{ mg}}{1.1 \text{ mL}} = \dfrac{80 \text{ mg}}{2.2 \text{ mL}}$ _____

3. Calculate the following dosages and express the answers to the nearest tenth. Assess your answers to determine if they are logical. Make sure to include the units of measure in your answers.

a. Ordered dosage:	24 mg
Solution strength available:	12.5 mg in 1.5 mL
Give:	_____
b. Ordered dosage:	30 mg
Solution strength available:	40 mg in 2.5 mL
Give:	_____
c. Ordered dosage:	0.3 mg
Solution strength available:	0.6 mg in 0.8 mL
Give:	_____
d. Ordered dosage:	24 mg
Solution strength available:	36 mg per 2 mL
Give:	_____
e. Ordered dosage:	52 mg
Solution strength available:	78 mg in 0.9 mL
Give:	_____
f. Ordered dosage:	150 mg
Solution strength available:	100 mg per mL
Give:	_____

g. Ordered dosage:	600 mcg
Solution strength available:	750 mcg in 3 mL
Give:	_____
h. Ordered dosage:	4 g
Solution strength available:	1.5 g per mL
Give:	_____
i. Ordered dosage:	0.25 mg
Solution strength available:	0.5 mg per mL
Give:	_____
j. Ordered dosage:	3 g
Solution strength available:	4 g in 2.7 mL
Give:	_____

Ratio and Proportion Expressed Using Colons

>>> **Remember**

It is easy to remember which numbers are the means and which are the extremes in a proportion. The means begin with the letter m, as does the *middle* of the equation. The extremes begin with the letter e, as do the *ends* of the equation.

Ratios and proportions may also be expressed using colons. For example,

$$\frac{3}{4} = \frac{15}{20}$$

$$3:4::15:20$$

In a proportion, the ratios also may be separated by an equal sign. When using colons instead of fractions for ratios and proportions, the numbers on the ends of the proportion (3 and 20 in the preceding example) are called the *extremes*. The numbers in the middle (4 and 15) are called the *means*. If you multiply the means and then the extremes, their products (answer) will be equal. However, you must never mix up the means and extremes in proportions, or the answer you obtain will be incorrect.

Dosage Calculations

■ Example 1:

Ordered: Biaxin® 0.5 g p.o. q8h
On hand: Biaxin® 250 mg
Desired dose = X

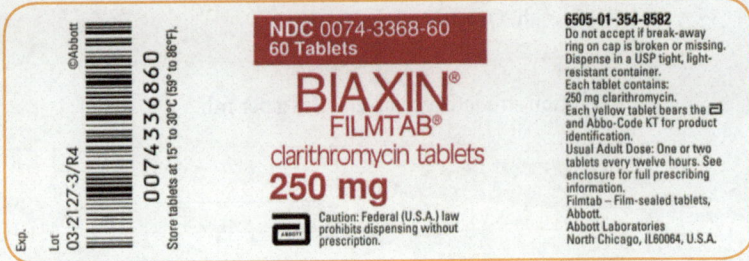

Biaxin 250 mg.
Courtesy of Abbott Laboratories.

> **Remember**
>
> • To find the desired dose:
>   Use the ratio and proportion method

■ Example 2:

1 tablet : 50 mg = 2 tablets : 100 mg

The means are 50 and 2, while the extremes are 1 and 100.

Therefore: 50 × 2 = 100 × 1
             100 = 100

meaning the ratios are equal and the proportion is true.

■ Example 3:

2 mL : 500 mg = 1 mL : 250 mg

Therefore: 500 × 1 = 2 × 250
             500 = 500

meaning the ratios are equal and the proportion is true.

■ Example 4:

1 mL : 10 units = 2 mL : 20 units

Therefore: 10 × 2 = 20
             20 = 20

This is a true proportion.

⬛ Stop and Review

Determine by calculations if these proportions are true.

1. 34 mg : 2 mL = 51 mg : 3 mL _____

2. 15 mg : 4 mL = 45 mg : 12 mL _____

3. 1.3 mL : 46 mg = 0.65 mL : 23 mg _____

4. 2.3 mL : 150 units = 1.9 mL : 130 units _____

5. 40 mg : 1.1 mL = 80 mg : 2.2 mL _____

Calculations Using Different Units of Measure

When units of measure are different, the ratio and proportion method may still be used. For example, a common situation is when the medication order is in grams and the dosage strength is available in milligrams per milliliter.

■ Example 1:

The order is for 0.15 g of medication. The dosage strength available is 200 mg per mL. Because the order unit and the dosage unit are different, conversion is required. Also, it is safer to use smaller units of measure to eliminate or avoid decimal points. Therefore, convert the 0.15 gram to milligrams (150 milligrams). To better show the math in this example, the ratios and proportions are shown as common fractions.

$$\frac{200 \text{ mg}}{1 \text{ mL}} = \frac{0.15 \text{ g}}{X \text{ mL}}$$

Change grams to milligrams.

$$\frac{200 \text{ mg}}{1 \text{ mL}} = \frac{150 \text{ mg}}{X \text{ mL}}$$

Therefore,

$$200X = 1 \times 150$$

So,

$$X = \frac{150}{200} = 0.75 \text{ or } 0.8 \text{ mL}$$

To check, because 150 mg is smaller than 200 mg, it must be contained in a smaller volume than 1 mL. Therefore, the answer, 0.8 mL, is logical.

■ Example 2:

The dosage ordered is 0.5 mg. You have a dosage strength of 200 mcg per mL.

$$\frac{200 \text{ mcg}}{1 \text{ mL}} = \frac{0.5 \text{ mg}}{X \text{ mL}}$$

Change mg to micrograms (mcg).

$$\frac{200 \text{ mcg}}{1 \text{ mL}} = \frac{500 \text{ mcg}}{X \text{ mL}}$$

Therefore,

$$200X = 500$$

So,
$$X = 2.5 \text{ mL}$$

Because 500 mcg is larger than 200 mcg, it must be contained in a quantity larger than 1 mL. Therefore, the answer, 2.5 mL, is logical.

■ Example 3:

In this example, ratio and proportion are used to solve a calculation for unit and mEq dosages. The order is for 1200 units. The available dosage strength is 1000 units per 1.5 mL.

$$\frac{1000 \text{ units}}{1.5 \text{ mL}} = \frac{1200 \text{ units}}{X \text{ mL}}$$

Therefore,
$$1000X = 1.5 \times 1200$$

So,
$$X = \frac{1.5 \times 1200}{1000}$$

The answer is 1.8 mL. Because 1200 units is a larger dosage than 1000 units, the answer (in mL) should be larger than 1.5 mL, which is logical.

■ Example 4:

A drug has a dosage strength of 2 mEq per mL. You are to prepare 10 mEq.

$$\frac{2 \text{ mEq}}{1 \text{ mL}} = \frac{10 \text{ mEq}}{X \text{ mL}}$$

Therefore,
$$2X = 10$$

So,
$$X = 5 \text{ mL}$$

Because 10 mEq is larger than 2 mEq, the answer should also be significantly larger, and therefore it is logical.

Stop and Review

Solve the following dosage calculations and express answers to the nearest tenth. Make sure to include the units of measure.

1. Ordered:	0.4 mg
Drug label reads:	1000 mcg in 2 mL
Give:	_____

2. Ordered:	275 mg
Drug label reads:	0.5 g per 2 mL
Give:	_____
3. Ordered:	0.15 mg
Drug label reads:	0.2 mg in 1.5 mL
Give:	_____
4. Ordered:	600 mg
Drug label reads:	1 g in 3.6 mL
Give:	_____
5. Ordered:	10,000 units
Drug label reads:	8000 units in 1 mL
Give:	_____
6. Ordered:	15 mEq
Drug label reads:	20 mEq per 20 mL
Give:	_____
7. Ordered:	200,000 units
Drug label reads:	150,000 units per 2 mL
Give:	_____

Test Your Knowledge

Use the ratio and proportion method to calculate the following parenteral dosages. Answers should be in milliliters and expressed to the nearest tenth or hundredth as needed. Check each answer to make sure it is logical. Measure the dosages on the syringes provided.

Dosage Ordered	mL required
1. Depo-Provera® 0.3 g 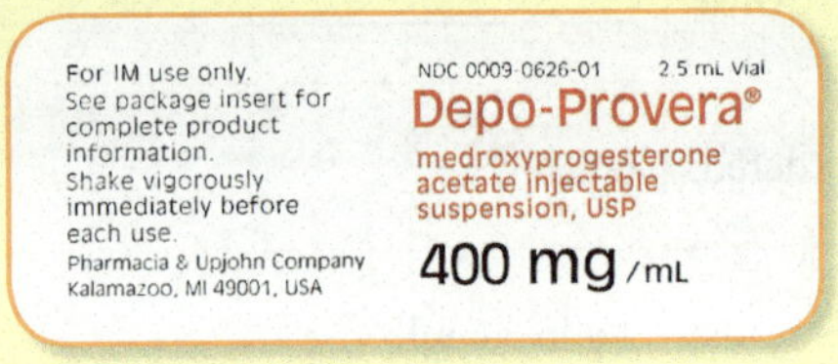 Depo-Provera 400 mg/mL. *Used with permission from Pharmacia Corporation, Peapack, NJ.*	_____
2. furosemide 15 mg 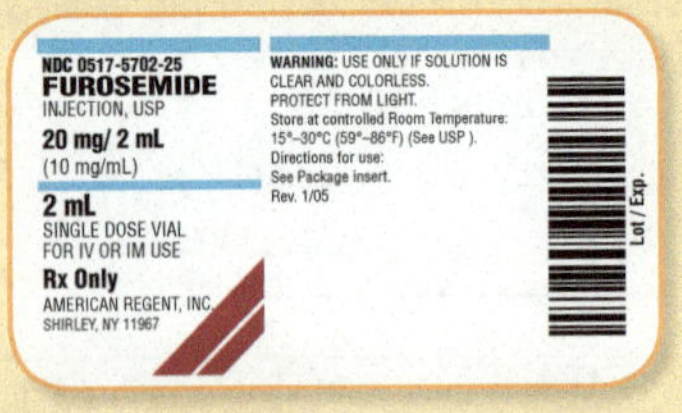 Furosemide 20 mg/mL. *Used with permission of American Regent, Inc.*	_____
3. heparin sodium 2000 units 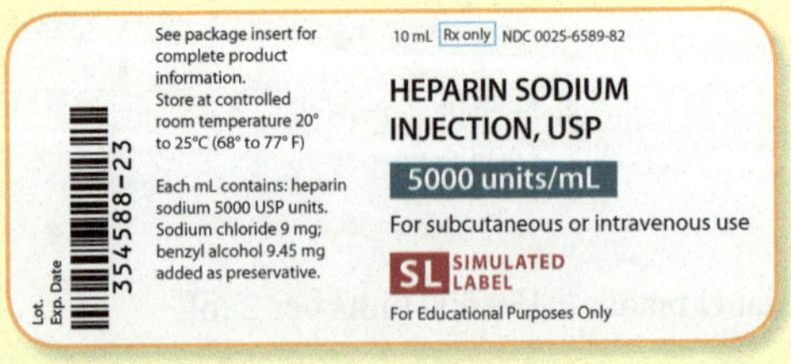 Heparin Sodium Injection, USP. © Cengage Learning 2013.	_____

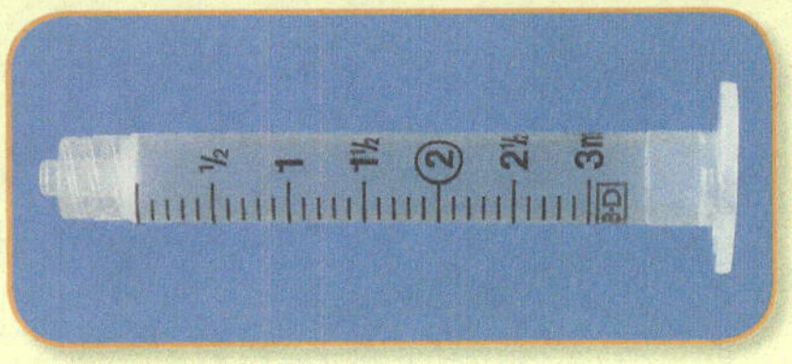

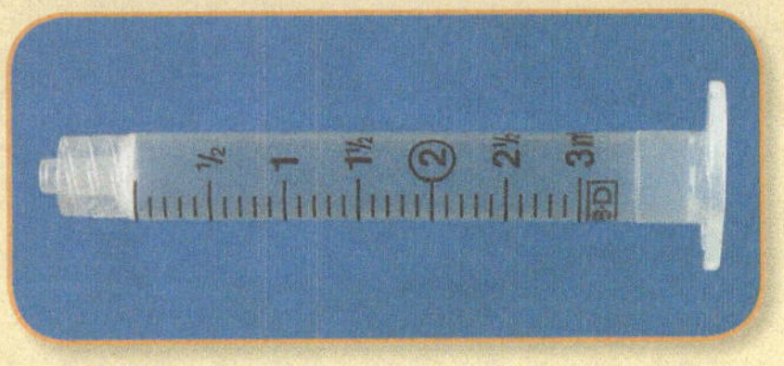

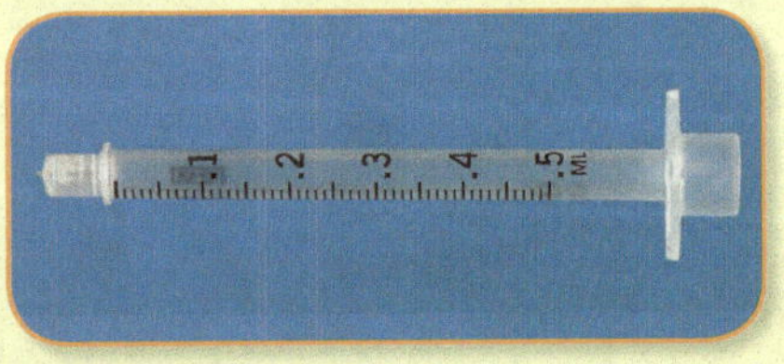

Chapter 6 • Ratio and Proportion Method   101

Dosage Ordered	mL required
4. Cleocin® 0.75 g for an IV additive Cleocin Phosphate 900 mg. *Used with permission from Pharmacia Corporation, Peapack, NJ.*	_____
5. naloxone 350 mcg Narcan® *Used with permission from Endo Pharmaceuticals Inc.*	_____
6. clindamycin 225 mg Clindamycin 150 mg/mL. *Used with permission from Bedford Laboratories.*	_____
7. Robinul® 75 mcg (calculate to the nearest hundredth) Robinul® 75 mcg. *Copyright Baxter International Inc. Robinul is a trademark of Wyeth Pharmaceuticals Division of Wyeth.*	_____

Dosage Ordered	mL required
8. midazolam HCl 4 mg Midazolam 25 mg/5 mL. *Used with permission from Bedford Laboratories.*	_____
9. benztropine mesylate 2.4 mg Benztropine mesylate 2 mg per 2 mL. © *Cengage Learning 2013.*	_____
10. cyanocobalamin 800 mcg Cyanocobalamin 1000 mcg/mL. *Used with permission of American Regent, Inc.*	_____
11. potassium chloride 16 mEq for IV additive Potassium Chloride 40 mEq. *Used with permission from Abraxis BioScience, Inc.*	_____

Dosage Ordered	mL required
12. calcium gluconate 0.93 mEq for an IV additive 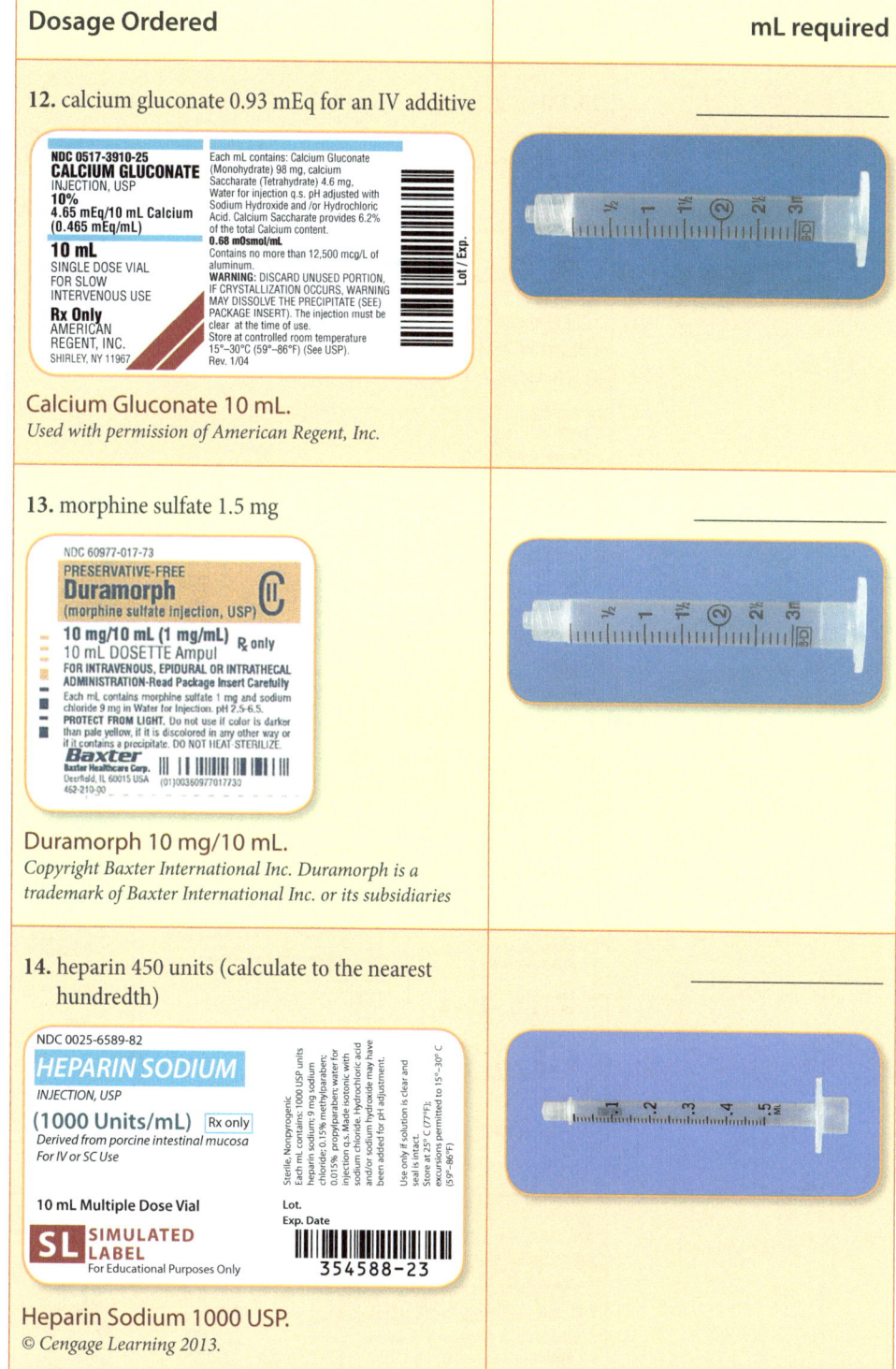 Calcium Gluconate 10 mL. *Used with permission of American Regent, Inc.*	_____
13. morphine sulfate 1.5 mg Duramorph 10 mg/10 mL. *Copyright Baxter International Inc. Duramorph is a trademark of Baxter International Inc. or its subsidiaries*	_____
14. heparin 450 units (calculate to the nearest hundredth) Heparin Sodium 1000 USP. © *Cengage Learning 2013.*	_____

Dosage Ordered	mL required
15. Dilantin® 0.1 g Dilantin 250 mg/5 mL. *Labels reproduced with permission of Pfizer, Inc.*	_____
16. gentamicin 70 mg Gentamicin 40 mg/mL. *Used with permission from Abraxis BioScience, Inc.*	_____
17. sodium chloride 60 mEq for an IV additive Sodium Chloride. © Cengage Learning 2013.	_____
18. meperidine 75 mg Meperidine 100 mg/mL. *Copyright Baxter International Inc.*	_____

Dosage Ordered	mL required
19. betamethasone sodium phosphate and betamethasone acetate 10 mg Betamethasone sodium phosphate and Betamethasone acetate, USP 5 mL multiple-Dose Vial, 6 mg per mL. © Cengage Learning 2013.	_____
20. gentamicin 0.1 g Gentamicin 40 mg/mL. *Reprinted with permission of Abraxis BioScience, Inc.*	_____
21. doxorubicin HCl 16 mg for an IV additive Doxorubicin HCl 20 mg. *Used with permission from Bedford Laboratories, Bedford, Ohio.*	_____
22. methotrexate 40 mg Methotrexate 200 mg. © Cengage Learning 2013.	_____

Dosage Ordered	mL required
23. haloperidol decanoate 75 mg Haldol 50 mcg/mL. © Cengage Learning 2013.	_____
24. chlorpromazine HCl 40 mg Thorazine 25 mg/mL. *Reprinted with permission from GlaxoSmithKline.*	_____
25. nalbuphine HCl 30 mg Nubain 20 mg/mL. *Used with permission from Endo Pharmaceuticals, Inc.*	_____

Dosage Ordered	mL required
26. cyanocobalamin 750 mg Cyanocobalamin 1000 mcg/mL. *Used with permission of American Regent, Inc.*	_____
27. naloxone HCl 0.5 mg Naloxone 400 mcg/mL. *Copyright Baxter Healthcare Corporation.*	_____
28. chlorpromazine (Thorazine®) 60 mg Thorazine 25 mg/mL. *Reprinted with permission from GlaxoSmithKline.*	_____

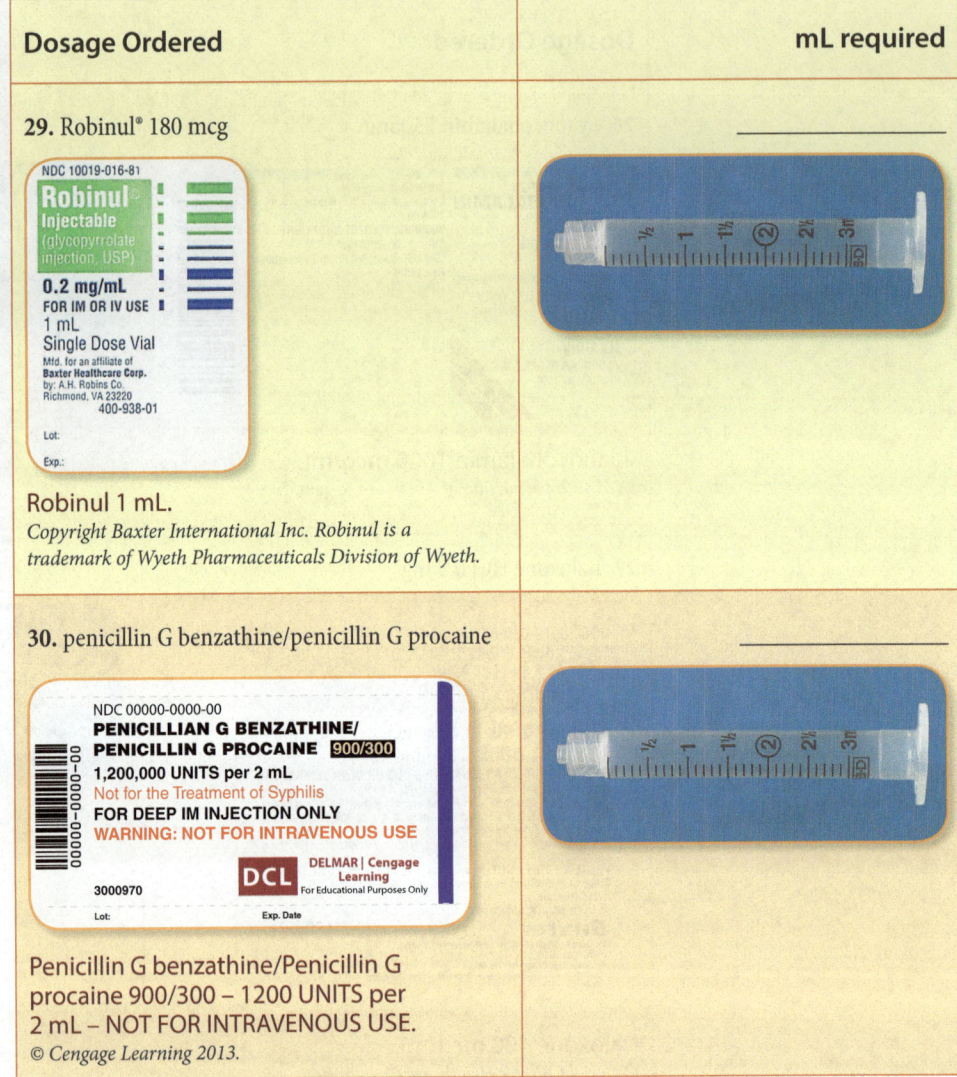

Dosage Ordered	mL required
29. Robinul® 180 mcg Robinul 1 mL. *Copyright Baxter International Inc. Robinul is a trademark of Wyeth Pharmaceuticals Division of Wyeth.*	_____
30. penicillin G benzathine/penicillin G procaine Penicillin G benzathine/Penicillin G procaine 900/300 – 1200 UNITS per 2 mL – NOT FOR INTRAVENOUS USE. © Cengage Learning 2013.	_____

Critical Thinking

A solution strength of 20 mg per mL is needed to prepare a dosage of 30 mg. The solution strength available is 20 mg per mL, which provides the known ratio. The dosage to be given is the incomplete ratio (30 mg).

1. How should the technician write the ratio in a proportion in the same sequence of measurement units?

   _____

2. What are the correct steps to make the calculation?

   _____

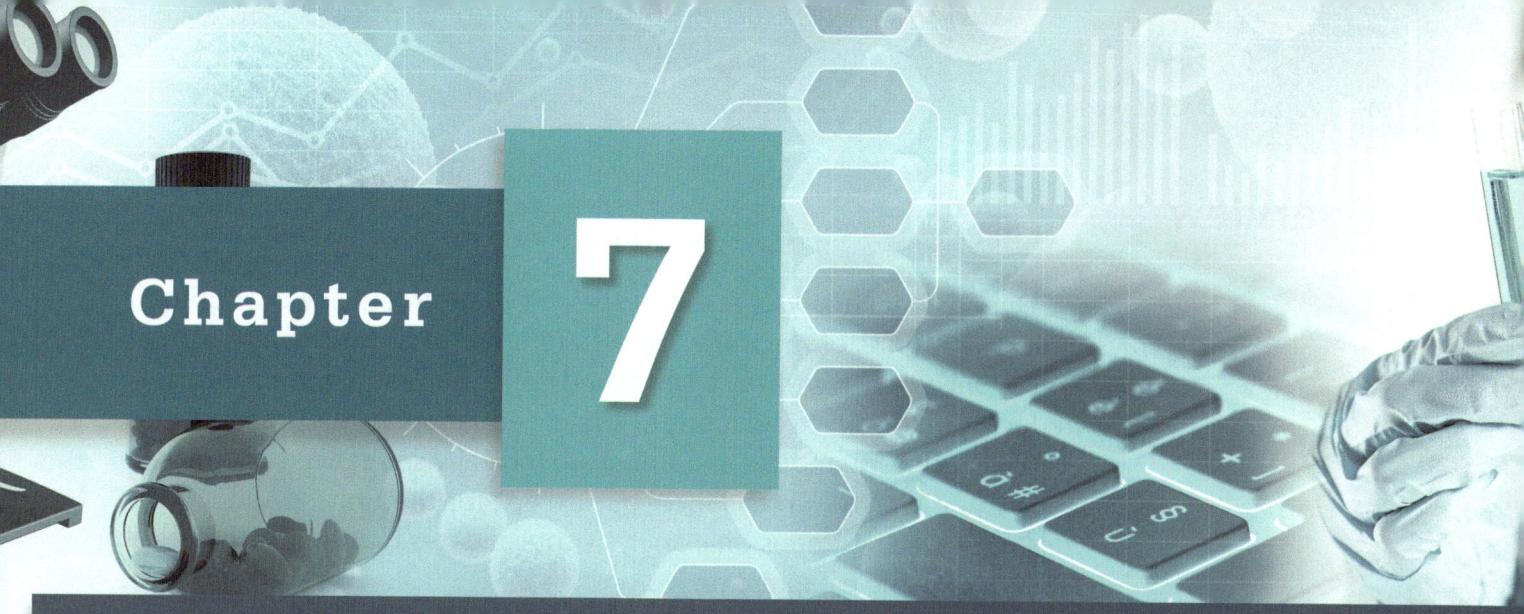

Chapter 7

Dimensional Analysis

Outline

Overview
Basic Dimensional Analysis
Equations Requiring Metric Conversions
Dosage Calculations Using Dimensional Analysis

Objectives

Upon completion of this chapter, you should be able to:

1. Use dimensional analysis to calculate dosages.
2. Round dosage calculations performed with dimensional analysis to the nearest tenth or hundredth.
3. Solve equations that require metric conversions.

Key Terms

clinical ratios
dimensional analysis
metric conversion
unit conversion

Overview

Dimensional analysis is the process of mathematically changing or converting units of measure. It is also referred to as **unit conversion** or *units conversion*. It utilizes a simplified version of ratio and proportion, reducing multistep calculations to a single equation. In this process, arithmetical terms (quantities and units) are logically sequenced and placed into equations. All units cancel out except for the unit or units of the desired answer. Dimensional analysis consolidates multiple arithmetical steps into a single expression.

To understand dimensional analysis, you must first understand clinical ratios. Dimensional analysis consolidates many steps of arithmetic into a single expression. It is used widely in chemistry, and pharmacists and pharmacy technicians often prefer it to the ratio-proportion method. In dimensional analysis, **clinical ratios** are written as common fractions, such as the following:

$$\frac{1 \text{ tablet}}{250 \text{ mg}} \quad \frac{2 \text{ grams}}{1.5 \text{ mL}} \quad \frac{1 \text{ mL}}{10 \text{ units}}$$

Basic Dimensional Analysis

To set up an equation for **dimensional analysis**, you must follow these steps:

1. Write the unit of measure being calculated, such as milliliters (mL). This eliminates confusion over which measure is being calculated and determines how the first clinical ratio is entered into the equation.

2. Identify the complete clinical ratio that contains the milliliters, as provided by the dosage strength available. This should be entered as a common fraction.

3. All additional ratios are entered so that each denominator matches with its successive numerator. If the first ratio denominator is milligrams, then the next numerator also must be in milligrams.

4. Cancel the alternate denominator/numerator measurement units (but not their quantities). They must match. If so, all clinical ratios were entered correctly. After cancellation, only the unit of measure being calculated can remain in the equation.

5. Calculate the equation now that all components are in place.

> **Remember**
>
> The unit of measure being calculated is written first, followed by an equal sign. It is then matched in the numerator of the first clinical ratio entered. The unit of measure in each denominator is matched in the successive numerator entered.

Example 1:

The available drug strength is 500 mg in 2 mL. How many mL are needed to prepare a 300 mg dosage?

$$mL = \frac{2\ mL}{500\ mg}$$

Therefore, based on the desired 300 mg dosage:

$$mL = \frac{2\ mL}{500\ mg} \times \frac{X\ mL}{300\ mg}$$

Therefore, by cross-multiplying, 2 mL × 300 mg = 600 mg. This amount, when divided by 500 mg, gives an answer of 1.2 mL, which contains the desired 300 mg of medication.

This type of equation works the same way for every calculation, no matter how many ratios are entered. There are no complicated rules to remember.

Example 2:

Because 1 liter (L) is equal to 1000 milliliters (mL), how many fluid ounces (fl oz) are in 2.5 liters? Approximately 30 milliliters are in 1 fluid ounce. Use ratio and proportion as follows:

$$\frac{2.5\ L}{1\ L} \times \frac{X\ mL}{1000\ mL}$$

Therefore, $X = 2500$ mL. So,

$$\frac{1\ fl\ oz}{X\ fl\ oz} \times \frac{30\ mL}{2500\ mL}$$

Therefore, $X = 83.3$ fl oz, which may be rounded to 83 fl oz.

Example 3:

To solve the same equation by dimensional analysis, you would do the following:

$$\frac{1\ fl\ oz}{30\ mL} \times \frac{1000\ mL}{1\ L} \times 2.5\ L$$

Therefore, the same answer, 83.3 fl oz., can be easily found.

Example 4:

If 1000 mL of dextrose is needed intravenously, to be infused over 8 hours, and an IV set delivering 10 drops per mL is used, how many drops per minute should be delivered to the patient? Using ratio and proportion.

Because 8 hours = 480 minutes:

$$\frac{1000 \text{ mL}}{X \text{ mL}} \times \frac{480 \text{ minutes}}{1 \text{ minute}}$$

Therefore, $X = 2.1$ mL/minute.

Then

$$\frac{2.1 \text{ mL/minute}}{1 \text{ mL}} \times \frac{X \text{ drops/minute}}{10 \text{ drops}}$$

Therefore, $X = 21$ drops per minute.

■ Example 5:

To solve the same equation by dimensional analysis, you would do the following (the terms should have "drops" in the numerator and "minutes" in the denominator to give the desired answer in drops per minute):

$$\frac{10 \text{ drops}}{1 \text{ mL}} \times \frac{1}{480 \text{ minutes}} \times 1000 \text{ mL}$$

Therefore, the same answer is easily found: 21 drops per minute.

Stop and Review

Using dimensional analysis, perform the following dosage calculations, expressing answers in mL, rounded to the nearest tenth.

1. A dosage strength of 0.4 mg in 2.5 mL is available. How many milliliters should be administered if a dose of 0.15 mg is required?

   _____

2. A pharmacy technician must prepare a 200,000 unit dosage from an available solution containing 150,000 units in 2 mL. How many milliliters should be administered to contain the correct dosage?

   _____

3. A dosage strength of 0.8 mg in 2 mL must be used to prepare a 0.5 mg dosage.

   _____

4. An IV additive has a dosage strength of 20 mEq per 20 mL. A dosage of 15 mEq has been ordered. How many mL will be needed?

   _____

5. A dosage of 0.3 g has been prescribed. The strength available is 0.4 g in 1.5 mL. How many mL will be needed?

   _____

Equations Requiring Metric Conversions

Dimensional analysis allows multiple ratios to be entered into a single equation. It is sometimes easier to do the conversion before the equation is set up. For instance, if a medication is available in milligrams (mg) but is labeled in another amount, such as grams or micrograms, **metric conversion** must be done.

■ Example 1:

The IM dosage ordered is 250 mg. The drug available is labeled 1 g per 2 mL. How many mL must you give?

$$mL = \frac{2\ mL}{1\ g}$$

Because the dosage ordered is in milligrams and the drug available is in grams, a conversion ratio is needed: 1 gram equals 1000 milligrams. Therefore, you can change "1 g" to "1000 mg":

$$mL = \frac{2\ mL}{1000\ mg}$$

Next, you must add the dosage ordered into the equation:

$$mL = \frac{2\ mL}{1000\ mg} \times \frac{250\ mg}{1}$$

Then remove the "milligrams" and carry out the multiplication:

$$mL = \frac{2 \times 250}{1000}$$

This leaves:

$$mL = \frac{500}{1000}$$

The result is ½ mL. Therefore, ½ mL contains the desired dosage of 250 mg.

■ Example 2:

An intramuscular medication order is for 0.5 mg of medication in solution. The drug label reads "750 mcg in 2 mL." Enter the mL to be calculated followed by an equal sign to the left of the equation. Locate the ratio containing mL, 750 mcg in 2 mL. Enter 2 mL as the numerator to match the mL being calculated. The denominator becomes 750 mcg.

$$mL = \frac{2\ mL}{750\ mcg}$$

Because the medication order was for milligrams, a conversion ratio is needed. Enter the 1000 mcg = 1 mg conversion ratio. The numerator is 1000 mcg, matching the mcg of the previous denominator. The denominator becomes 1 mg.

$$mL = \frac{2 \text{ mL}}{750 \text{ mcg}} \times \frac{1000 \text{ mcg}}{1 \text{ mg}}$$

The mg denominator is now matched by the 0.5 mg dosage to be administered, completing the equation.

$$mL = \frac{2 \text{ mL}}{750 \text{ mcg}} \times \frac{1000 \text{ mcg}}{1 \text{ mg}} \times 0.5 \text{ mg}$$

Cancel the alternate denominator–numerator mcg/mcg and mg/mg units of measure, which checks for the correct ratio entry. Only the mL being calculated should remain. Do the math as follows:

$$mL = \frac{2 \text{ mL}}{750} \times \frac{1000}{1} \times 0.5 = 1.33$$

To give a dosage of 0.5 mg from the available 2 mL per 750 mcg strength, you must prepare 1.33 mL.

■ Example 3:

Prepare a 0.5 mg dosage from an available strength of 200 mcg per mL. Enter the mL being calculated to the left of the equation followed by an equal sign. Enter the 1 mL in 200 mcg dosage as the starting ratio, with 1 mL as the numerator to match the mL being calculated; 200 mcg becomes the denominator.

$$mL = \frac{1 \text{ mL}}{200 \text{ mcg}}$$

A mcg to mcg conversion ratio is needed. Enter 1000 mcg as the numerator to match the mcg in the previous denominator; 1 mg becomes the new denominator.

$$mL = \frac{1 \text{ mL}}{200 \text{ mcg}} \times \frac{1000 \text{ mcg}}{1 \text{ mg}}$$

The mg denominator is now matched by the 0.5 mg dosage ordered to complete the equation.

$$mL = \frac{1 \text{ mL}}{200 \text{ mcg}} \times \frac{1000 \text{ mcg}}{1 \text{ mg}} \times 0.5 \text{ mg}$$

Cancel the alternate mcg/mcg and mg/mg units of measure to double-check for correct ratio entry. Only the mL unit being calculated remains in the equation. Do the math.

$$mL = \frac{1 \text{ mL}}{200} \times \frac{1000}{1} \times 0.5 = 2.5 \text{ mL}$$

A 0.5 dosage requires a 2.5 mL volume of the 200 mcg per mL strength solution available.

>>> Remember

For calculations using dimensional analysis:

- The unit of measure being calculated is written first to the left of the equation.
- The unit of measure is followed by an equal sign.
- All ratios entered must include the quantity and the unit of measure.
- The numerator in the starting ratio must be in the same measurement unit as the unit of measure being calculated.
- The unit of measure in each denominator must be matched in the numerator of each successive ratio entered.
- Metric system conversions can be made by incorporating a conversion ratio directly into the dimensional analysis equation.
- The unit of measure in each alternate denominator and numerator must cancel. This leaves only the unit of measure being calculated remaining in the equation.
- The numerator of the starting ratio is never cancelled.

■ Example 4:

The medication has a strength of 0.5 mg in 1.5 mL. The order is for 750 mcg. Therefore, how many mL should be given?

Enter the mL to be calculated to the left of the equation followed by an equal sign. Enter the starting ratio, the 1.5 mL in 0.5 mg dosage available, with 1.5 mL as the numerator, to match the mL being calculated; 0.5 mg becomes the denominator.

$$mL = \frac{1.5 \text{ mL}}{0.5 \text{ mg}}$$

The problem has no "milligram" dosage, but asks for micrograms, which signals the need for a conversion ratio. Enter the 1 mg = 1000 mcg conversion ratio, with 1 mg as the numerator, to match the milligrams denominator of the starting ratio; 1000 mcg becomes the new denominator.

$$mL = \frac{1.5 \text{ mL}}{0.5 \text{ mg}} \times \frac{1 \text{ mg}}{1000 \text{ mcg}}$$

Enter the dosage ordered (750 mcg) as the final numerator to match the mcg in the previous denominator. The equation is complete.

$$mL = \frac{1.5 \text{ mL}}{0.5 \text{ mg}} \times \frac{1 \text{ mg}}{1000 \text{ mcg}} \times 750 \text{ mcg}$$

Cancel the alternate mg/mg and mcg/mcg units of measure to check the accuracy of ratio entry, and then complete the math.

$$mL = \frac{1.5 \text{ mL}}{0.5} \times \frac{1}{1000} \times 750 = 2.25 = 2.3 \text{ mL}$$

Therefore, a 750 mcg dosage requires 2.3 mL of the 0.5 mg in 1.5 mL medication.

Test Your Knowledge

Calculate the following dosages using dimensional analysis.

1. A prescriber ordered 0.2 g tablets. On hand are tablets labeled "80 mg." How many tablets should be given to the patient?
   _____

2. A physician ordered a dosage of 85 mg. The drug on hand is labeled "0.1 g in 1.5 mL." How many mL should be given to the patient?
   _____

3. A pharmacy technician prepares 0.1 g of an IM medication from a strength of 200 mg per mL. How many mL must be administered?
   _____

4. The prescriber ordered 0.5 mg of a medication. The dosage strength on hand is 200 mcg per mL. How many mL should be administered to the patient?

   _____

5. A pharmacy technician is preparing a 0.75 mg dosage. The strength available is 500 mcg in 1.5 mL. How many mL should be given?

   _____

6. If you want to prepare a 130 mg dosage of a drug labeled "0.1 g in 2 mL," how many mL must be given?

   _____

7. A physician ordered a dosage of 1500 mcg (1.5 mg). The solution available is 0.5 mg per mL. How many mL should be administered?

   _____

8. A technician prepares 500 mg for IM injection from an available strength of 1 g per 3 mL. How many mL must be administered?

   _____

9. An oral solution has a dosage of 500 mg in 5 mL. If a 0.7 g dosage is required, how many mL must be given?

   _____

10. A technician prepares a 0.75 g dosage from a 250 mg per mL strength solution. How many mL are needed?

    _____

Dosage Calculations Using Dimensional Analysis

Using dimensional analysis, calculate the dosages from the medication labels provided. Your answers should be in mL, rounded to the nearest tenth or hundredth. Use the syringes that are shown to measure your dosages.

Dosage Ordered	mL Needed
1. terbutaline sulfate 800 mcg 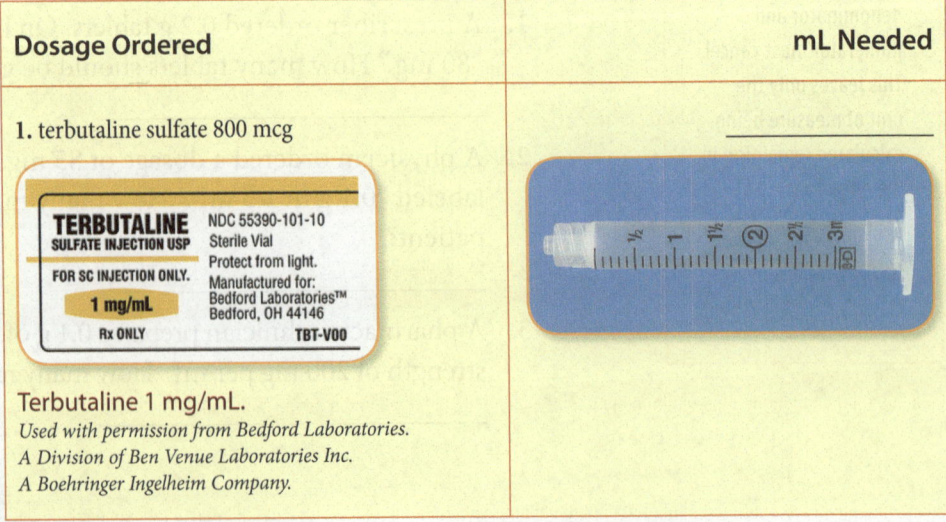 Terbutaline 1 mg/mL. *Used with permission from Bedford Laboratories. A Division of Ben Venue Laboratories Inc. A Boehringer Ingelheim Company.*	_____

Chapter 7 • Dimensional Analysis 117

Dosage Ordered	mL Needed
2. Vistaril® 70 mg Vistaril 50 mg/mL. Used with permission from Pfizer, Inc.	_____
3. fentanyl citrate 0.15 mg Fentanyl 250 mcg/5 mL. Copyright Baxter Healthcare Corporation.	_____
4. naloxone 350 mcg Narcan® 1 mL. Used with permission from Endo Pharmaceuticals, Inc.	_____
5. clindamycin 225 mg Clindamycin 150 mg/mL. Used with permission from Bedford Laboratories. A Division of Ben Venue Laboratories Inc. A Boehringer Ingelheim Company.	_____

Dosage Ordered	mL Needed
6. Robinul® 75 mcg (calculate to the nearest hundredth) 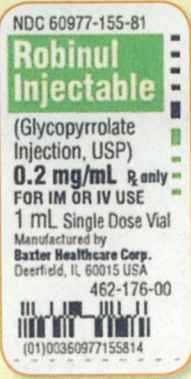 **Robinul Injectable.** *Copyright Baxter International Inc. Robinul is a trademark of Wyeth Pharmaceuticals Division of Wyeth.*	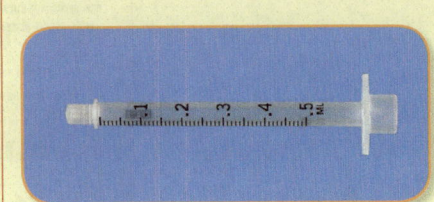 _____
7. midazolam HCl 4 mg 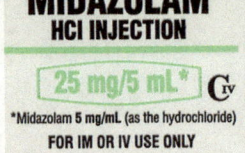 **Midazolam 25 mg/mL.** *Used with permission from Bedford Laboratories. A Division of Ben Venue Laboratories Inc. A Boehringer Ingelheim Company.*	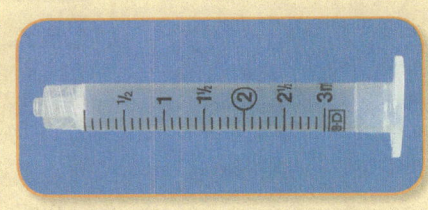 _____
8. Inapsine® 3 mg 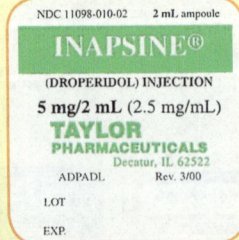 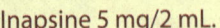 **Inapsine 5 mg/2 mL.** *Used with permission from Akorn Inc., and Taylor Pharmaceuticals.*	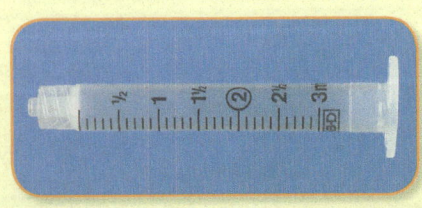 _____

Chapter 7 • Dimensional Analysis

Dosage Ordered	mL Needed
9. morphine sulfate 1.5 mg Duramorph 10 mg/10 mL. *Copyright Baxter International Inc. Duramorph is a trademark of Baxter International Inc. or its subsidiaries.*	_____
10. heparin sodium 450 units (calculate to the nearest hundredth) Heparin Sodium 1000 Units/mL. *© Cengage Learning 2013.*	_____
11. droperidol 4 mg Inapsine 5 mg/2 mL. *Used with permission from Akorn Inc., and Taylor Pharmaceuticals.*	_____

120 Part 2 • Dosage Calculations

Dosage Ordered	mL Needed
12. Dilantin® 0.1 g Dilantin 250 mg. *Used with permission from Pfizer Inc.*	_____
13. medroxyprogesterone 0.9 g Depo-Provera® 400 mg. *Used with permission from Pfizer, Inc.*	_____
14. Vistaril® 120 mg Vistaril 50 mg/mL. *Used with permission from Pfizer, Inc.*	_____
15. sodium chloride 60 mEq for an IV additive Sodium Chloride 100 mL. © Cengage Learning 2013.	_____

Dosage Ordered	mL Needed
16. atropine sulfate 150 mcg	
17. meperidine 75 mg	
18. fentanyl citrate 80 mcg	

Atropine Sulfate 0.1 mg/mL.
1 mg per 10 mL – For IV use/Single Dose.
© Cengage Learning 2013.

Meperidine 100 mg/mL.
Copyright Baxter Healthcare Corporation.

Fentanyl Citrate 250 mcg/5 mL.
Copyright Baxter Healthcare Corporation.

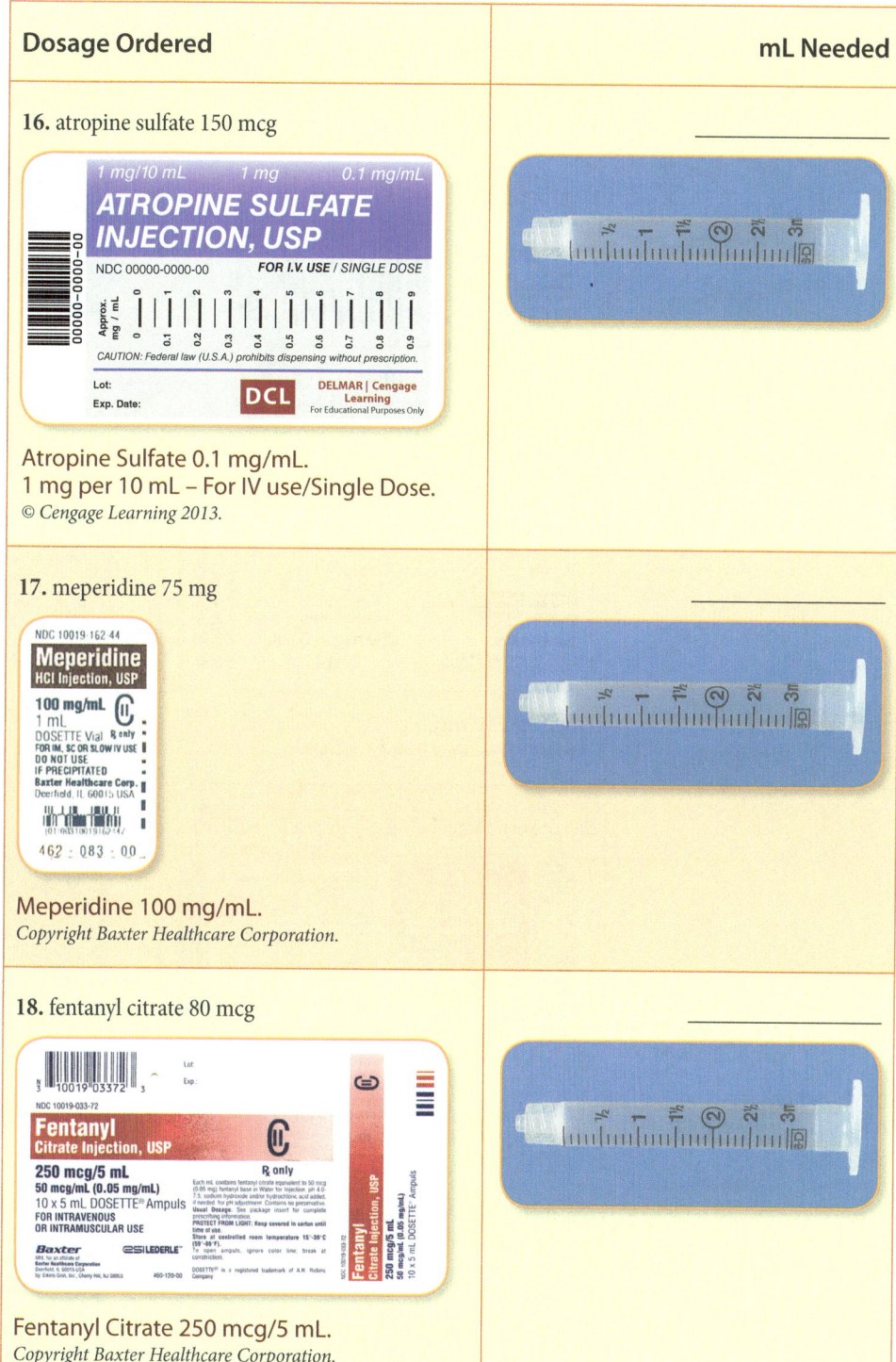

Dosage Ordered	mL Needed
19. gentamicin 0.1 g Gentamicin 40 mg/mL. *Used with permission of Abraxis BioScience, Inc.*	
20. Dilantin® 0.15 g Dilantin 250 mg. *Used with permission from Pfizer, Inc.*	
21. doxorubicin HCl 16 mg for an IV additive Doxorubicin Hydrochloride Injection. *Used with permission from Bedford Laboratories.* *A Division of Ben Venue Laboratories Inc.* *A Boehringer Ingelheim Company.*	
22. meperidine HCl 30 mg Meperidine 25 mg/mL. *Copyright Baxter Healthcare Corporation.*	

Chapter 7 • Dimensional Analysis

Dosage Ordered	mL Needed
23. methotrexate 40 mg Methotrexate 200 mg. *Copyright Baxter Healthcare Corporation.*	_____
24. midazolam HCl 3 mg Midazolam 25 mg/mL. *Used with permission from Bedford Laboratories.* *A Division of Ben Venue Laboratories Inc.* *A Boehringer Ingelheim Company.*	_____
25. ondansetron 3 mg Ondansetron 4 mg/2 mL. *Used with permission from Bedford Laboratories.* *A Division of Ben Venue Laboratories Inc.* *A Boehringer Ingelheim Company.*	_____
26. hydroxyzine HCl 40 mg Vistaril 25 mg/mL. *Used with permission from Pfizer, Inc.*	_____

Part 2 • Dosage Calculations

Dosage Ordered	mL Needed
27. ketorolac tromethamine 20 mg Ketorolac 15 mg/mL. *Used with permission from Bedford Laboratories.* *A Division of Ben Venue Laboratories Inc.* *A Boehringer Ingelheim Company.*	
28. nalbuphine HCl 30 mg Nubain 20 mg/mL. *Used with permission from Endo Pharmaceuticals, Inc.*	
29. morphine 15 mg Morphine 10 mg/mL. *Copyright Baxter Healthcare International Inc.*	
30. Dilantin® 125 mg Dilantin 250 mg. *Used with permission from Pfizer Inc.*	

Dosage Ordered	mL Needed
31. ketorolac 25 mg Ketorolac 15 mg/mL. Used with permission from Bedford Laboratories. A Division of Ben Venue Laboratories Inc. A Boehringer Ingelheim Company.	_____
32. Vistaril® 50 mg Vistaril 25 mg/mL. Used with permission from Pfizer, Inc.	_____
33. Robinul® 180 mcg Robinul Injectable 1 mL. Copyright Baxter International Inc. Robinul is a trademark of Wyeth Pharmaceutical Division of Wyeth.	_____
34. hydroxyzine HCl 70 mg Vistaril 50 mg/mL. Used with permission from Pfizer Inc.	_____

Part 2 • Dosage Calculations

Dosage Ordered	mL Needed
35. potassium chloride 20 mEq for an IV additive Potassium Chloride 30 mEq. © Cengage Learning 2013.	_____
36. Inapsine® 4.5 mg Inapsine 5 mg/2 mL. *Used with permission from Akron Inc. and Taylor Pharmaceuticals.*	_____
37. Nubain® 15 mg Nubain 20 mg/mL. *Used with permission from Endo Pharmaceuticals, Inc.*	_____
38. phenytoin Na 0.1 g Dilantin 250 mg. *Used with permission from Pfizer, Inc.*	_____

Dosage Ordered	mL Needed
39. lidocaine HCl 15 mg 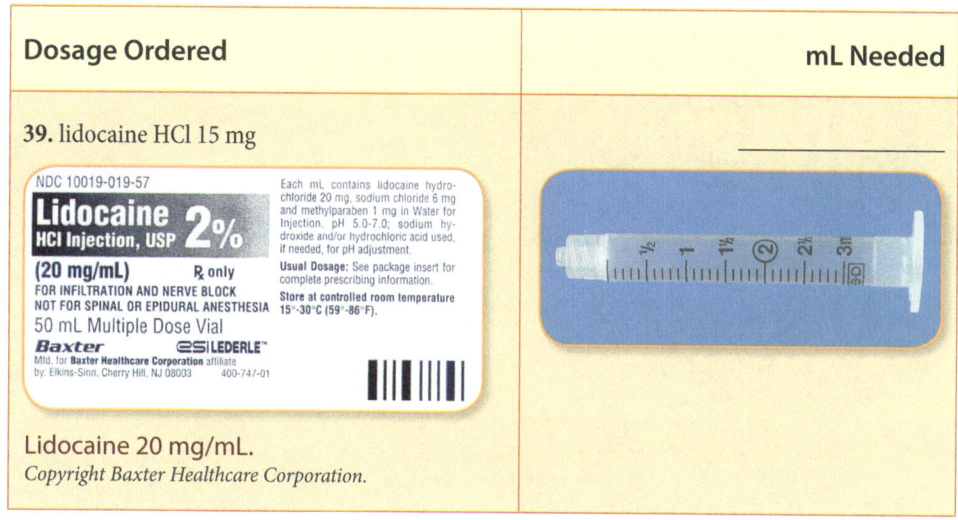 Lidocaine 20 mg/mL. Copyright Baxter Healthcare Corporation.	_____

Critical Thinking

A physician ordered 100 mg of a medication for a patient. The pharmacy had the medication available as 125 mg in 5 mL.

1. Using dimensional analysis, how many mL would be administered?

   _____

2. If the same 100 mg was ordered, but the pharmacy had the medication available as 125 mg in 2 mL, how many mL would be administered?

   _____

A pharmacy technician received a prescription for Lanoxin 0.25 mg. The pharmacy had Lanoxin available in tablets containing 0.125 mg.

1. Using dimensional analysis, how many tablets would be administered?

   _____

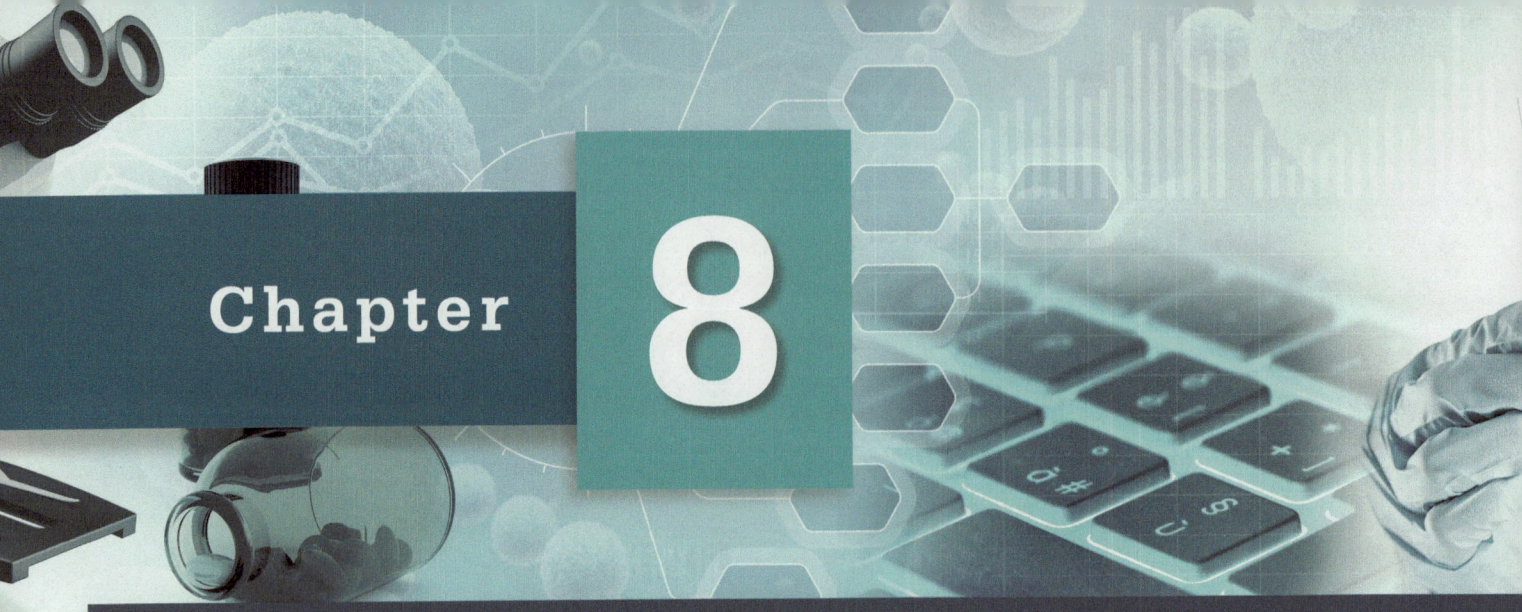

Chapter 8

Formula Method

Outline

Overview
Basic Formula
Use with Metric Conversions
Use with Units and Milliequivalent Calculations

Objectives

Upon completion of this chapter, you should be able to:

1. Use the formula method with metric conversions.
2. Round calculations and conversions made with the formula method to the nearest tenth.
3. Use the formula method to calculate dosages expressed as decimal fractions rounded to the nearest tenth.

Key Terms

desired dosage   dosage ordered   dosage strength available

Overview

The *formula method* is used for simple, one-step dosage calculations. It is a variation of ratio and proportion. Various initials are used to represent the components used in the formula method. In this book, the initials used are *D*, *H*, *Q*, and *X*. It is not important which initials are used, as long as the answer achieved is correct.

Basic Formula

The following initials are usually used in the formula method:

$$\frac{D}{H} \times Q = X$$

These initials mean:

D = "desired" (**dosage ordered** in milligrams, grams, and so forth)

H = "have" (**dosage strength available** in mg, g, and so forth)

Q = "quantity" (the mL volume that the dosage strength available is contained in)

X = "unknown" (the mL volume that the **desired dosage** will be contained in)

The "unknown" (*X*) is always expressed in the same units of measure as the "quantity" (*Q*), which is the mL volume that the dosage available is contained within.

> **Remember**
>
> You must memorize the formula used in the formula method. Always double-check calculations. Determine if answers are logical. Ask for help if you doubt the accuracy of your calculations.

■ Example 1:

You have on hand a dosage strength of 80 mg in 2 mL. A dosage of 60 mg is ordered. How many mL are necessary to administer this dosage?

Desired dosage (*D*) = 60 mg

On hand (*H*) = 80 mg in (*Q*) 2 mL

Remember that *X* must be expressed in the same units of measure as *Q*, which is mL in this example. Always include the units of measure in the formula.

$$\frac{(D)\ 60\ mg}{(H)\ 80\ mg} \times (Q)\ 2\ mL = X\ mL$$

$$\frac{60}{80} \times 2 = X = 1.5\ mL$$

Therefore, to give a dosage of 60 mg, 1.5 mL must be administered.

Because 60 mg is required, which is a smaller dosage than the dosage strength available of 80 mg in 2 mL, the answer, 1.5 mL, is smaller, and because of this, logical.

■ Example 2:

A dosage of 0.5 mg is ordered. On hand is 0.45 mg in 1.2 mL. So, $D = 0.4$ mg. $H = 0.45$ mg in (Q) 1.2 mL.

$$\frac{0.5 \text{ mg}}{0.45 \text{ mg}} \times 1.2 \text{ mL} = X \text{ mL}$$

$$\frac{0.5}{0.45} \times 1.2 = X = 1.33 = 1.3 \text{ mL}$$

Therefore, to give 0.5 mg, you must administer 1.3 mL. Because 0.5 mg ordered is larger than the 0.45 mg strength available and the volume containing it must be larger; 1.3 mL is larger, so it is logical.

■ Example 3:

The strength available is 1000 mcg per mL. A dosage of 660 mcg has been ordered.

$$\frac{660 \text{ mg}}{1000 \text{ mcg}} \times 1 \text{ mL} = X \text{ mL}$$

$$\frac{660}{1000} \times 1 = X = 0.66 = 0.7 \text{ mL}$$

Therefore, to give a dosage of 660 mcg, you must administer 0.7 mL. The answer must be a smaller quantity than 1 mL, and it is.

Stop and Review

Calculate the dosages and express your answers to the nearest tenth.

1. Ordered:	0.6 g
Strength available:	1 g in 2.5 mL
Give:	_____
2. Ordered:	150 mg
Strength available:	250 mg in 1.5 mL
Give:	_____
3. Ordered:	0.4 g
Strength available:	1 g in 3 mL
Give:	_____

Chapter 8 • Formula Method   131

4. Ordered:	275 mcg
Strength available:	600 mcg in 1.2 mL
Give:	_____

Use with Metric Conversions

When drug strengths are in different units of measure, one of them must be changed before a dosage can be determined. The drug strengths (*D* and *H*) must always be expressed in the same units of measure.

■ Example 1:

A dosage (*D*) of 200 mcg is ordered. However, the strength available (or "dose on hand") is 0.4 mg in 1.5 mL. This is labeled as "*H*". First, you must convert mg to mcg to eliminate the decimal point:

$$0.4 \text{ mg} = 400 \text{ mcg}$$

Then use the formula for the calculation as follows:

$$\frac{200 \text{ mcg}}{400 \text{ mcg}} \times 1.5 \text{ mL} = X \text{ mL}$$

The result is 0.75 mL.

Therefore, to give 200 mcg, you must administer 0.75 mL. of 0.4 mg medication. Remember that your answer must be smaller than 1.5 mL (which it is) because the dosage ordered is smaller than the strength available. Therefore, this answer is logical.

■ Example 2:

On hand is a strength of 1000 mg in 1.5 mL. A dosage of 0.8 g has been ordered. First, convert g to mg to eliminate the decimal point:

$$0.8 \text{ g} = 800 \text{ mg}$$

Then use the formula for calculation:

$$\frac{800 \text{ mg}}{1000 \text{ mg}} \times 1.5 \text{ mL} = X \text{ mL}$$

The result is 1.2 mL.

Therefore, to give 0.8 g, you must administer 1.2 mL. The answer must be less than 1.5 mL (which it is) because the 800 mg ordered is less than the 1000 mg strength available.

Stop and Review

Calculate the dosages and express your answers to the nearest tenth.

1. Ordered:	870 mcg
Strength available:	1 mg per mL
Give:	_____
2. Ordered:	450 mg
Strength available:	0.1 g per mL
Give:	_____
3. Ordered:	0.6 mg
Strength available:	1000 mcg per 2 mL
Give:	_____
4. Ordered:	0.4 g
Strength available:	500 mg per 1.3 mL
Give:	_____

Use with Units and Milliequivalent Calculations

The same as with metric conversions, it also is easy to convert dosages expressed in units or milliequivalents (mEq).

■ **Example 1:**

If a dosage of 6500 units is ordered, and the available strength is 10,000 units per mL, first do the following:

$$\frac{6500 \text{ units}}{10{,}000 \text{ units}} \times 1 \text{ mL} = X \text{ mL}$$

Therefore, to give 6500 units, you must administer 0.7 mL (which is rounded to the nearest tenth from the answer of 0.65 mL). Because the dosage ordered (6500 units) is less than the strength available (10,000 units), it must be contained in less solution than 1 mL (which it is).

Example 2:

If a dosage of 40 mEq is ordered, and the available strength is 70 mEq in 5 mL, first do the following:

$$\frac{40 \text{ mEq}}{70 \text{ mEq}} \times 5 = X \text{ mL}$$

Therefore, to give 40 mEq, you must administer 3.75 mL (which is rounded to the nearest tenth from the answer of 2.86 mL). Because the dosage ordered (40 mEq) is less than the dosage strength available (70 mEq), it must be contained in a smaller volume than 5 mL, and it is.

Stop and Review

Calculate the dosages and express the answers to the nearest tenth.

1. Ordered:	1250 units	
Strength available:	1000 units per 1.5 mL	
Give:	_____	
2. Ordered:	45 units	
Strength available:	80 units per mL	
Give:	_____	
3. Ordered:	50 mEq	
Strength available:	200 mEq per 20 mL	
Give:	_____	
4. Ordered:	30 mEq	
Strength available:	80 mEq per 5 mL	
Give:	_____	

Test Your Knowledge

After calculating the following dosages, express your answers as decimal fractions, rounding to the nearest tenth.

1. A 50 mg dosage is ordered. Strength available is 60 mg in 1.5 mL. _____

2. A 300 mcg dosage is ordered. Strength available is 0.4 mg per mL. _____

3. Prepare a 0.45 g dosage. Strength available is 300 mg per mL. _____

4. An 8 mg dosage has been ordered. The medication is labeled 5 mg per mL. _____

5. A 70 mg dosage must be prepared from a solution labeled 250 mg in 5 mL. _____

6. A dosage of 30 mg has been ordered. The drug is labeled 25 mg per mL. _____

7. Prepare a 60 mg dosage. The label reads 50 mg per mL. _____

8. The vial is labeled 5 mg per mL. The order is for 12 mg. _____

9. The vial label reads 10 mg per mL. A dosage of 7 mg has been ordered. _____

10. A dosage of 8 mg has been ordered. The dosage strength is 10 mg in 1 mL. _____

11. A medication is labeled 900 mg per 6 mL. Prepare a 0.3 g dosage. _____

12. A vial is labeled 0.5 g in 20 mL. Prepare a 300 mg IV dosage. _____

13. A dosage of 750 mg has been ordered. The vial is labeled 0.5 g per 2 mL. _____

14. An available dosage is 250 mcg in 5 mL. Prepare a dosage of 0.2 mg. _____

15. A single-use ampule is labeled 0.1 g per 2 mL. The order is for 130 mg. _____

16. A vial is labeled 15 mg in 5 mL. Draw up a 12 mg dosage. _____

17. Prepare 14 mg. The ampule is labeled 20 mg in 2 mL. _____

18. Draw up an 800 mg dosage for IV administration from a container labeled 1.2 g per 30 mL. _____

19. Prepare an 80 mg dosage of a medication. The container is labeled 100 mg in 2 mL. _____

20. A dosage of 300 mcg is ordered. The solution strength is 0.4 mg per mL. _____

21. An available dosage strength is 0.4 g per mL. Prepare a 600 mg dosage. _____

22. A solution is labeled 40 mEq per 20 mL. Draw up a 60 mEq dosage for addition to an IV. _____

23. A dosage of 0.6 mg has been ordered. The label reads 400 mcg per mL. _____

24. A 60 mg dosage must be prepared from a 75 mg per mL strength. _____

25. A vial is labeled 40 mg per mL. Prepare a 0.1 g dosage. _____

26. The order is for 8 mg. The drug is labeled 50 mg in 10 mL. _____

27. An available strength is 1000 mcg per mL. Measure a 0.8 mg dosage. _____

28. A vial is labeled 25 mg per mL. Prepare 40 mg. _____

29. You have an available strength of 4000 mcg per mL. A dosage of 10 mg has been ordered. _____

30. A medication is labeled 0.25 g per 25 mL. Prepare 200 mg for IV use. _____

31. A dosage of 10 mg has been ordered. The dosage strength available is 15 mg in 1 mL. _____

32. An available strength is 5 mg per mL. Prepare a 4 mg dosage. _____

33. An available strength is 90 units in 1.5 mL. A dosage of 75 units has been ordered. _____

34. The solution available is labeled 80 mEq per 20 mL. You are to prepare 100 mEq for addition to an IV solution. _____

35. The solution is 0.15 g in 1 mL, and you must prepare a dosage of 180 mg. _____

36. An available strength is 1000 units per mL. Prepare a 750 unit dosage. _____

37. A vial is labeled 40 mEq in 20 mL. Draw up a 60 mEq dosage for addition to an IV solution. _____

38. A dosage of 400,000 units has been ordered. The available strength is 300,000 units in 1 mL. _____

39. Prepare a 250 mcg dosage. A dosage of 0.2 mg per 2 mL is available. _____

40. The solution is labeled 50 mEq per 50 mL. A dosage of 35 mEq has been ordered. _____

Critical Thinking

A physician ordered 200 mcg of a medication. The drug strength available is 0.4 mg in 1.5 mL.

1. What is the first step that the pharmacy technician needs to take?
   _____
   _____

2. How many mL of the medication should be administered?
   _____

A physician ordered 40 mEq of a medication. In the pharmacy, a strength of 70 mEq in 5 mL is available.

1. How many mL must be administered?
   _____
   _____

2. If a dosage of 80 mEq was ordered, how many mL must be administered?
   _____

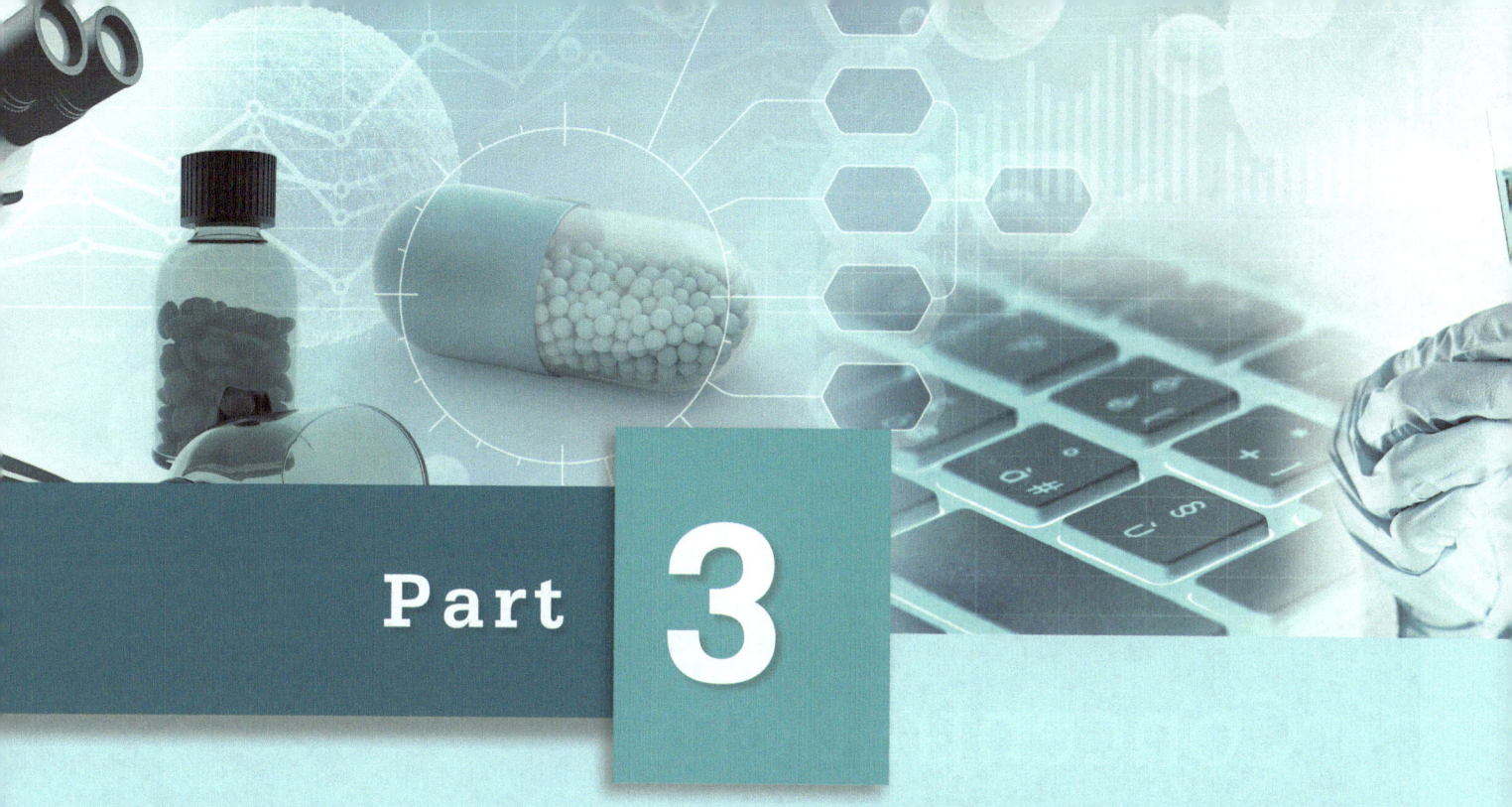

Part 3

Concentrations and Dilutions

Chapter 9 Concentrations

Chapter 10 Dilutions and Solutions

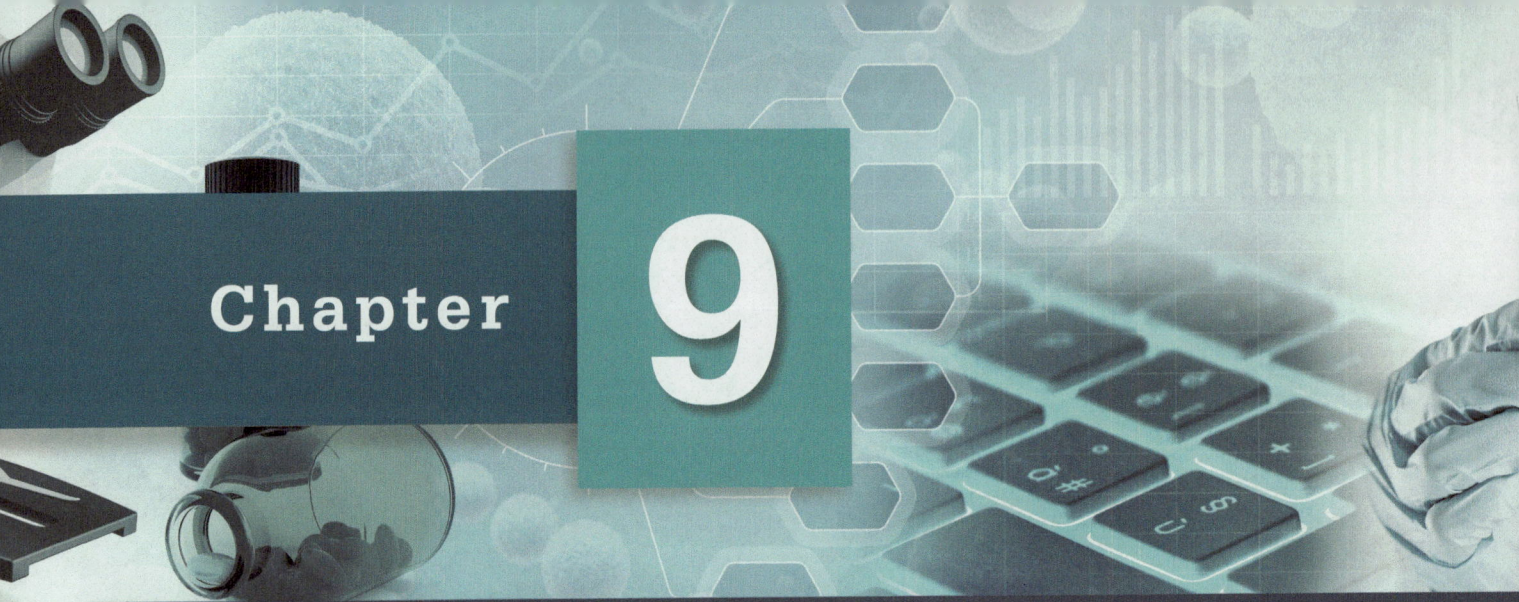

Chapter 9

Concentrations

Outline

Overview
    Concentrations and Volumes of Solutions
Weight/Weight
Volume/Volume
Weight/Volume
Ratio Strength

Objectives

Upon completion of this chapter, you should be able to:

1. Determine a final concentration from an original concentration and a dilution.
2. Use the formula $V_1 \times C_1 = V_2 \times C_2$ to solve dilution problems.
3. Solve problems using percentages of weight/weight, volume/volume, and weight/volume.

Key Terms

concentrate
concentration

normal saline
ratio strength

solute

Overview

When a solution is diluted, it will have a decreased concentration as well as an increased volume. Two volumes and two concentrations may be related by using the formula:

$$V_1 \times C_1 = V_2 \times C_2$$

In this formula, V_1 and C_1 represent the original volume and concentration. Likewise, V_2 and C_2 represent the volume and concentration of the diluted solution.

The term **concentration** refers to the amount of a particular substance in a given volume. The greater the substance in a given volume, the more concentrated the solution becomes. Therefore, the less the amount of a substance in a given volume, the less concentrated the solution becomes. For example, in a 15% solution, the entire solution consists of 15% of a certain substance in 100 mL of the solution. To dilute this into a one-third solution, the dilution would be referred to as $\frac{1}{3}$ or 1:3. It is easy to see that $\frac{1}{3}$ of 15% is 5%. This can also be represented as the following formula:

$$15\% \times \frac{1}{3} =$$

$$\frac{15\%}{1} \times \frac{1}{3} = \frac{15\%}{3} = 5\%$$

Therefore, the original concentration × the dilution = the final concentration.

> **Remember**
>
> Original concentration × dilution = final concentration

Example 1:

Find the final concentration if a solution consisting of 20% of a substance is diluted using a 1:5 dilution.

$$20\% \text{ solution} \times \frac{1}{5} = \frac{20\%}{5} = 4\% \text{ solution}$$

Example 2:

Find the final concentration if a solution consisting of 25% is diluted using a 1:10 dilution.

$$25\% \text{ solution} \times \frac{1}{10} = \frac{25\%}{10} = 2.5\% \text{ solution}$$

Example 3:

If a 15% solution is diluted 1:30, what is the final concentration?

$$15\% \text{ solution} \times \frac{1}{30} = \frac{15\%}{30} = 0.5\% \text{ solution}$$

> **Remember**
>
> One of the most common ways of expressing a concentration is as a percent. This tells you how many grams of a solute are found in every 100 mL of a solution.

■ **Example 4:**

If a solution has an original concentration of 40% and is diluted so that the final concentration is 10%, what amount of dilution was performed?

Original concentration	Dilution	Final concentration
(40%)	× (X) =	(10%)

When this equation is rewritten, we have 40X = 10. After dividing by 40, we find:

$$X = \frac{10}{40} = \frac{1}{4}$$

Therefore, a dilution of 1:4 was performed.

Concentrations and Volumes of Solutions

The mathematical formula used to determine concentrations and volumes of two solutions is the following:

$$\frac{V_1}{V_2} = \frac{C_2}{C_1}$$

When this formula is cross-multiplied, it becomes

$$V_1 \times C_1 = V_2 \times C_2$$

This formula can be used to find the volumes and concentrations of original and resulting solutions when they change as a result of adding a diluent.

■ **Example 5:**

If V_1 = 10 mL, V_2 = 15 mL, and C_1 = 30%, find C_2 using the following equation:

$$V_1 \times C_1 = V_2 \times C_2$$

After substituting the given values, we have:

$$10 \text{ mL} \times 30\% = 15 \text{ mL} \times C_2$$

When the left side of the equation is simplified, we have:

$$3 = 15 \times C_2$$

Dividing both sides by 15 results in:

$$\frac{3}{15} = C_2$$

Simplifying, we find that:

$$C_2 = 0.20 \text{ or } 20\%$$

Therefore, the concentration of the diluted solution is 20%.

■ **Example 6:**

12 mL of a 3% solution are added to water to make a total volume of 60 mL. What is the concentration of the 60 mL solution? Use the equation $V_1 \times C_1 = V_2 \times C_2$. V_1 = 12 mL, C_1 = 3%, and V_2 = 60 mL.

Therefore, we begin with:

$$12 \times 0.03 = 60 \times C_2$$

Simplifying the left side results in:

$$0.36 = 60 \times C_2$$

Dividing both sides by 60 results in:

$$C_2 = 0.006 = 0.6\%$$

Therefore, the concentration of the diluted solution is 0.6%.

■ Example 7:

10 mL of a 5% solution are added to water to make a total volume of 50 mL. What is the concentration of the 50 mL solution? Use the same equation as in the preceding examples. $V_1 = 10$ mL, $C_1 = 5\%$, and $V_2 = 50$ mL.

Therefore, we begin with:

$$10 \times 0.05 = 50 \times C_2$$

Simplifying the left side results in:

$$0.5 = 50 \times C_2$$

Dividing both sides by 50 results in:

$$C_2 = 0.01 = 1\%$$

Therefore, the concentration of the diluted solution is 1%.

■ Example 8:

An 8% solution must be diluted to achieve an ordered solution of 2% with a volume of 200 mL. How many milliliters of the 8% solution are needed? $V_2 = 200$, $C_2 = 2\%$, and $C_1 = 8\%$. In this example, remember that we are solving for V_1.

Therefore, we begin with:

$$V_1 \times 0.08 = 200 \times 0.02$$

Simplifying the left side results in:

$$V_1 \times 0.08 = 4$$

Dividing both sides by 0.08 results in:

$$V_1 = 50 \text{ mL}$$

Therefore, take 50 mL of the 8% solution and dilute it to a total of 200 mL by adding 150 mL of the desired diluent.

■ Example 9:

A pharmacy technician poured a 5% solution into a container that already held a solution of an unknown volume. If the total volume of the mixed solution in the container is 100 mL, and its concentration is 2%, how many milliliters of the 5% solution were poured into the container? In this example, $C_1 = 5\%$, $C_2 = 2\%$, and $V_2 = 100$ mL. We are trying to solve for V_1.

Therefore, we begin with:

$$V_1 \times 0.05 = 100 \times 0.02$$

Simplifying the right side results in:

$$V_1 \times 0.05 = 2$$

Dividing both sides by 0.05 results in:

$$V_1 = 40 \text{ mL}$$

Therefore, 40 mL of the 5% solution were poured into the container.

Stop and Review

Find the missing values in the following equations.

1. A physician prescribed an antibiotic to be mixed in white petrolatum to produce a 25% antibiotic preparation. The physician later changed the prescription to be only for 12.5%. How much white petrolatum must be mixed with each 6 oz ointment container of 25% preparation to make the new 12.5% preparation? Calculate your answer in grams.

2. How much silver nitrate (in grams) must be used in preparing 600 mL of a solution such that 20 mL diluted to 1 L will yield a 1:5000 solution?

3. A pharmacy technician needs to prepare 3 L of 15% neomycin solution by diluting the stock solution with sterile water. If a 25% stock solution of neomycin is available, how much stock solution and how much sterile water do they need?

Weight/Weight

The term *percent* means "per 100." A *percent weight per unit weight* is abbreviated as *% w/w*. A percent weight per unit weight is defined as:

$$\frac{\text{Unit weight of solute}}{100 \text{ unit weight of solution}} = \frac{\text{Grams of solute}}{100 \text{ grams of solution}}$$

A **solute**, as described in the preceding equation, is the substance being dissolved in the solution. A solute is often a medication. Therefore, the phrase *5% w/w* means that 5% of the total mass of an entire solution is the mass of the solute or medication itself.

Example 1:

150 grams of a medication in a 20% w/w solution are required. How would this be made? Use the *% w/w* formula.

Therefore, we begin with:

$$0.20 = \frac{X \text{ g solute}}{100 \text{ g solution}}$$

If we multiply both sides by 100, we have:

$$X = 20 \text{ g}$$

To make a solution containing 100 g of medication, you need to have 20 g of solute. To find out how to make a solution containing 150 g of medication, use the following proportions:

$$\frac{20 \text{ g solute}}{100 \text{ g solution}} = \frac{X \text{ g solute}}{150 \text{ g solution}}$$

After cross-multiplying, we have:

$$100X = 3000$$

After dividing by 100, we have:

$$X = 30$$

Therefore, to make the solution containing 150 g of medication (such as an ointment or cream), you would mix 30 g of solute (active ingredient) with 120 g of diluent (base) to get a total of 150 g.

Stop and Review

Find the missing value in the following:

1. A pharmacist added 15 g of 20% w/w calamine cream to 300 g of Aquaphor®. What is the percent strength w/w of the final calamine product?

   _____

Volume/Volume

A *percent volume per unit volume* is abbreviated % *v/v* and defined as:

$$\frac{\text{mL concentrate}}{100 \text{ mL solution}} = \frac{\text{mL concentrate}}{100 \text{ mL solution}}$$

The term **concentrate** refers to a concentrated solution. A 25% v/v solution means that 25% of the entire solution is the solute itself.

■ Example 1:

If a solution of 50 mL of 60% v/v solution of hydrogen peroxide in water is required, how would it be made? Use the % v/v formula.

Therefore, we begin with:

$$0.60 = \frac{X \text{ mL hydrogen peroxide}}{100 \text{ mL solution}}$$

Multiplying both sides by 100 results in X = 60. Therefore, 60 mL of hydrogen peroxide should be added to 40 mL water to get a 100 mL solution that has a 60% v/v. Since 50 mL is desired, use proportions to solve this:

$$\frac{60 \text{ mL}}{100 \text{ mL}} = \frac{X \text{ mL}}{50 \text{ mL}}$$

By cross-multiplying, we find that X = 30. Therefore, 30 mL of hydrogen peroxide should be added to 20 mL water to get a 50 mL solution with a 60% v/v.

■ Example 2:

How many milliliters of alcohol are in 40 mL of a 60% v/v solution? The concentration remains the same, so you can solve this with proportions:

$$\frac{60 \text{ mL alcohol}}{100 \text{ mL solution}} = \frac{X \text{ mL alcohol}}{40 \text{ mL solution}}$$

Cross-multiplying results in 100X = 2400. Dividing by 100, we have X = 24.

Therefore, 24 mL alcohol are in 40 mL of a 60% v/v solution.

Stop and Review

Calculate the following.

1. 1000 mL of a 7% solution are needed, but only a 10% solution is in stock. How many mL of the 10% solution are required to make 1000 mL of the 7% solution?

   _____

2. A 5% solution has been poured into a container already containing some solution. The total volume is now 300 mL and its concentration is 4.5%. How many mL of the 5% solution were poured in?

   _____

3. A 10% solution has been poured into a container already containing some solution. The total volume is now 400 mL and its concentration is 6%. How many mL of the 10% solution were poured in?

   _____

4. A 9% solution was poured into a test tube already containing some solution. The total volume is now 300 mL and its concentration is 5%. How many mL of the 9% solution were poured in?

   _____

5. A 7% solution was poured into a flask already containing some solution. The total volume is now 200 mL and its concentration is 5.5%. How many mL of the 7% solution were poured in?

_____

Weight/Volume

A *percent weight per unit volume* is abbreviated *% w/v* and defined as:

$$\frac{\text{Grams of solute}}{100 \text{ mL solution}} = \frac{\text{Grams of solute}}{100 \text{ mL solution}}$$

>>> **Remember**

Weight/volume is also expressed as a function of grams per 100 mL.

Therefore, 5% w/v means that a 100 mL solution would contain 5 g solute. This type of calculation is probably the most common type used in the pharmacy setting. Many medications are solutions prepared as a ratio of the amount of medicine (as weight) to the volume of solution.

■ **Example 1:**

If 350 mL of a 12% w/v Duramorph solution are required, how would it be made? Use the *% w/v* formula.

Therefore, we begin with:

$$0.12 = \frac{X \text{ grams}}{100 \text{ mL}}$$

Multiply by 100, which gives us: X = 12. Therefore, 12 g of Duramorph would be dissolved in 100 mL of diluent (usually water) to get 100 mL. However, 350 mL are desired. Use proportions to solve this:

$$\frac{12 \text{ g}}{100 \text{ mL}} = \frac{X \text{ g}}{350 \text{ mL}}$$

By cross-multiplying, we have: 100X = 4200. Dividing by 100 results in X = 42. Therefore, for this example, dissolve 42 g of Duramorph in 350 mL diluent. This is a 12% solution.

■ **Example 2:**

If 200 mL of a 70% w/v lidocaine solution are desired, how would it be made? Use the same formula as that used in Example 1.

Therefore, we begin with:

$$0.70 = \frac{X \text{ g}}{100 \text{ mL}}$$

We then have: X = 70. Therefore, 12 g lidocaine would be dissolved in 100 mL water to get 100 mL. However, 200 mL are needed. Use proportions to solve this:

$$\frac{70 \text{ g}}{100 \text{ mL}} = \frac{X \text{ g}}{200 \text{ mL}}$$

Cross-multiplying gives us: 100X = 14,000. Dividing by 100 gives us X = 140. Therefore, for this example, dissolve 140 g of lidocaine in 200 mL water. This is a 70% solution.

Example 3:

If 1000 mL of a 5% dextrose w/v solution are desired, how would it be made? Use the same formula as that used in Example 1.

Therefore, we begin with:

$$0.05 = \frac{X \text{ g}}{100 \text{ mL}}$$

We then have: X = 5. Therefore, for this example, dissolve 5 g dextrose in 100 mL water to get 100 mL. However, 1000 mL are desired. Use proportions to solve this:

$$\frac{5 \text{ g}}{100 \text{ mL}} = \frac{X \text{ g}}{1000 \text{ mL}}$$

Cross-multiplying gives: 100X = 5000. Dividing by 100 gives: X = 50. Therefore, dissolve 50 g dextrose in 1000 mL water. This is a 5% solution.

Example 4:

How many grams of sodium chloride (NaCl) are in 25 mL of a 0.9% w/v solution (known as a **normal saline** solution)? This solution contains 0.9 gram of sodium chloride in every 100 mL. Use proportions to solve this:

$$\frac{0.9 \text{ g NaCl}}{100 \text{ mL solution}} = \frac{X \text{ g NaCl}}{25 \text{ mL solution}}$$

Cross-multiplying gives: 100X = 22.5, and dividing by 100 gives: X = 0.225.

Therefore, there is 0.225 g NaCl in 25 mL of a 0.9% w/v NaCl solution. Note that this is less than a 1% solution.

Example 5:

A 500 mL solution contains 50 g ibuprofen. What is the percentage of ibuprofen in this solution?

$$\text{The ratio is } \frac{50 \text{ g ibuprofen}}{500 \text{ mL solution}}$$

Because the percent formula is % w/v =

$$\frac{\text{Grams of solute}}{100 \text{ mL solution}}$$

Set up the following proportion:

$$\frac{X \text{ grams of ibuprofen}}{100 \text{ mL solution}} = \frac{50 \text{ grams of ibuprofen}}{500 \text{ mL solution}}$$

Cross-multiplying gives: 500X = 5000. Dividing by 500 gives: X = 10 (the percentage of drug in the solution). Observe that $\frac{50}{500} = 0.1 = 10\%$.

Example 6:

How many mL of a 5% dextrose w/v solution can be made by using 20 grams of dextrose? A 5% dextrose w/v solution is made up of:

$$\frac{5 \text{ g dextrose}}{100 \text{ mL}}$$

Use proportions to find the number of mL that can be made by using 20 g dextrose:

$$\frac{5 \text{ g dextrose}}{100 \text{ mL}} = \frac{20 \text{ g dextrose}}{X \text{ mL}}$$

Cross-multiplying gives: 5X = 2000. Dividing by 5 gives: X = 400. So, 400 mL of a 5% dextrose w/v solution can be made from 20 g dextrose. Observe that $\frac{20}{400} = 0.05 = 5\%$.

Stop and Review

Calculate the following.

1. Prepare one dose of 0.6 mg kanamycin in 2 mL diluted from a stock solution of 20 mg/mL. How much kanamycin and how much diluent are used?

2. Furosemide is packaged as 10 mg/mL. A pharmacy technician must make a preparation totaling 25 mL of 2 mg/mL concentration. How much drug and how much diluent are used?

3. Bactocill comes packaged as a powder for reconstitution at 250 mg/mL. You must prepare 20 mL of a 25 mg/mL dilution. How many milligrams of the drug are needed, and what volume of diluent is needed?

4. You are asked to prepare 20 mL of a 50 mg/mL drug dilution from a stock of 2 g/5 mL. How many milliliters of diluent will be needed?

5. You must prepare 10 mL of a 4 mcg/mL solution of magnesium sulfate. You have 10 mcg/mL on hand. How much concentrate will you need?

6. You need 5 mL of heparin 100 units/mL. In stock are 10,000 units/mL in a 20 mL vial. How much concentrate will you need?

7. Tobramycin 2 mL of 80 mg/mL is ordered. The pharmacy has 160 mg/mL tobramycin in stock. How much concentrate will you need?

8. A patient needs 50 mL of 5% dextrose. You have 70% dextrose 1000 mL on hand. How much concentrate will you need?

9. What is the w/v % concentration of 250 mL of aqueous sodium chloride solution that contains 5 g of NaCl?

10. 2 liters of an aqueous solution of potassium chloride contains 45 g of KCl. What is the w/v % concentration of this solution in grams per 100 mL?

Ratio Strength

The term **ratio strength** is defined as the concentration of weak solutions. All percentages are a ratio of parts per hundred. In a ratio, the numerator expresses the strength of an active ingredient, and the denominator expresses the strength of a whole preparation. A ratio strength is commonly used to express the concentration of weak solutions or liquid preparations. It is another way of expressing the percentage strength of solutions or liquid preparations, and sometimes mixtures of solids. For example, 10% means that 10 parts per 100 can be expressed as 10:100, which can be reduced to 1:10.

To calculate the ratio strength of a solution obtained by diluting or concentrating it, the following example contains several steps:

■ **Example 1:**

If 500 mL of a 15% v/v solution are diluted to 1500 mL, what is the percentage strength?

Begin with:

$$500 \text{ mL} \times 15\% = 1500 \text{ mL} \times X\%$$

Calculate the left side first:

$$75 = 1500 \times X\%$$

Divide both sides by 1500:

$$0.05 = X\%$$

Therefore, X = 5%. This can also be solved by *inverse proportion*:

$$\frac{1500 \text{ mL}}{500 \text{ mL}} = \frac{15\%}{X\%}$$

This also can be solved by *calculating the active ingredient*:

$$\frac{1500 \text{ mL}}{75 \text{ mL}} = \frac{100\%}{X\%}$$

By any method of calculation, the preceding answer is still 5%.

Example 2:

50 mL of 1:20 w/v solution is diluted to 1000 mL. What is the ratio strength w/v?

Begin with:
$$1:20 = 5\%$$

Therefore,
$$50 \text{ (mL)} \times 5 \text{ (\%)} = 1000 \text{ (mL)} \times X \text{ (\%)}$$

This gives:
$$2.5 = 1000 \times X\%$$

Dividing by 1000 produces the following answer:
$$X = 0.25\% \text{ or } 1:400$$

Again, this example may also be solved by inverse proportion or by calculating the active ingredient.

Test Your Knowledge

Calculate the following concentrations.

1. What is the final concentration of a 15% solution diluted 1:10?

2. What is the final concentration of an 8% solution diluted 1:10?

3. What is the final concentration of a 25% solution diluted 1:5?

4. What is the final concentration of a 50% solution diluted 1:2?

5. What is the final concentration of a 12% solution diluted 1:8?

6. A 10% solution was diluted to a 2% solution. Determine the dilution ratio used.

7. A 20% solution was diluted to a 10% solution. Determine the dilution ratio used.

8. An 8% solution was diluted to a 2% solution. Determine the dilution ratio used.

9. A 12% solution was diluted to a 4% solution. Determine the dilution ratio used.

10. A 20% solution is diluted by $\frac{1}{10}$. It is diluted again by $\frac{1}{10}$. What is the final concentration?

11. An 8% solution is diluted by $\frac{1}{2}$. It is diluted again by $\frac{1}{4}$. What is the final concentration?

12. A 40% solution is diluted by $\frac{1}{2}$. It is diluted again by $\frac{1}{2}$. What is the final concentration?

Calculate the following concentrations and volumes of solutions.

1. If $V_1 = 16$ mL, $V_2 = 20$ mL, and $C_1 = 6\%$, find C_2.

2. If $V_1 = 10$ mL, $V_2 = 20$ mL, and $C_1 = 15\%$, find C_2.

3. If $V_1 = 30$ mL, $C_1 = 60\%$, and $C_2 = 20\%$, find V_2.

4. If $V_1 = 150$ mL, $C_1 = 7\%$, and $C_2 = 12\%$, find V_2.

5. If $V_2 = 200$ mL, $C_1 = 80\%$, and $C_2 = 50\%$, find V_1.

6. If $V_2 = 80$ mL, $C_1 = 25\%$, and $C_2 = 30\%$, find V_1.

7. If 60 mL of a 2.5% solution are diluted to 120 mL, what is its concentration?

8. If 50 mL of a 3% solution are diluted to 300 mL, what is its concentration?

9. If 80 mL of a 3.5% solution has another 80 mL added to make a total of 160 mL, what is this concentration?

10. A 40 mL medication has a 4.5% concentration. It is diluted to 240 mL. What is its concentration?

11. On hand are 100 mL of a 2% solution. It is diluted to 500 mL. What is its concentration?

12. You need 500 mL of a 4% solution, and a 5% solution must be added to do this. How many mL of the 5% solution are required?

13. You need 200 mL of a 6% solution. Because only 7% solution is in stock, how many mL of the stock solution are needed to make 200 mL of the 6% solution?

14. You need 300 mL of a 7% solution. A 9% solution must be used to dilute it. How many mL of the 9% solution are required?

15. You need 1200 mL of a 7% solution. Only a 12% solution is in stock. How many mL of the 12% solution are needed to make 1200 mL of the 7% solution?

Calculate the w/w, v/v, or w/v equations.

1. Calculate how to make 125 g of an 18% w/w NaOH solution.

2. Calculate how to make 250 g of a 15% w/w NaOH solution.

3. Calculate how to make 75 g of a 9% w/w NaCl solution.

4. Calculate how to make 300 g of a 30% w/w NaCl solution.

5. Calculate how to make 250 mL of an 18% v/v solution of isopropyl alcohol in water.

6. Calculate how to make 200 mL of a 20% v/v solution of isopropyl alcohol in water.

7. Calculate how to make 225 mL of a 10% v/v solution of isopropyl alcohol in water.

8. Calculate how to make 70 mL of a 70% v/v solution of isopropyl alcohol in water.

9. Calculate how to make 150 mL of a 25% w/v NaCl solution.

10. Calculate how to make 200 mL of a 6% w/v ampicillin solution.

11. Calculate how to make 50 mL of a 2% w/v NaCl solution.

12. Calculate how to make 125 mL of a 12% w/v cephapirin solution.

13. Calculate how to make 150 mL of a 14% w/v cephapirin solution.

14. How many grams of dextrose are contained in 10 dL of a 15% w/v NaCl solution?

15. How many grams of dextrose are contained in 45 dL of a 30% w/v NaCl solution?

16. How many grams of NaCl are in 20 mL of a 10% w/v solution?

17. How many grams of NaCl are in 250 mL of an 8% w/v solution?

18. How many mL of a 5% dextrose w/v solution can be produced by using 30 g of dextrose?

19. How many mL of a 5% dextrose w/v solution can be produced by using 50 g of dextrose?

20. How many mL of a 6% dextrose w/v solution can be produced by using 35 g of dextrose?

21. How many mL of a 6% dextrose w/v solution can be produced by using 15 g of dextrose?

22. If a 1000 mL solution contains 30 g of a drug, what is the percentage of the drug in this solution?

23. If a 1000 mL solution contains 80 g of kanamycin, what is the percentage of kanamycin in this solution?

24. If a 200 mL solution contains 12 g of a drug, what is the percentage of the drug in this solution?

25. If a 300 mL solution contains 25 g of a drug, what is the percentage of the drug in this solution?

26. If a 500 mL solution contains 100 g of acetaminophen, what is the percentage of acetaminophen in this solution?

27. If an 800 mL solution contains 150 g of ibuprofen, what is the percentage of ibuprofen in this solution?

Critical Thinking

A pharmacy technician poured a 5% solution into a container that already held a solution of an unknown volume. If the total volume of the mixed solution in the container is 100 mL, and its concentration is 2%, how would you answer the following questions?

1. How many milliliters of the 5% solution were poured into the container?

2. If the pharmacy technician poured a 20% solution in, instead of a 5% solution, how many milliliters could be poured into the container?

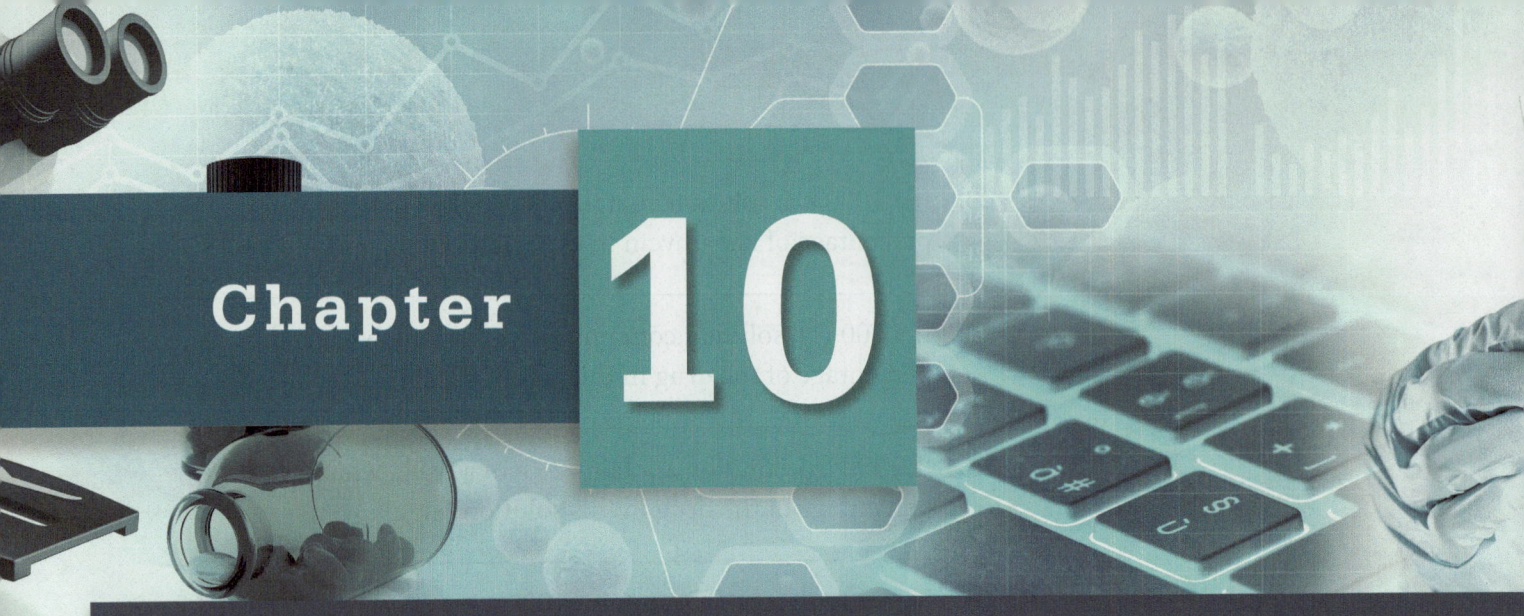

Chapter 10

Dilutions and Solutions

Outline

Overview
Dilutions
Stock Solutions for Solids
   Stock Vials and Ampules
Liquid Dilutions
Alligation

Objectives

Upon completion of this chapter, you should be able to:

1. Define the term *stock solution*.
2. Calculate the appropriate solution strength using alligation methods.
3. Demonstrate how to calculate the volume of a stock solution needed to prepare a given solution for a patient.
4. Describe the components of the X-shaped diagram that is used in alligation.
5. Determine various dilution ratios, such as from serum to water and alcohol to water.

Key Terms

alligation
diluents
dilutions
solvents

Overview

Pharmacy technicians should be familiar with dilutions because many stock solutions must be diluted in order to prepare patient-specific doses. Diluted solutions have decreased concentrations and increased volumes. Pharmacy technicians often calculate mixtures of substances by using **alligation**. This is a mathematical process that allows for calculation of amounts of substances based on their different percentage strengths.

Dilutions

>>> **Remember**

The total volume = the parts of the concentrate + the parts of the diluent.

Solutions must often be diluted by adding water or a saline solution. **Solvents** are referred to as **diluents**. They decrease a solution's concentration and increase its volume. The formula $V_1 \times C_1 = V_2 \times C_2$ applies to dilutions with its V_2 and C_2 values, which usually represent the diluted solution. Often, powdered medications are diluted with normal saline or sterile water. **Dilutions** represent parts of concentrate in *total volume*.

Stock Solutions for Solids

Stock solutions are solutions of known concentration prepared by the pharmacist or pharmacy technician for convenience in dispensing. Dilute solutions are usually made from them. Stock solutions enable pharmacists to obtain the small quantities of medicinal substances that are to be dispensed in solution. They are usually prepared on a weight-in-volume basis. Their concentration is expressed as a ratio strength, or less frequently, as a percentage strength.

■ **Example 1:**

How many milliliters of a 1:400 w/v stock solution are needed to make 4 L of a 1:2000 w/v solution? Remember that 4 L = 4000 mL. A 1:400 stock solution = 0.25%, while a 1:2000 solution = 0.05%. Using the standard formula to calculate this dilution,

$$X \text{ mL} \times 0.25\% = 4000 \text{ mL} \times 0.05\%$$

Therefore, by inverse proportion:

$$\frac{0.25\%}{0.05\%} = \frac{4000 \text{ mL}}{X \text{ mL}}$$

Or:

$$\frac{\frac{1}{400}}{\frac{1}{2000}} = \frac{4000 \text{ mL}}{X \text{ mL}}$$

The answer is 800 mL.

Stock Vials and Ampules

Vials and ampules are commonly labeled with concentrations as milligrams per milliliter (mg/mL) or micrograms per milliliter (mcg/mL). Often, injectable products are mixed into concentrations intended for oral administration based on physician orders. The same method is usually used to calculate the amount of stock solution and diluent as is used to calculate the amount of active ingredient.

Liquid Dilutions

A stock solution often contains a concentrate, such as a medication, and a diluent, such as saline or sterile water. If 1 microliter of serum were mixed with 6 microliters of saline, the ratio would be 1:7. This means that there is 1 part concentrate out of a total of 7 parts (6 of which are the diluent). Remember that *dilution* is defined as parts concentrate in total volume.

■ **Example 1:**

We need to make a 1 in 10 dilution of serum in saline. The total volume must be 150 microliters. What volume of serum and what volume of diluent are needed?

First, set up a proportion:

$$\frac{1 \text{ part serum}}{10 \text{ parts total volume}} = \frac{X \text{ parts serum}}{150 \text{ parts total volume}}$$

Cross-multiplying gives: 10X = 150. Dividing both sides by 10 gives: X = 15.

Therefore, 15 parts serum are needed. Because the units are microliters, 15 microliters of serum are needed.

To determine how much diluent is needed, remember that parts concentrate plus parts diluent equal the total volume. Therefore,

$$15 \text{ (parts serum)} + X = 150$$

Solve by subtracting 15 from both sides, which gives: X = 135.

Therefore, we need 135 microliters of saline to make this solution. Notice that:

$$\frac{\text{Part serum}}{\text{Total volume}} = \frac{15 \text{ microliters}}{150 \text{ microliters}} = \frac{15}{150} = \frac{1}{10}$$

Therefore, a 1 in 10 dilution was achieved, which is what was required.

■ **Example 2:**

Make a 1 in 8 dilution of insulin in normal saline. The total volume must be 220 mL. What volume of insulin is needed?

Set up a proportion:

$$\frac{1 \text{ part insulin}}{8 \text{ parts total volume}} = \frac{X \text{ parts insulin}}{220 \text{ parts total volume}}$$

Cross-multiplying gives: 8X = 220. Dividing both sides by 8 gives: X = 27.5.

What volume of diluent is needed? We need 27.5 mL of insulin, and insulin plus diluent equals total volume, so 27.5 + X = 220. Subtracting 27.5 from both sides gives X = 192.5. Therefore, 192.5 mL of diluent is needed.

■ Example 3:

Find the quantity of hydrogen peroxide in water in a 150 mL solution if the dilution is 1:6.

$$\frac{1 \text{ hydrogen peroxide}}{6 \text{ total volume}} = \frac{X \text{ hydrogen peroxide}}{150 \text{ total volume}}$$

Cross-multiplying gives: 6X = 150. Dividing by 6 gives: X = 25. Therefore, for a 1:6 mixture, 25 mL of hydrogen peroxide are needed, mixed with 125 mL of water to reach the total volume of 150 mL.

■ Example 4:

Find the quantity of liquid penicillin in a 50 mL solution if the dilution is $\frac{1}{5}$.

$$\frac{1 \text{ penicillin}}{5 \text{ total volume}} = \frac{X \text{ penicillin}}{50 \text{ total volume}}$$

Cross-multiplying gives: 5X = 50. Dividing by 5 results in X = 10. Therefore, for a 1:5 mixture, 10 mL penicillin are needed, mixed with 40 mL water to reach the total volume of 50 mL.

■ Example 5:

For a 4 in 10 dilution, what is the ratio of serum to saline? Remember that serum plus diluent equals total volume. Therefore,

$$\frac{\text{Parts serum}}{\text{Total volume}} = \frac{4}{10}$$

So, 4 + X = 10, resulting in X = 6. This means that there are 6 parts of saline. The serum-to-saline ratio is $\frac{4}{6}$.

■ Example 6:

For a 3 in 18 dilution, what is the ratio of ammonia to water? Remember that ammonia plus water equals total volume. Therefore,

$$\frac{\text{Parts ammonia}}{\text{Total volume}} = \frac{3}{18}$$

So, 3 + X = 18, resulting in X = 15. This means that there are 15 parts of water. The ammonia to water ratio is $\frac{3}{15}$.

Stop and Review
Fill in the blanks and calculate the dilutions or stock solutions.

1. Solutions must often be diluted by adding _____ or a _____ solution.

2. Diluents are also known as _____.

3. Dilutions represent parts of concentrate in _____ volume.

4. Solutions of known concentration prepared for convenience in dispensing are known as _____ solutions.

5. If one microliter of serum was mixed with 6 microliters of saline, the ratio would be _____ : _____.

6. To make 4000 mL of a 1:2000 w/v solution using a 1:400 w/v stock solution, you need _____ mL of the stock solution.

7. To make 3000 mL of a 1:1000 w/v solution using a 1:500 w/v stock solution, you need _____ mL of the stock solution.

8. If a 1 in 5 dilution of insulin in normal saline is required, and the total volume must be 200 mL, the volume of insulin needed is _____ mL.

9. For a 3 in 10 dilution, the ratio of serum to saline is _____ to _____.

10. 15 parts serum to 150 parts total volume signifies a dilution of _____ to _____.

Alligation

Alligation is defined as a method of arithmetic that involves the mixing of solutions or of solids possessing different percentage strengths. Sometimes it is necessary to obtain the desired strength of a medication by compounding, mixing higher and lower concentrations of medications to be able to fill a specific prescription or medication order. This method is known as "alligation alternate" and offers a rapid method of calculation that is useful to pharmacists and pharmacy technicians.

All concentrations must be in a percentage form, and the strength of the desired solution must lie between the stronger and weaker solutions available. In other words, the final mixture will be an average of the individual strengths. These will be calculated as proportional parts. If the concentration is not expressed in the percentage form, it must be converted to the percentage form. For example, a solution strength expressed as 1:200 must be converted to a percentage.

$$\frac{1}{200} \times 100 = 0.5\%$$

By using alligation, the number of parts of each component needed to prepare the final percentage concentration may be calculated. Lines are drawn during calculation to bind quantities together. The substance with a higher value than what is required is the one with the lower amount. The increase in the value or amount of one of the substances balances the decrease in value or amount of the other substances.

■ Example 1:

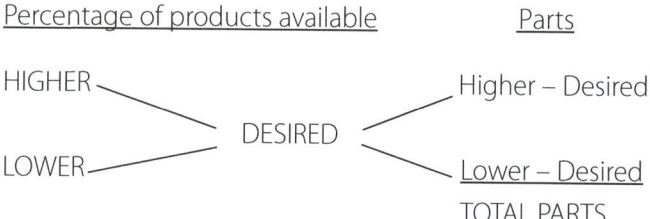

The upper-right and lower-right corners of the X-shaped diagram are achieved by calculating the difference between the higher percentage (shown in the upper-left corner of the preceding example) and the desired percentage, as well as between the lower percentage (shown in the lower-left corner of the preceding example) and the desired percentage. The difference between these two figures is placed in the upper-right corner of the X. Then the total number of parts is calculated by adding the higher and lower parts.

Alligation is useful in solving any type of dilution or concentration problem. Concentrations expressed in mg/mL, ratios, and even mixtures of liquids of known specific gravities may be solved using alligation. The strengths of the preparations being mixed, as well as the final mixture, have to be expressed in a common denomination when the alligation formula is being set up. When diluting a preparation, the diluent's strength is considered to be 0%. When the strength of a mixture is increased by adding more drug, the strength of this component is 100%. The final proportion allows a distinct correlation between the parts in the mixture and any specific denomination needed.

The quantities of the higher and lower percentages of products may be achieved by using the following formula:

$$\text{HIGHER quantity: } \frac{\text{Number of HIGHER Parts}}{\text{Total Number of Parts}} = \frac{X}{\text{Total Quantity for Compounding}}$$

$$\text{LOWER quantity: } \frac{\text{Number of LOWER Parts}}{\text{Total Number of Parts}} = \frac{X}{\text{Total Quantity for Compounding}}$$

>>> **Remember**

- Use alligation to determine the proper mixtures of solutions or solids with different percentage strengths.

- By using alligation, the final mixture will be an average of the individual strengths expressed as a percentage.

- The substance with a higher value (percentage) than what is required is the substance with the lower amount (strength).

- The increase in value of one of the substances balances the decrease in value of the other substances.

- Calculate the upper-right and lower-right corners by subtracting the desired amount from the higher concentration substance, and then subtracting the lower concentration substance from the desired amount.

- Add the higher and lower parts to determine the total number of parts.

> **Remember**
>
> Higher concentration
> parts = 35 − 20 = 15
>
> Lower concentration
> parts = 70 − 35 = 35

■ Example 2:

To find what proportion is required for a 1000 mL preparation containing 70% alcohol mixed with another that contains 20% alcohol, to produce a mixture of 35% strength, the following steps are taken:

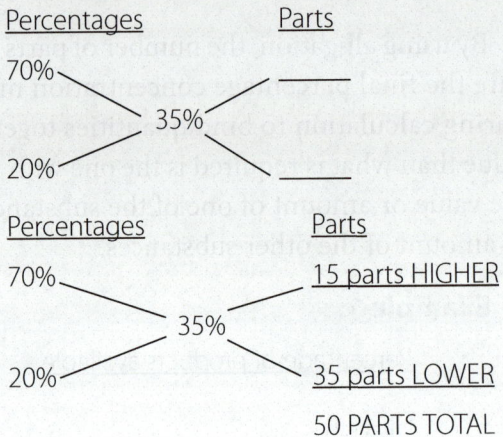

Therefore, the result will be as follows:

Amount of 70% solution:

$$\frac{15}{50} = \frac{X \text{ mL}}{1000 \text{ mL}} \quad X = 300 \text{ mL of 70% solution}$$

Amount of 20% solution:

$$\frac{35}{50} = \frac{X \text{ mL}}{1000 \text{ mL}} \quad X = 700 \text{ mL of 20% solution}$$

■ Example 3:

To find what proportion is required for a preparation containing 10% of a drug mixed with another that contains 15% of a drug, to produce a mixture of 12% strength, the following steps are taken:

1. Understand that the 10% drug is 2% too weak. The 15% drug is 3% too strong. The excess strength of 3 parts of the stronger drug can be calculated to balance the deficient strength of 2 parts of the weaker drug, as follows:

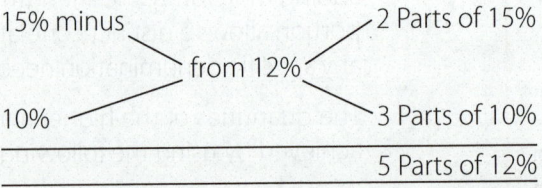

The figure obtained from 12% − 10% is placed in the upper-right side of the equation. This is labeled as "2 parts of 15%."

The figure obtained from 15% − 12% is placed in the lower-right side of the equation. This is labeled as "3 parts of 10%."

This calculation produces a drug mixture of "5 parts of 12%," which is the desired strength.

Alligation calculations used to mix solutions may be checked by using the following formula:

$$\text{milliliters} \times \text{percent (as a decimal)} = \text{grams}$$

■ Example 4:

Prepare 250 mL of dextrose 7.5%. To do this, you are required to use dextrose 5% (D_5W) and dextrose 50% ($D_{50}W$). Determine how many milliliters of each will be required.

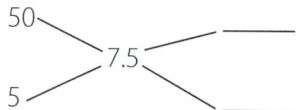

As discussed previously, subtract the center number from the upper-left number and put it at the lower right. Then subtract the lower-left number from the center number, and put it at the upper right.

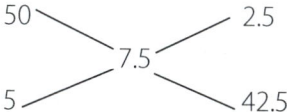

The sum of the two numbers written at the right side of the equation, 2.5 + 42.5, equals 45, which is the total number of parts of the 7.5% final solution. Put in the terms of ratios, the ratio of the 5% solution to the 7.5% solution is 42.5:45. The ratio of the 50% solution to the 7.5% solution is 2.5:45. Therefore, much less of the 50% solution is needed to make the 7.5% solution.

To calculate the volume needed of each dextrose solution, use the following equations:

50% Dextrose

$$\frac{X \text{ mL}}{2.5 \text{ parts}} = \frac{250 \text{ mL}}{45 \text{ parts}}$$

$$X \text{ mL} = \frac{(2.5 \text{ parts}) \times 250 \text{ mL}}{45 \text{ parts}}$$

$$X \text{ mL} = 13.89 \text{ mL } D_{50}W$$

5% Dextrose

$$\frac{X \text{ mL}}{42.5 \text{ parts}} = \frac{250 \text{ mL}}{45 \text{ parts}}$$

$$X \text{ mL} = \frac{(42.5) \times 250 \text{ mL}}{45 \text{ parts}}$$

$$X \text{ mL} = 236.11 \text{ mL } D_5W$$

Add the volumes of the two solutions. The sum should equal the required volume of 7.5% dextrose.

$$\begin{array}{r} 236.11 \text{ mL} \\ + 13.89 \text{ mL} \\ \hline 250.00 \text{ mL} \end{array}$$

Check your answer using the following formula. The number of grams of solute should equal the sum of the grams of the solutes of the 50% solution and the 5% solution.

$$mL \times \% 5 g$$
$$250 \text{ mL} \times 0.075 = 18.75 \text{ g} \qquad 13.89 \text{ mL} \times 0.5 = 6.945 \text{ g}$$
$$236.11 \text{ mL} \times 0.05 = 11.805 \text{ g}$$

Now, add:

$$\begin{array}{r} 11.805 \text{ g} \\ + \ 6.945 \text{ g} \\ \hline 18.75 \text{ g} \end{array}$$

Stop and Review

Use alligation to calculate.

1. Ammoniated mercury ointment is available in 10% and 3%. A technician needs to prepare 450 g of a 5% ointment. How many grams of each of the 10% and 3% ointments will be needed?

   _____

2. How many mL of each of a 20% stock solution and a 30% stock solution will a technician need to make 500 mL of a 28% solution?

   _____

3. An order for 6 liters of 0.9% sodium chloride solution is to be prepared from 23.4% concentrated NaCl solution and sterile water for injection. How many milliliters of each will be used?

   _____

4. A technician is to prepare 250 mL of a 40% solution from a 60% stock solution and purified water. How many milliliters of each are needed?

   _____

5. A liter of $\frac{1}{3}$ NS is to be prepared from 0.9% concentrated sodium chloride solution and sterile water for injection. How many milliliters of each are to be used?

   _____

6. Stock solutions of 27% and 31% are available in the pharmacy. How many milliliters of each stock solution are needed to prepare 2 L of a 29% solution?

   _____

7. From two stock solutions, 18% and 42%, you are to prepare 1.5 L of a 34% solution. How many milliliters of each of the stock solutions do you need?

   _____

Test Your Knowledge

1. To create a desired concentration, we must have a 2 mg substance for each 6 mL solution. How much substance is needed to make a 10 mL solution?

2. To create a desired concentration, we must have a 3 mg substance for each 10 mL solution. How much substance is needed to make a 50 mL solution?

3. To create a desired concentration, we must have 4 mg substance for every 60 mL solution. How much substance is needed to make a 100 mL solution?

4. To create a desired concentration, we must have 8 mg substance for every 20 mL solution. How much substance is needed to make 250 mL solution?

5. For a 2 in 7 dilution, what is the ratio of serum to saline? What is the ratio of serum to total volume?

6. For a 3 in 10 dilution, what is the ratio of urine to water? What is the ratio of water to total volume?

7. For a 4 in 15 dilution, what is the ratio of urine to water? What is the ratio of water to total volume?

8. For a 5 in 12 dilution, what is the ratio of serum to saline? What is the ratio of saline to total volume?

9. One microliter serum is added to 6 microliters diluent. Give the dilution of the solution. What is the serum-to-total volume ratio?

10. Three milliliters urine are added to 11 mL diluent. Give the dilution of the solution. What is the urine-to-total volume ratio?

11. Two milliliters urine are added to 15 mL diluent. Give the dilution of the solution. What is the urine-to-total volume ratio?

12. Five milliliters serum are added to 18 mL diluent. Give the dilution of the solution. What is the serum-to-total volume ratio?

13. The serum-to-water ratio is 2:3. Determine the dilution ratio of serum to total volume.

14. The alcohol-to-water ratio is 5:8. Determine the dilution ratio of alcohol to total volume.

15. The alcohol-to-water ratio is 1:10. Determine the dilution ratio of alcohol to total volume.

16. The serum-to-water ratio is 3:10. Determine the dilution ratio of serum to total volume.

17. Explain how a healthcare professional would make a 270 mL urine in water solution if the dilution is to be $\dfrac{9}{15}$.

18. Explain how a healthcare professional would make a 100 mL urine in water solution if the dilution is to be $\frac{2}{5}$.

_____
_____

19. Explain how a healthcare professional would make an 80 mL urine in water solution if the dilution is to be $\frac{5}{8}$.

_____
_____

20. Three parts serum are added to nine parts water. Find the solution dilution.

_____
_____

21. Two parts urine are added to 12 parts water. Find the solution dilution.

_____
_____

22. Two parts serum are added to 5 parts water. Find the solution dilution.

_____
_____

23. A technician needs to make a 1 in 8 dilution of serum. The total volume must be 120 microliters. What volume of serum is needed? What volume of diluent is needed?

_____
_____

24. Four milliliters urine are to be used to make a 2 in 9 dilution. What will be the total volume of the solution? What volume of diluent is needed?

_____
_____

25. A technician needs to make a 1 in 15 dilution of serum. The total volume is to be 150 microliters. What volume of serum is needed? What volume of diluent is needed?

_____
_____

26. Three milliliters urine are to be used to make a 2 in 8 dilution. What will be the total volume of the solution? What volume of diluent is needed?

27. How would a scientist make 500 mL of a $\frac{3}{5}$ dilution of concentrate?

28. How would a scientist make 400 microliters of a $\frac{2}{5}$ dilution of concentrate?

29. We have 50 microliters of a $\frac{1}{4}$ dilution of serum. How much serum would be present?

30. How would a scientist make 250 microliters of a $\frac{1}{2}$ dilution of concentrate?

31. We have 20 microliters of a $\frac{1}{10}$ dilution of serum. How much serum would be present?

32. Five milliliters concentrate will make how much of a $\frac{2}{5}$ dilution?

33. How many grams of 20% and 15% stock ichthammol ointments are needed to prepare 60 g of a 12.5% ichthammol ointment?

34. Rx: zinc oxide 10% ointment 60 g
    How many grams of zinc oxide 20% ointment and zinc oxide 5% ointment should you mix to prepare the order?

35. Rx: coal tar 5% ointment 160 g
    You have coal tar 10% ointment and coal tar 2% ointment. How many grams of each will you use to prepare the final product?

36. Rx: benzocaine 5% ointment 4 oz
    How many grams of benzocaine 2% ointment should you mix with 25 g of benzocaine 10% ointment to prepare the order?

37. How much 10% hydrocortisone cream and 0.5% hydrocortisone cream will you need to prepare 90 g of 2.5% hydrocortisone cream?

38. How would a pharmacy technician prepare 2 L of a 20% alcohol solution using a 90% alcohol and a 10% alcohol?

39. You are asked to prepare 4 L of a 30% strength solution. Your pharmacy stocks the active ingredient in 8 oz bottles of 60%. How many bottles of the active ingredient will you need to open to complete the order?

40. Prepare 1 L of a 7.5% dextrose solution using sterilized water for injection (SWFI) and dextrose 10% in water ($D_{10}W$).

41. How many grams of petrolatum should you add to 60 g of hydrocortisone 2.5% ointment to reduce its strength to 2%? The percent strength of petrolatum is zero.

42. Prepare 480 mL of a 1:20 solution using a 1:10 solution and a 1:50 solution.

Critical Thinking

You must prepare 400 mL of a solution that requires a 1:8 dilution. The diluent to be used is sterile water.

1. How would you calculate this dilution?

   _____

2. How many milliliters of sterile water must be added to the solution to achieve the desired dilution?

   _____

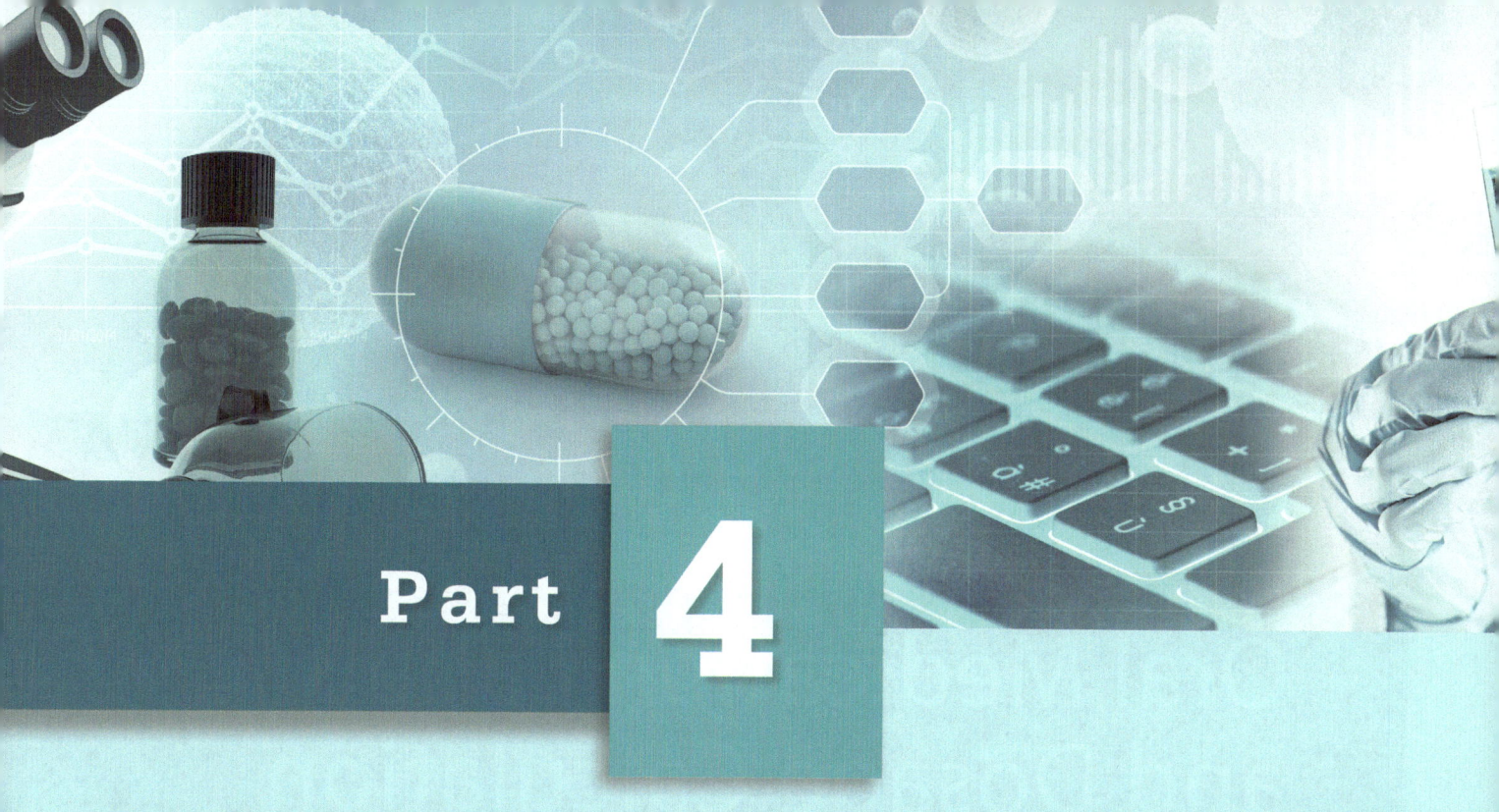

Part 4

Medication Preparation

Chapter 11 Oral Medication Labels and Dosage Calculation

Chapter 12 Reconstitution of Powdered Drugs

Chapter 13 Parenteral Medication Labels and Dosage Calculation

Chapter 14 Intravenous Flow Rate Calculations

Chapter 15 Pediatric Drug Administration

Chapter 16 Business Math for Pharmacy Technicians

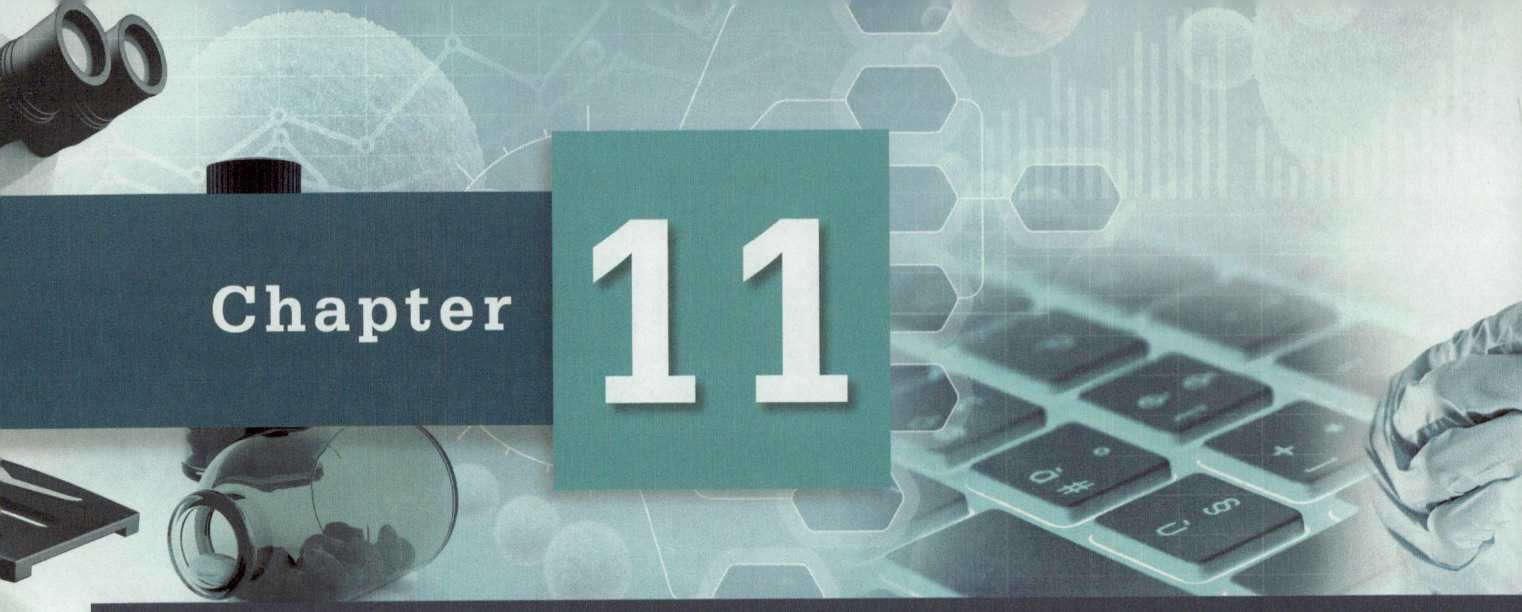

Chapter 11

Oral Medication Labels and Dosage Calculation

Outline

Overview
Tablet and Capsule Labels and Calculations
Oral Solution Labels
Measurement of Oral Solutions

Objectives

Upon completion of this chapter, you should be able to:

1. Determine if the strength or concentration of a drug on hand is the same as the dosage ordered.
2. Calculate doses for tablets and capsules using available strengths.
3. Calculate doses for liquid drug preparations using available concentrations and explain their measurement.

Key Terms

capsules
National Formulary
scored
tablets
United States Pharmacopeia (USP)

Overview

It is vital to understand the information on drug labels. This information includes the drug's name, dosage strength, form, total amount contained, route of administration, storage requirements, warnings, manufacturing information, and references. The **United States Pharmacopeia (USP)** sets official public standards for all prescription and OTC medications, dietary supplements, and other health care products. The **National Formulary** is part of the USP. The *United States Pharmacopeia–National Formulary (USP-NF)* is a book containing public pharmacopeia standards. It contains standards for medicines, dosage forms, drug substances, excipients, biologics, compounded preparations, medical devices, dietary supplements, and other therapeutics.

Tablet and capsule labels contain information about the drug contained. To calculate tablet and capsule dosages, you must know the desired dose, the available drug quantity, and the dosage unit. Oral solutions are often ordered for children, the elderly, and patients who have trouble swallowing. Pharmacy technicians must calculate the volume of these solutions so that the prescribed dosage of the drug is administered.

Tablet and Capsule Labels and Calculations

When a prescriber orders medications in tablet or capsule form, the pharmacy technician must determine if the strength or concentration of the drug on hand is the same as the dosage ordered or in multiples of the dosage ordered. Sometimes patients should divide the tablet in half or, less commonly, into quarters. **Figure 11-1** shows Biaxin **tablets** in two different strengths (**scored** and nonscored).

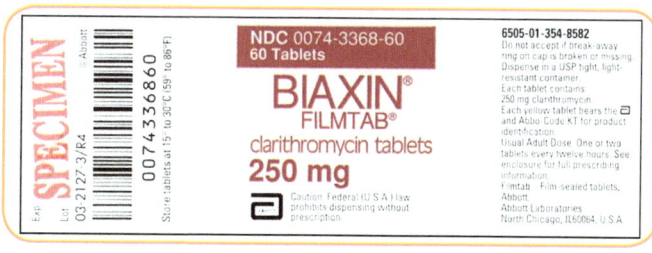

(a)

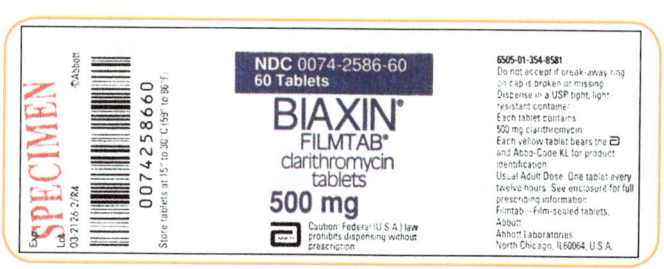

(b)

Figure 11-1 (a) Biaxin 250 mg, (b) Biaxin 500 mg.
(a) and (b) Courtesy of Abbott Laboratories

■ **Example 1:**

The doctor's order reads: *Biaxin 500 mg p.o. q12h.*

Biaxin comes in tablet strengths of 250 milligrams per tablet (or filmtab) and 500 milligrams per tablet. When both strengths are available, the pharmacy technician should select the 500 milligram strength, and give one whole tablet for each dose.

■ **Example 2:**

The order reads: *Clonazepam 1.5 mg p.o. t.i.d.*

Clonazepam comes in strengths of 0.5 mg, 1 mg, and 2 mg tablets (**Figure 11-2**). When the three strengths are available, the pharmacy technician should select one 1 mg tablet and one 0.5 mg tablet (1 mg + 0.5 mg = 1.5 mg). This provides the ordered dose of 1.5 mg and is the least number of tablets (2 tablets total) for the patient to swallow. However, another option would be to give three 0.5 mg tablets, which will also equal 1.5 mg.

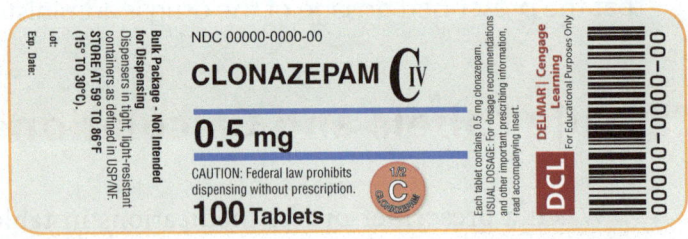
(a)

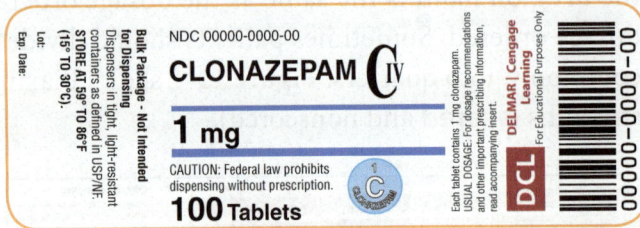
(b)

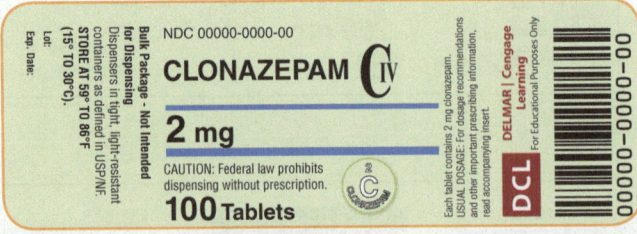
(c)

Figure 11-2 (a) Clonazepam 0.5 mg, (b) Clonazepam 1 mg, (c) Clonazepam 2 mg.
(a), (b), and (c) © Cengage Learning 2013

Another option for the pharmacy technician is to halve the 2 mg tablets to obtain two 1 mg parts, and pair one half tablet with a 0.5 mg tablet. This would also equal 1.5 mg, and would amount to $1\frac{1}{2}$ tablets. However, cutting any tablet in half may produce slightly unequal halves. It is preferable to give whole, undivided tablets when they are available. In practice, only scored tablets should be cut in half.

In some instances it may be necessary to convert between systems of measurement to accurately calculate the dosage. Previously, you learned a formula for dosage calculations, as follows:

$$\frac{D}{H} \times Q = X$$

$$\frac{D \text{ (desired)}}{H \text{ (have)}} \times Q \text{ (quantity)} = X \text{ (amount)}$$

To convert dosages, ensure that all measurements are in the same system of measurement and the same size unit of measurement. If not, convert before proceeding.

■ Example 3:

The drug order reads: *Ampicillin 0.5 g p.o. q6h*.

Available on hand: *Ampicillin 500 mg per capsule*

This medication order is written and supplied in the same system (metric) but in different size units (g and mg). A drug order written in grams but supplied in milligrams will have to be converted to the same size unit. You must convert 0.5 gram to milligrams, as follows:

$$1 \text{ g} = 1000 \text{ mg}$$

Remember, you are converting from a larger to a smaller unit. Therefore, you will multiply by the conversion factor of 1000 or move the decimal point three places to the right.

$$0.5 \text{ g} = 0.5 \times 1000 = 500 \text{ mg, or } 0.5 \text{ g} = 0.500 = 500 \text{ mg}$$

Order: *Ampicillin 500 mg p.o. q6h*

On hand: *Ampicillin 500 mg per capsule*

You would give the patient one ampicillin 500 mg capsule by mouth every 6 hours.

■ Example 4:

The drug order reads: *Lopressor 100 mg p.o. b.i.d.*

The medication container is labeled "Lopressor 50 mg per tablet."

Calculate one dose:

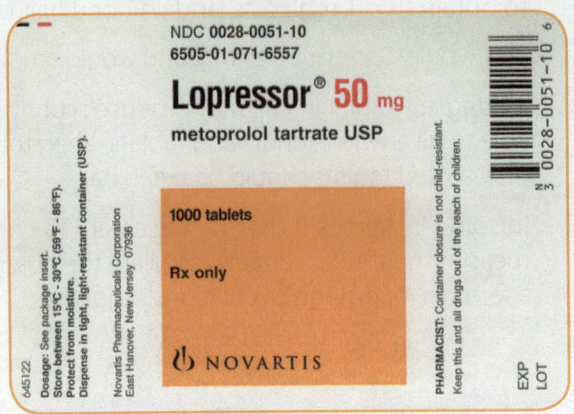

Lopressor 50 mg.
Courtesy of Novartis

$$\frac{D}{H} \times Q = \frac{100 \text{ mg}}{50 \text{ mg}} \times 1 \text{ tablet}$$

$$\frac{100 \text{ mg}}{50 \text{ mg}} = \frac{2 \text{ mg}}{1 \text{ mg}} \times 1 \text{ tablet} = 2 \times 1 \text{ tablet}$$

$$= 2 \text{ tablets, given orally, twice daily}$$

■ Example 5:

The drug order reads: *V-Cillin K 0.5 g p.o. q.i.d.*

Available on hand: *V-Cillin K 250 mg per tablet*

How many tablets should you give to the patient per dose?

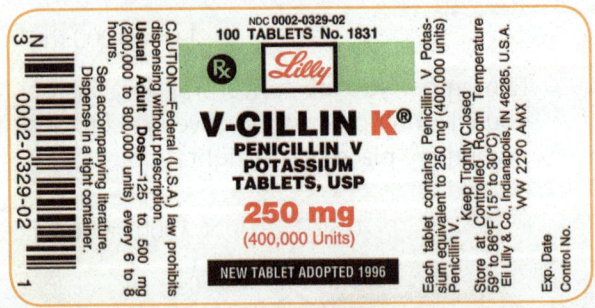

V-Cillin K 250 mg.
© Eli Lilly and Company. Used with permission

As you know, 1 g = 1000 mg.

$$0.5 \text{ g} = 0.5 \times 1000 = 0.500 = 500 \text{ mg}$$

Now you have the ordered drug and the on-hand drug measured in the same size units.

Ordered: *V-Cillin K 0.5 g = 500 mg*

On hand: *V-Cillin K 250 mg tablets*

$$\frac{500 \text{ mg}}{250 \text{ mg}} \times 1 \text{ tablet} = 2 \times 1 \text{ tablet} = 2 \text{ tablets, given orally 4 times daily}$$

■ Example 6:

The drug order reads: *Codeine sulfate gr $\frac{3}{4}$ p.o. q4h p.r.n., pain.*

The drug on hand is: *Codeine sulfate 30 mg per tablet*

Calculate one dose.

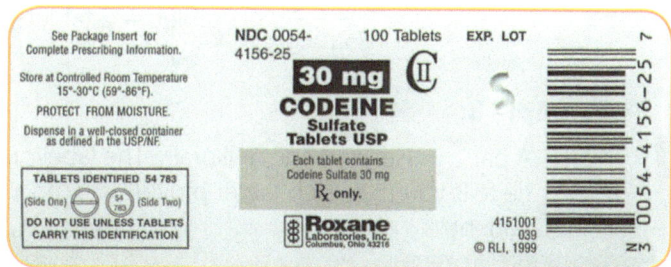

Codeine 30 mg.
Used with permission of Roxane Laboratories, Inc.

$$\text{gr I} = 60 \text{ mg}$$

$$\text{gr} = \frac{3}{4} = \frac{3}{4} \times 60 = \frac{3 \times 60}{4} = 45 \text{ mg}$$

Therefore, order: Codeine gr $\frac{3}{4}$ = 45 mg

Then calculate:

$$\frac{D}{H} \times Q = \frac{45}{30} \times 1 \text{ tablet} = \frac{3}{2} \text{ tablets}$$

$$= 1\frac{1}{2} \text{ tablets}$$

Therefore, $1\frac{1}{2}$ tablets are to be given every 4 hours as needed for pain.

■ Example 7:

The order is: *Synthroid 0.05 mg p.o. q.d.*

The tablets available are 25 mcg. How many tablets will you give?

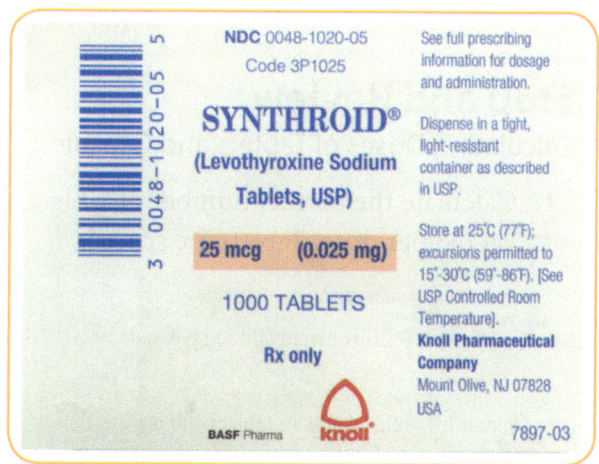

Synthroid 25 mcg.
Courtesy of Abbott Laboratories, 2002

1 mg = 1000 mcg. Conversion factor is 1000.

$$0.05 \text{ mg} = 0.05 \times 1000 = 0.050 = 50 \text{ mcg}$$

Ordered: *Synthroid 0.05 mg = 50 mcg*

On hand: *Synthroid 25 mcg tablets*

$$\frac{D}{H} \times Q = \frac{50 \text{ mcg}}{25 \text{ mcg}} \times 1 \text{ tablet} = 2 \text{ tablets, given orally once a day}$$

■ Example 8:

A patient uses codeine gr ii orally. The label on the available codeine bottle tells you that each tablet provides 30 mg. How much will you give the patient?

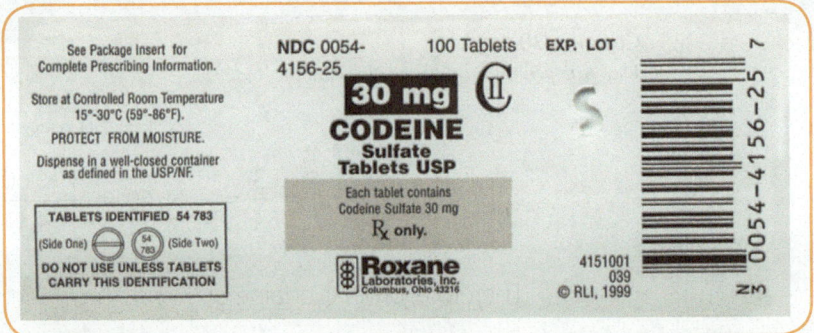

Codeine 30 mg.
Used with permission of Roxane Laboratories, Inc.

Approximate equivalent gr 1 = 60 mg. The conversion factor is 60.

$$\text{gr}\frac{1}{60} \times 60 = \frac{60}{60} = 1 \text{ mg}$$

Ordered: Codeine gr ii orally p.r.n., pain

On hand: Codeine 30 mg tablet

Calculate how much you will give as needed for pain:

$$\frac{D}{H} \times Q = \frac{120 \text{ mg}}{30 \text{ mg}} = 4 \text{ tablets}$$

 ## Stop and Review
Calculating Doses of Tablets and Capsules.

1. Calculate the correct number of tablets or **capsules** to be administered per dose. Tablets are scored.

a. Ordered:	Telithromycin 800 mg p.o. q.d.
On hand:	Telithromycin tablets 400 mg
Give:	_____

b. Ordered:	Pravachol 20 mg p.o. q.h.s.
On hand:	Pravachol 10 mg tablets
Give:	_____
c. Ordered:	Ferrous sulfate 300 mg p.o. q.d.
On hand:	Ferrous sulfate tablets 5 gr (324 mg)
Give:	_____
d. Ordered:	Codeine 60 mg p.o.; q3h p.r.n.
On hand:	Codeine tablets 15 mg ($\frac{1}{4}$ gr)
Give:	_____
e. Ordered:	Nitroglycerin $\frac{1}{150}$ gr S.L. p.r.n.
On hand:	Nitrostat tablets 0.4 mg ($\frac{1}{150}$ gr)
Give:	_____
f. Ordered:	Quinidine 0.6 g p.o. q4h
On hand:	Quinidine 200 mg tablets
Give:	_____
g. Ordered:	Prednisone 7.5 mg p.o. q.d.
On hand:	Prednisone 5 mg scored tablets
Give:	_____
h. Ordered:	Aldomet 250 mg p.o. b.i.d.
On hand:	Aldomet 125 mg tablets
Give:	_____

i. Ordered:	Duricef 0.5 g p.o. b.i.d.	
On hand:	Duricef 500 mg tablets	
Give:	_____	
j. Ordered:	Coumadin 5 mg p.o. q.d.	
On hand:	Coumadin 2 mg scored tablets	
Give:	_____	

2. Calculate one dose for each of the medication orders in questions a through i. The labels lettered A through I are the drugs you have available. Indicate the letter corresponding to the label you select.

a. Order:	*verapamil sustained release 240 mg p.o. q.d.*	
Select:	_____	
Give:	_____	
b. Order:	*carbamazepine 0.2 g p.o. t.i.d.*	
Select:	_____	
Give:	_____	
c. Order:	*Lopressor 50 mg p.o. b.i.d.*	
Select:	_____	
Give:	_____	
d. Order:	*potassium chloride 16 mEq p.o. q.d.*	
Select:	_____	
Give:	_____	

e. Order:	procainamide hydrochloride 1 g p.o. q6h
Select:	_____
Give:	_____
f. Order:	cephalexin 0.5 g p.o. q.i.d.
Select:	_____
Give:	_____
g. Order:	levothyroxine sodium 0.2 mg p.o. q.d.
Select:	_____
Give:	_____
h. Order:	digoxin 0.5 mg p.o. q.d.
Select:	_____
Give:	_____
i. Order:	allopurinol 0.1 g p.o. t.i.d.
Select:	_____
Give:	_____
j. Order:	procainamide hydrochloride 1000 mg q6h
Select:	_____
Give:	_____

Part 4 • Medication Preparation

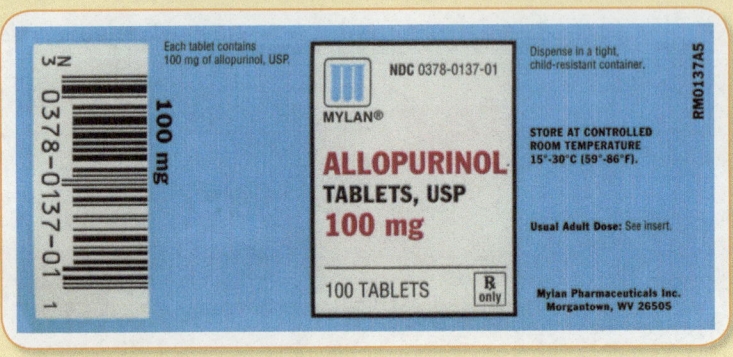

Label A

Allopurinol 100 mg.
Courtesy of Mylan Pharmaceuticals Inc.

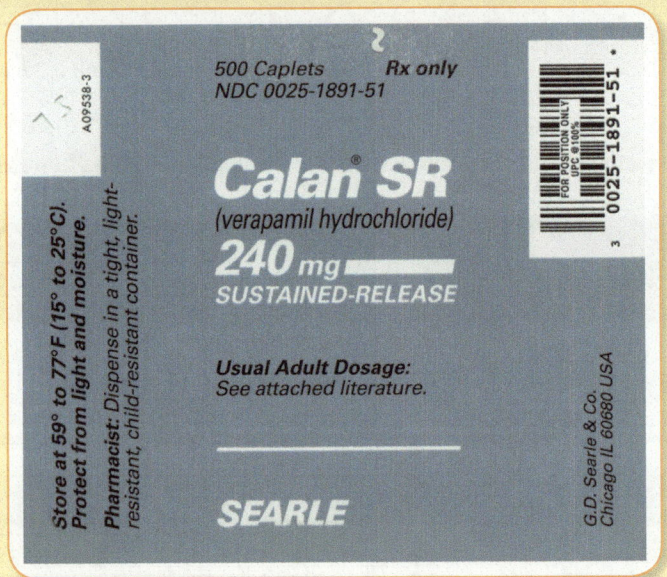

Label B

Calan SR 240 mg.
Courtesy of Pharmacia Corporation, Peapack, NJ

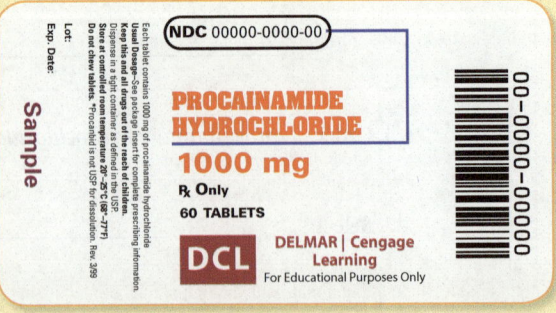

Label C

Procainamide hydrochloride 1000 mg.
© *Cengage Learning 2013*

Chapter 11 • Oral Medication Labels and Dosage Calculation

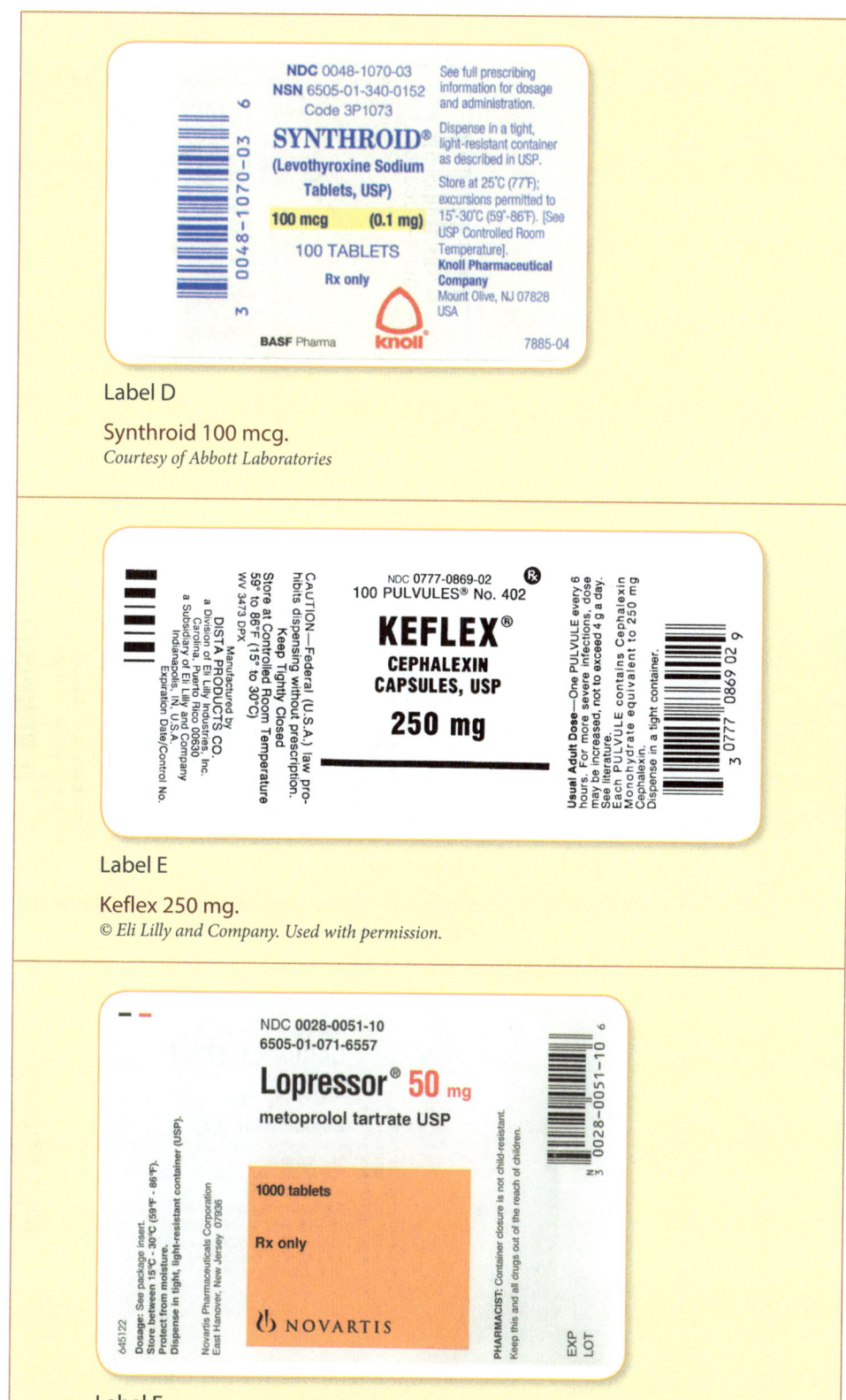

Label D

Synthroid 100 mcg.
Courtesy of Abbott Laboratories

Label E

Keflex 250 mg.
© *Eli Lilly and Company. Used with permission.*

Label F

Lopressor 50 mg.
Courtesy of Novartis

Label G

Digoxin 250 mcg.
© Cengage Learning 2013

Label H

Potassium Chloride extended release tablets USP, 100 tablets.
© Cengage Learning 2013

Label I

Carbamazepine USP 100 mg, chewable tablets.
© Cengage Learning 2013

Oral Solution Labels

Oral solutions are liquids usually ordered for children, elderly people, or patients who are not able to swallow tablets or capsules. Each oral solution contains a specific amount of medication in a given volume as written on the label (**Figures 11-3a** through **c**).

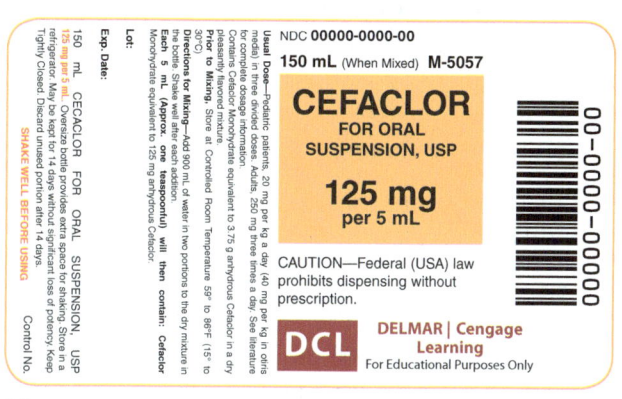

(a)

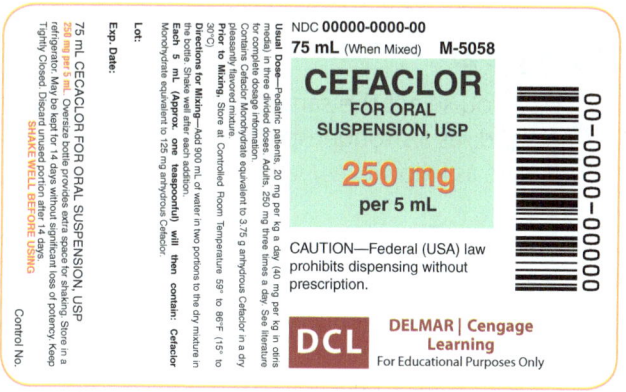

(b)

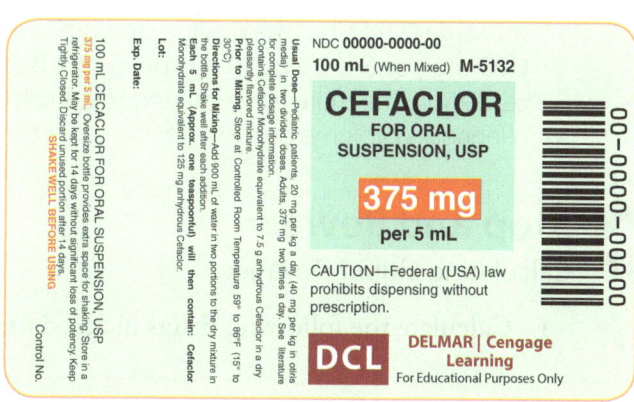

(c)

Figure 12-3 (a) Cefaclor 125 mg, (b) Cefaclor 250 mg, (c) Cefaclor 375 mg.
(a), (b), and (c) © Cengage Learning 2013

Measurement of Oral Solutions

When in solid form, the drugs can be calculated by the number of tablets or capsules that contain the prescribed dosage. When in liquid form, the volume of the liquid that contains the prescribed dosage of the drug must be calculated by the pharmacy technician. The supply strength is written on the label, indicating the amount of drug per 1 mL of solution; example amounts are as follows: 125 mg per 5 mL, 250 mg per 5 mL, 375 mg per 5 mL.

■ Example 1:

The prescriber orders *Cefaclor 100 mg p.o. q.i.d.*

To calculate this prescription, look at the label of Ceclor available in Figure 11-3a.

$$\frac{D}{H} \times Q = X$$

$$\frac{100 \text{ mg}}{125 \text{ mg}} \times 5 \text{ mL} = \frac{4}{5} \times 5 \text{ mL} = \frac{20}{5} = 4 \text{ mL}$$

given orally 4 times a day

■ Example 2:

If you select the same drug order as in Example 1, Cefaclor 100 mg p.o. q.i.d., as a stronger solution (Cefaclor 250 mg per 5 mL), you must calculate as follows:

$$\frac{D}{H} \times Q = \frac{100 \text{ mg}}{250 \text{ mg}} \times 5 \text{ mL}$$

$$\frac{2}{5} \times 5 \text{ mL} = 2 \text{ mL}$$

given orally 4 times a day

You realize that in both Example 1 and Example 2, the supply quantity is the same (5 mL), but the dosage strength (weight) of the drug is different (125 mg per 5 mL vs. 250 mg per 5 mL) because of each liquid's concentration. The more concentrated solution must be given to the patient, offering less volume per dose for the same dosage.

Stop and Review
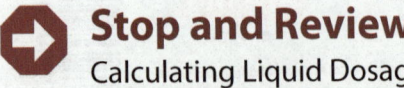
Calculating Liquid Dosages

1. Calculate the following drugs ordered for one dose.

a. Ordered:	Zovirax susp 400 mg p.o. b.i.d.
On hand:	Zovirax 200 mg/5 mL suspension 10 mL
Give:	_____ mL

b. Ordered:	Artane 3 mg p.o. t.i.d. a.c.	
On hand:	Artane Elixir 2 mg/5 mL	
Give:	_____ mL	
c. Ordered:	Depakene syrup 125 mg p.o. q12h	
On hand:	Depakene syrup 250 mg/5 mL	
Give:	_____ mL	
d. Ordered:	Amoxil 100 mg p.o. q.i.d.	
On hand:	80 mL bottle suspension (125 mg per 5 mL)	
Give:	_____ mL	
e. Ordered:	Zofran 8 mg p.o. b.i.d.	
On hand:	Zofran liquid 4 mg/5 mL	
Give:	_____ mL	
f. Ordered:	Compazine syr 10 mg p.o. t.i.d.	
On hand:	Compazine syrup 5 mg/5 mL	
Give:	_____ mL	
g. Ordered:	erythromycin suspension 600 mg p.o. q6h	
On hand:	erythromycin 400 mg/5 mL	
Give:	_____ mL	

h. Ordered:	Ceclor suspension 225 mg p.o. b.i.d.
On hand:	Ceclor suspension 375 mg per 5 mL
Give:	_____ mL
i. Ordered:	Dilantin-125 150 mg p.o. b.i.d.
On hand:	Dilantin-125 suspension 125 mg/5 mL
Give:	_____ mL
j. Ordered:	digoxin elixir 0.25 mg p.o. q.d.
On hand:	digoxin elixir 50 mcg/mL
Give:	_____ mL
k. Ordered:	Pepcid 20 mg p.o. q.i.d.
On hand:	Pepcid 80 mg/10 mL
Give:	_____ mL
l. Ordered:	Grifulvin V 500 mg p.o. b.i.d.
On hand:	Grifulvin V suspension 125 mg/5 mL
Give:	_____ mL
m. Ordered:	Mycostatin 250,000 units p.o. q.i.d.
On hand:	Mycostatin 100,000 units per mL
Give:	_____ mL
n. Ordered:	dicloxacillin: 100 mg q.i.d.
On hand:	dicloxacillin 62.5 mg per 5 mL
Give:	_____ mL

o. Ordered:	Augmentin 0.5 g, p.o. t.i.d.	
On hand:	Augmentin 250 mg/5 mL	
Give:	_____ mL	
p. Ordered:	Vistaril 10 mg p.o. q.i.d.	
On hand:	25 mg/5 mL	
Give:	_____ mg	

Vistaril 25 mg/5 mL.
Label reproduced with permission of Pfizer Inc.

q. Ordered:	Cephalexin 50 mg p.o. q.i.d.	
On hand:	125 mg/5 mL	
Give:	_____ mg	

Cephalexin 125 mg.
© Cengage Learning 2013

r. Ordered:	Digoxin elixir 0.25 mg p.o. q.d.
On hand:	0.05 mg/mL
Give:	_____ mL

Digoxin 50 mcg.
© Cengage Learning 2013

s. Ordered:	OxyFast (oral solution concentrate) 15 mg p.o. q.i.d. p.r.n.
On hand:	20 mg/mL
Give:	_____ mL

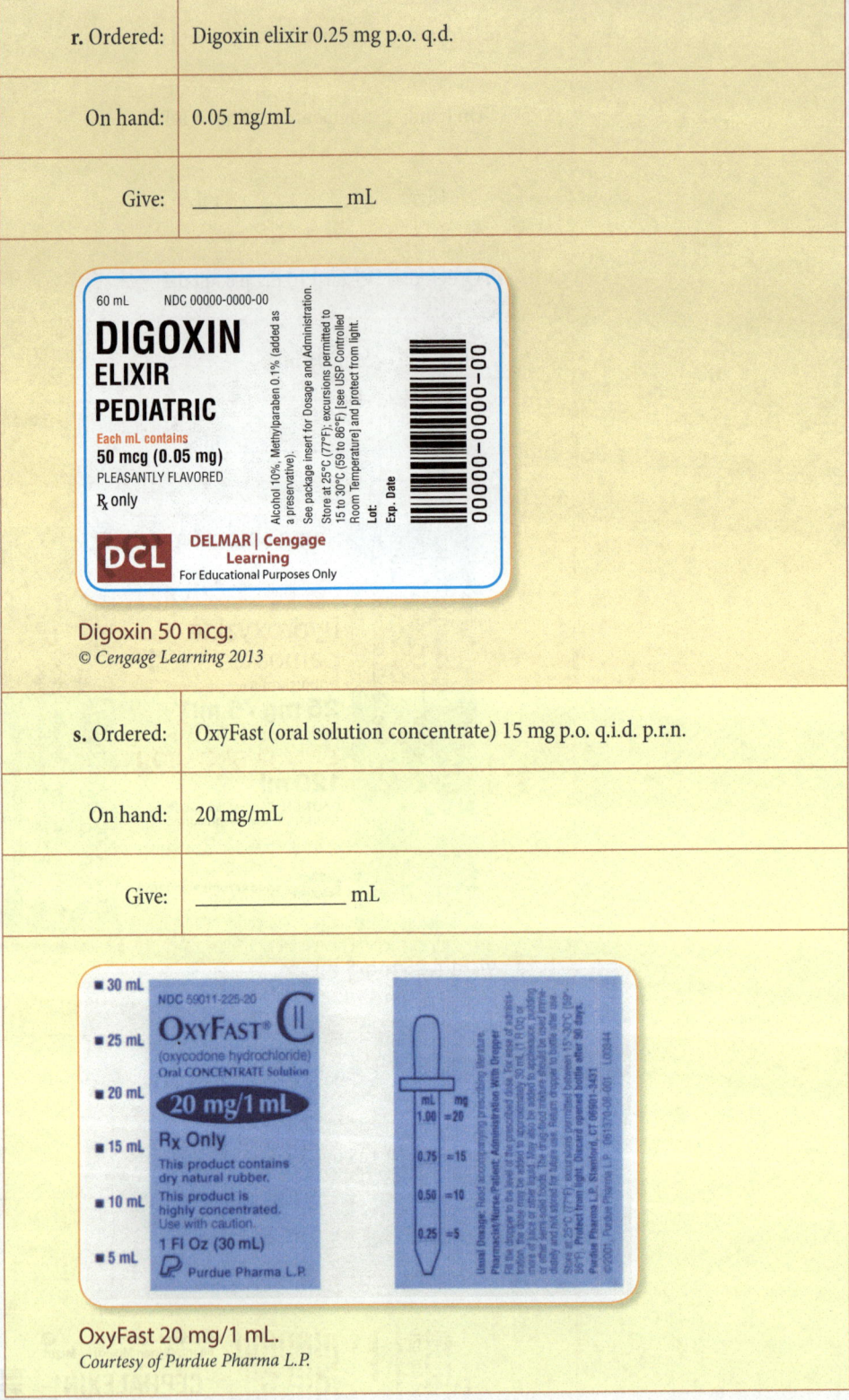

OxyFast 20 mg/1 mL.
Courtesy of Purdue Pharma L.P.

t. Ordered:	Valproic acid 0.5 g p.o. t.i.d.
On hand:	250 mg/5 mL
Give:	_____ mL

Valproic acid syrup, USP 250 mg per 5 mL.
© Cengage Learning 2013

u. Ordered:	Biaxin 75 mg p.o. b.i.d.
On hand:	125 mg/5 mL
Give:	_____

Biaxin granules 125 mg per 5 mL.
Courtesy of Abbott Laboratories

Test Your Knowledge

Calculating oral medication dosages.

1. Ordered: calcium carbonate 1.5 grams P.O. t.i.d.
   On hand: calcium carbonate labeled "750 mg capsules"
   Give: _____

2. Ordered: allopurinol 0.6 gram P.O. every day
   On hand: allopurinol 300 mg tablets
   Give: _____

3. Ordered: anastrozole 1000 mcg P.O. once daily
   On hand: anastrozole 1 mg tablets
   Give: _____

4. Ordered: levothyroxine sodium 0.15 mg by mouth each morning
   On hand: levothyroxine sodium 150 mcg tablets
   Give: _____

5. Ordered: acetaminophen 160 mg P.O. b.i.d.
   On hand: acetaminophen 325 mg tablets
   Give: _____

6. Ordered: cefaclor 0.5 gram P.O. t.i.d.
   On hand: cefaclor 250 mg capsules
   Give: _____

7. Ordered: oxcarbazepine 600 mg b.i.d.
   On hand: oxcarbazepine 150 mg tablets
   Give: _____

8. Ordered: busulfan 8000 mcg per day as a single oral dose
   On hand: busulfan 2 mg tablets
   Give: _____

9. Ordered: zidovudine 0.1 gram every 4 hours
   On hand: zidovudine 100 mg capsules
   Give: _____

10. Ordered: OxyContin $\frac{1}{3}$ grain P.O., b.i.d. for 7 days
    On hand: OxyContin 20 mg tablets
    Give: _____

11. Ordered: zafirlukast 0.020 gram P.O. b.i.d.
    On hand: zafirlukast 10 mg tablets
    Give: _____

12. Ordered: codeine sulfate 1 grain P.O. q.i.d., p.r.n.
    On hand: codeine sulfate 30 mg tablets
    Give: _____

13. Ordered: clonidine hydrochloride 200 mcg
    On hand: clonidine hydrochloride 0.2 mg extended-release tablets
    Give: _____

14. Ordered: clonazepam 0.25 mg P.O. every morning
    On hand: clonazepam 125 mcg tablets
    Give: _____

15. Ordered: triamcinolone hexacetonide 0.004 gram P.O. t.i.d.
    On hand: triamcinolone hexacetonide 2 mg tablets
    Give: _____ per dose

16. Ordered: clorazepate dipotassium 7.5 mg P.O. b.i.d.
    On hand: clorazepate dipotassium 3.75 mg tablets
    Give: _____

17. Ordered: pyridoxine 0.2 gram P.O. every day
    On hand: pyridoxine 50 mg tablets
    Give: _____ per dose

18. Ordered: naproxen sodium 0.75 gram P.O. every day
    On hand: naproxen sodium 375 mg tablets
    Give: _____

19. Ordered: propylthiouracil 200 mg P.O. q.i.d.
    On hand: propylthiouracil 50 mg tablets
    Give: _____

20. Ordered: nitroglycerin sublingual 300 mcg at first sign of chest pain
    On hand: sublingual nitroglycerin 0.3 mg tablets
    Give: _____

21. Ordered: gatifloxacin 400 mg P.O. daily for 5 days
    On hand: gatifloxacin oral suspension with a concentration of 200 mg/5 mL
    Give: _____

22. Ordered: haloperidol 3 mg P.O. at bedtime
    On hand: haloperidol oral concentrate 2 mg/mL
    Give: _____ at bedtime

23. Ordered: oxycodone elixir 5 mg every 4 hours for pain
    On hand: oxycodone elixir concentration of 5 mg/5 mL
    Give: _____

24. Ordered: furosemide 100 mg P.O.
    On hand: furosemide oral solution 40 mg/5 mL
    Give: _____

25. Ordered: guaifenesin oral liquid 300 mg every 4 hours
    On hand: guaifenesin oral liquid concentration 200 mg/5 mL
    Give: _____

26. Ordered: ibuprofen oral suspension 75 mg P.O., q.i.d. for fever
    On hand: ibuprofen oral suspension concentration 50 mg/1.25 mL
    Give: _____

27. Ordered: haloperidol 0.5 mg P.O. b.i.d.
    On hand: haloperidol oral solution 2 mg/2 mL
    Give: _____

28. Ordered: isoniazid 300 mg P.O. once daily
    On hand: isoniazid syrup 50 mg/5 mL
    Give: _____ per dose

29. Ordered: lansoprazole 15 mg P.O. solution daily
    On hand: lansoprazole 2.5 mg/mL oral solution
    Give: _____

30. Ordered: memantine 5 mg P.O. per day
    On hand: memantine 2 mg/2 mL oral solution
    Give: _____

31. Ordered: vancomycin 0.125 gram P.O. q.i.d.
    On hand: vancomycin 250 mg/5 mL of oral solution
    Give: _____

32. Ordered: methadone 2.5 mg P.O. every 3–4 hours p.r.n.
    On hand: methadone 5 mg/5 mL
    Give: _____

33. Ordered: mycophenolate mofetil 1 gram P.O., b.i.d.
    On hand: mycophenolate mofetil oral suspension concentration 200 mg/mL
    Give: _____

34. Ordered: tetracycline 500 mg P.O., q.i.d.
    On hand: tetracycline syrup 125 mg/5 mL
    Give: _____

35. Ordered: amoxicillin 275 mg P.O.
    On hand: amoxicillin suspension 250 mg/5 mL
    Give: _____

36. Ordered: azithromycin 300 mg P.O. for 5 days
    On hand: azithromycin 450 mg in 5 mL
    Give: _____

37. Ordered: amprenavir 1350 mg P.O., b.i.d.
    On hand: amprenavir oral liquid 15 mg/mL
    Give: _____ per dose

38. Ordered: amoxicillin/clavulanate potassium 100 mg P.O. b.i.d.

    On hand: amoxicillin/clavulanate potassium 150 mg in a 5 mL suspension

    Give: _____

39. Ordered: cetirizine 2.5 mg daily

    On hand: cetirizine syrup containing 1 mg/mL

    Give: _____

40. Ordered: clindamycin 300 mg P.O., q.i.d.

    On hand: clindamycin 75 mg/5 mL oral solution

    Give: _____

Critical Thinking

1. The physician ordered Inderal 120 mg P.O. q.d. for 10 days. The pharmacy technician dispensed sixty 20 mg tablets. The nurse mistook "q.d." for "q.i.d." and then calculated the dosage for a 24-hour period as follows:

$$\frac{\text{Desired}}{\text{Have}} \times \text{Quantity} = \text{Amount}$$

So,

$$\frac{120 \text{ mg}}{20 \text{ mg}} \times 4 = 24 \text{ tablets (incorrect)}$$

If the nurse gave the patient 24 tablets of 20 mg per tablet Inderal, how many milligrams will the patient receive over a 24-hour period? Is it the correct dosage?

_____

_____

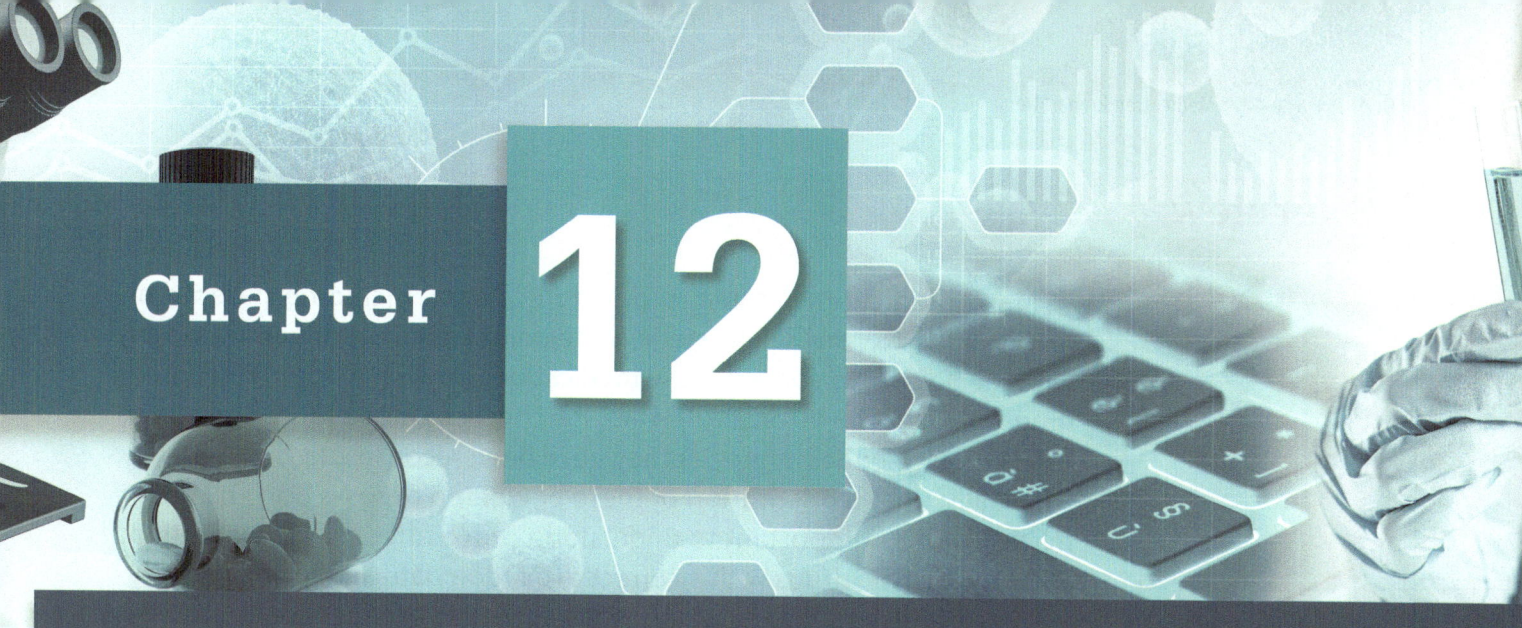

Chapter 12

Reconstitution of Powdered Drugs

Outline

Overview
Reconstitution of a Single-Strength Solution
Reconstitution of Multiple-Strength Solutions

Objectives

Upon completion of this chapter, you should be able to:

1. Interpret the information provided on powdered drug labels and package inserts.
2. Calculate the volume of reconstituted medication that is required when the medication is supplied in powdered form.
3. Determine whether an in-stock vial contains enough medication to fill an order.
4. Demonstrate reconstitution of single- and multiple-strength solutions.
5. Calculate amounts of solutes and solvents needed to prepare various strengths and quantities.
6. Demonstrate reconstitution by following package insert directions.
7. Reconstitute and label medications supplied in powdered or dry form.

Key Terms

diluent
reconstitution
solute
solution

Overview

Many medications come in powdered form, including parenteral medications. Normal saline, sterile water, or some other **diluent** is mixed with the powder to convert these medications into liquid form. Powdered drugs that must be reconstituted are used because in this form they retain their potency longer than after they have been reconstituted.

Usually, the **reconstitution** of these powdered drugs is done by pharmacies, but it is important to understand procedures for reconstitution and how to label drugs with a correct expiration date and time once they are reconstituted. Drug labels and instructional package inserts provide this specific information. You must understand the properties of various types of solutions.

Reconstitution of a Single-Strength Solution

Using the label shown in **Figure 12-1**, notice that the directions for reconstituting this single-strength **solution** are on the left side of the label. A **solute** is the substance dissolved in a solvent to form a solution.

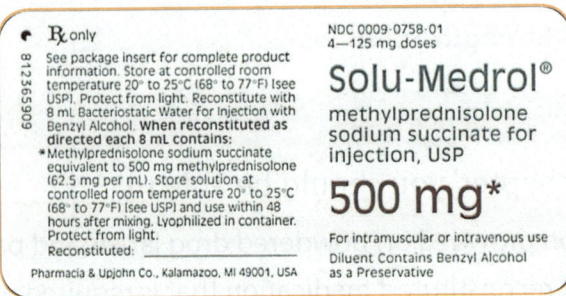

Figure 12-1 Solu-Medrol 500 mg.
Used with permission from Pharmacia Corporation, Peapack, NJ.

>>> **Remember**

After *reconstitution*, it is important to understand how long the reconstituted solution may be stored and the correct storage conditions.

An order is given to "Reconstitute with 8 mL Bacteriostatic Water for injection with Benzyl Alcohol." In this example, the *diluent* is the bacteriostatic water. In **Figure 12-1**, notice that the reconstituted medication can be stored at room temperature, but it must be used within 48 hours after reconstitution.

Once you have reconstituted a medication, print your initials on the label to identify yourself as the person who reconstituted the drug. Add the expiration date and time to the label.

The total vial strength is 500 mg. The individual dose strength is four 125 mg doses. Because 8 mL of diluent has been injected, this is approximately 2 mL for each 125 mg dose. However, as you should in every instance,

> **Remember**
>
> Most reconstituted volumes are not exactly equal to the amount of diluent added. The medication itself has a certain volume, so combined, the final volume could be larger than the amount of diluent injected.

check the small print on the label. It says that the strength of the diluted solution is 62.5 mg per mL. Therefore, if 62.5 mg are ordered, you need 1 mL. If 125 mg are ordered, you must have 2 mL. If 250 mg are ordered, you must have 4 mL. If 500 mg are ordered, you must have 8 mL.

■ Example 1:

A physician orders 400 mg of Zithromax IV. The vial in stock lists the following instructions: "Reconstitute to 100 mg/mL with 4.8 mL of Sterile Water for Injection." The single-dose vial contains 500 mg. What volume must be given?

Apply the dosage formula, based on the following:

Desired dose (D) is 400 mg

On-hand amount (H) is 100 mg

Vehicle (V) is 1 mL

Therefore,

$$\frac{D}{H} \times V = A$$

So,

$$\frac{400 \text{ mg}}{100 \text{ mg}} \times 1 \text{ mL} = 4 \times 1 \text{ mL} = 4 \text{ mL}$$

Apply proportions by substituting given values into the formula $D/A = H/V$:

$$\frac{400 \text{ mg}}{A} = \frac{100 \text{ mg}}{1 \text{ mL}}$$

Cross-multiply, which gives:

$$A \times 100 \text{ mg} = (400 \text{ mg})(1 \text{ mL})$$

Divide by 100, which gives:

$$A = \frac{(400)(1 \text{ mL})}{100} = \frac{400 \text{ mL}}{100} = 4 \text{ mL}$$

Apply dimensional analysis to determine the quantity in milliliters:

$$\frac{100 \text{ mg}}{\text{mL}} \text{ as } \frac{1 \text{ mL}}{100 \text{ mg}}$$

Therefore,

$$400 \, (1 \text{ mL}/100) = \frac{400 \text{ mL}}{100} = 4 \text{ mL}$$

Therefore, add 4.8 mL sterile water to the vial contents and mix. Draw 4 mL of the reconstituted solution into a syringe for IV administration.

The vial contains 500 mg and the order is for 400 mg, so there is enough for a full dose. Notice, however, that there is not enough for a second dose.

■ Example 2:

An order is placed for 125,000 units penicillin for IM injection. If a vial on hand contains 50,000 units/mL penicillin, how many mL should be administered? Again, you can apply the dosage formula, apply proportions, or apply dimensional analysis to solve this example. Regardless of the method used, we find that:

$$\frac{125,000 \text{ units} \times 1 \text{ mL}}{50,000 \text{ units}} = \frac{125,000 \text{ mL}}{50,000} = 2.5 \text{ mL}$$

Therefore, from 3 single vials, you must draw 2.5 mL into a syringe for IM administration. Because one vial contains 50,000 units and the order is for 125,000 units, a total of 3 vials are needed. Notice that only ½ of the third vial will be used.

■ Example 3:

An order is placed for 250 mg of a medication for IM injection. On hand is a vial that contains 1 g of the powdered medication. The directions on the vial note that 2.5 mL diluent should be added, resulting in a concentration of 300 mg/mL. What volume should be administered? (Because the order is in mg, you must first convert 1 g to milligrams.) Regardless of the method of calculation, we find that:

$$\frac{250 \text{ mg}}{300 \text{ mg}} \times 1 \text{ mL} = 0.83 \times 1 \text{ mL} = 0.8 \text{ mL}$$

Therefore, you must add 2.5 mL diluent to the vial contents and mix. Draw 0.8 mL of the reconstituted solution into a 1 mL syringe for IM administration.

■ Example 4:

An order is placed for 2,000,000 units penicillin for IM injection. On hand is a vial containing 5,000,000 units penicillin. The vial instructions list the following:

- The concentration will be 250,000 units/mL if 18.2 mL diluent is added.
- The concentration will be 500,000 units/mL if 8.2 mL diluent is added.
- The concentration will be 1,000,000 units/mL if 3.2 mL diluent is added.

Because 3 mL is the maximum volume an adult should receive as an IM injection in a large muscle, which of the three sets of directions should be used for this order? Use the D/H × V formula.

- We will need 8 mL if 18.2 mL is added.
- We will need 4 mL if 8.2 mL is added.
- We will need 2 mL if 3.2 mL is added (the preferred dilution direction).

Because a 2 mL syringe is less than a 3 mL syringe, 2 mL is the syringe size that should be chosen. (However, a 3 mL syringe is often chosen because this size is more readily available.) Measure 2 mL of penicillin reconstituted to 1,000,000 units per milliliter for IM administration.

Stop and Review
Reconstitution of a Single-Strength Solution
LABEL 1:

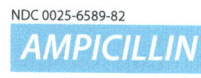

Ampicillin.
© Cengage Learning 2013

Using the ampicillin label, answer the following questions.

1. What types of diluent may be used for reconstitution?
   _____

2. What volume of diluent is specified for a 250 mg vial?
   _____

3. How much diluent is needed for a 500 mg vial?
   _____

4. How much diluent is needed for a 1 g vial? _____

5. How much diluent is needed for a 2 g vial? _____

6. What is the total volume in mL of all four reconstituted solutions?
   _____

7. How much diluent must be added to the 250 mg vial and to the 500 mg vial? _____

8. List the stipulation for direct IV administration of the 250 mg and 500 mg reconstituted solution. _____

9. Locate the caution pertaining to rapid IV administration. _____

LABEL 2:

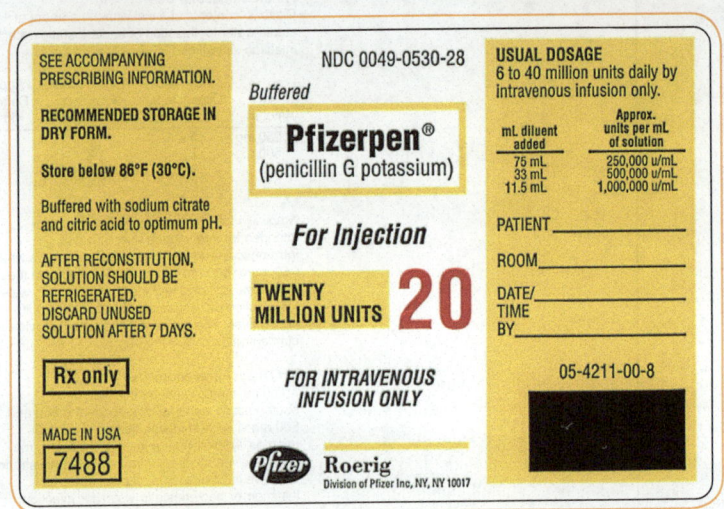

Pfizerpen 20 million units.
Used with permission from Pfizer, Inc.

Using the Pfizerpen label, answer the following questions.

1. If 75 mL of diluent is added, what dosage strength should be printed on the label? _____

2. Does this prepared solution need to be refrigerated? _____

3. If reconstituted at 2 p.m. on June 1, what expiration date and time must be printed on the label? _____

4. What is the vial's total dosage strength? _____

5. Besides the dosage strength, what else must be printed on the label? _____

6. Where can you find information on the diluent that should be used? _____

LABEL 3:

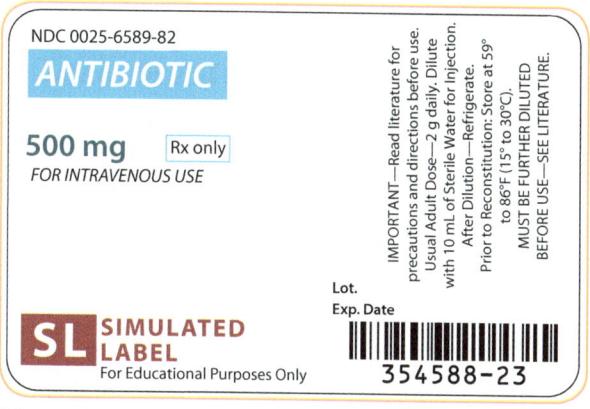

(a)

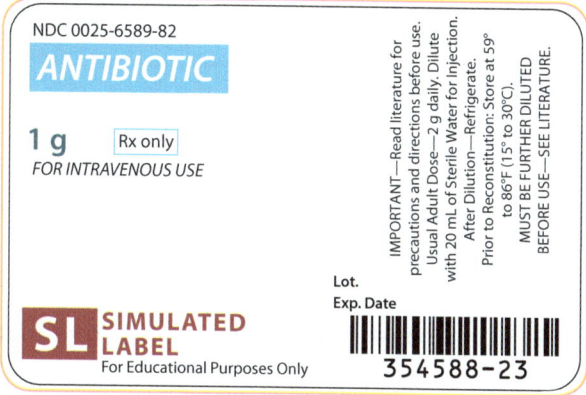

(b)

PREPARATION AND STABILITY
At the time of use, reconstitute by adding either 10 mL of Sterile Water for Injection to the 500-mg vial or 20 mL of Sterile Water for Injection to the 1-g vial of dry, sterile powder. Vials reconstituted in this manner will give a solution of 50 mg/mL. FURTHER DILUTION IS REQUIRED.
After reconstitution, the vials may be stored in a refrigerator for 14 days without significant loss of potency. Reconstituted solutions containing 500 mg must be diluted with at least 100 mL of diluent. Reconstituted solutions containing 1 g must be diluted with at least 200 mL of diluent, The desired dose, diluted in this manner, should be administered by intermittent intravenous infusion over a period of at least 60 minutes.

(c)

(a) Antibiotic 500 mg, (b) Antibiotic 1 g, (c) Preparation and Stability.
(a), (b), and (c) © Cengage Learning 2013

Using the three antibiotic labels, answer the following questions.

1. To reconstitute a 500 mg vial, how much diluent is needed?
   _____

2. For a 1 g vial, how much diluent is needed? _____

3. What kind of diluent is specified? _____

4. For both solutions, what is the reconstituted dosage per mL?
   _____

5. If refrigerated, how long can the solution be used? _____

6. If reconstituted at 1350 hours on May 4, what expiration date and time should be printed on the label? _____

7. What else must be printed on the label? _____

LABEL 4:

Ceftriaxone sodium 1 g.
© Cengage Learning 2013

Using the ceftriaxone sodium label, answer the following questions.

1. What is the vial's total strength? _____

2. For reconstitution, what volume of diluent is needed? _____

3. What is the dosage strength of 1 mL of reconstituted solution? _____

LABEL 5:

Levothyroxine 200 mcg.
Used with permission from Bedford Laboratories, A Division of Ben Venue Laboratories. A Boehringer-Ingelheim Company.

Using the levothyroxine label, answer the following questions.

1. What is this vial's total strength in mcg and mg? _____

2. To prepare the solution for use, what volume of diluent must be added? _____

3. What kind of diluent is required? _____

4. How long will this reconstituted solution be potent?
   _____

5. What is this reconstituted solution's per mL strength?
   _____

6. Where can you find average dosage instructions?
   _____

LABEL 6:

CYTARABINE FOR INJECTION USP
NDC 55390-133-01   LYOPHILIZED
See package insert for complete prescribing information.
Each vial contains cytarabine 1 g and, if necessary, hydrochloric acid and/or sodium hydroxide for pH adjustment.
When reconstituted with 10 mL Bacteriostatic Water for Injection USP with benzyl alcohol, each mL contains 100 mg cytarabine. **Do not use a diluent containing benzyl alcohol for intrathecal and high dose investigational use.**
Store both powder and reconstituted solution at 25°C (77°F); excursions permitted to 15° to 30°C (59° to 86°F) [see USP Controlled Room Temperature].
Use reconstituted solution within 48 hours. Discard solution if a slight haze develops.
FOR INTRAVENOUS, SUBCUTANEOUS, OR INTRATHECAL USE
1 gram
Rx ONLY
Manufactured for: Bedford Laboratories™ Bedford, OH 44146
Manufactured by: Ben Venue Laboratories, Inc. Bedford, OH 44146
CYB-VC05

Cytarabine 1 g.
Used with permission from Bedford Laboratories, A Division of Ben Venue Laboratories. A Boehringer-Ingelheim Company.

Using the Cytarabine label, answer the following questions.

1. How much diluent is needed for reconstitution?
   _____

2. What type of diluent should be used? _____

3. What is the total dosage of this vial? _____

4. What temperature should be used to store this medication?
   _____

5. What dosage will be contained in each mL? _____

6. What is this reconstituted solution's expiration time?
   _____

7. If reconstituted at 0840 hours on Feb. 14, what is the expiration date to be printed on the label? _____

LABEL 7:

Vfend® I.V. 200 mg.
Used with permission from Pfizer, Inc.

Using the Vfend IV label, answer the following questions.

1. How much diluent is required for reconstitution? _____

2. What diluent must be used? _____

3. What is the strength of each mL of the reconstituted solution? _____

4. What is this vial's total strength? _____

LABEL 8:

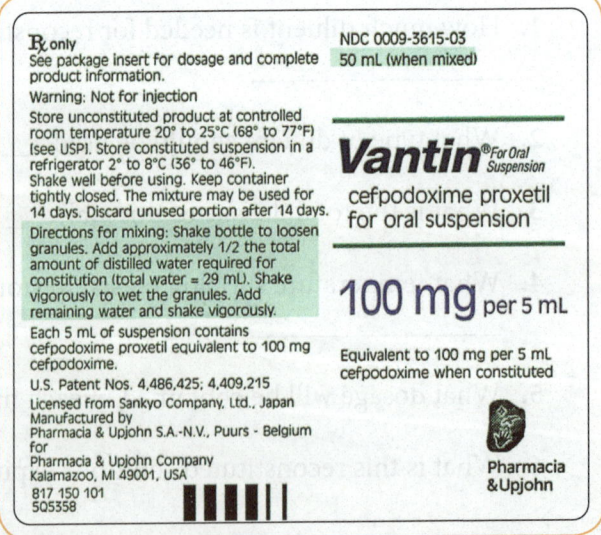

Vantin 100 mg per 5 mL.
Used with permission from Pharmacia Corporation, Peapack, NJ.

Using the Vantin label, answer the following questions.

1. To reconstitute this medication, how much diluent is required? _____

2. What type of diluent must be used? _____

3. How must the diluent be added? _____

4. What is the reconstituted suspension strength?
_____

5. How long will the reconstituted medication be potent?
_____

LABEL 9:

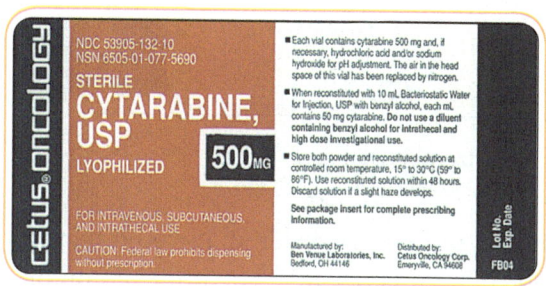

Cytarabine 500 mg.
Used with permission from Bedford Laboratories, A Division of Ben Venue Laboratories. A Boehringer-Ingelheim Company.

Using the Cytarabine label, answer the following questions.

1. What is this medication's total strength? _____

2. What diluent is needed for reconstitution? _____

3. How much diluent is needed? _____

4. What is the strength per mL after reconstitution?
_____

5. How long does this reconstituted medication remain potent at room temperature? _____

Drug package inserts contain much more information than do labels, including specific uses for diagnosed conditions, dosage recommendations if the vial label does not contain them, and information about untoward or adverse reactions. While no standard way is used to feature all of this information, it is included somewhere in the package insert and must be located and studied carefully.

Reconstitution of Multiple-Strength Solutions

Because some powdered drugs can be diluted to different solution strengths, you must understand how to choose the most appropriate strength for the dosage ordered. In **Figure 12-2**, the penicillin label shows the solution strengths on the right side. Three different strengths are listed: 250,000 units per mL; 500,000 units per mL; and 1,000,000 units per mL.

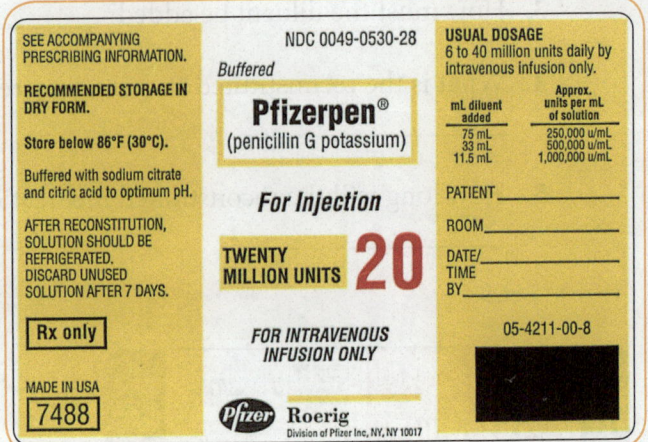

Figure 12-2 Pfizerpen 20 million units.
Used with permission from Pfizer, Inc.

> **Remember**
>
> After reconstituting a multiple-strength solution, to prevent dosing errors, you must include the strength you have just reconstituted to the label.

If 500,000 units were ordered, it would be most appropriate to reconstitute to 500,000 units per mL. The information on the label indicates that to achieve this, you should add 33 mL of diluent.

Test Your Knowledge

LABEL 1:

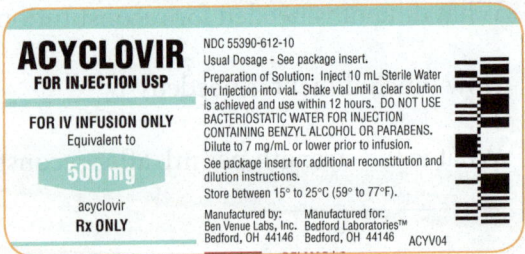

Acyclovir 500 mg.
Used with permission from Bedford Laboratories, A Division of Ben Venue Laboratories. A Boehringer-Ingelheim Company.

Based on the Acyclovir label, answer the following questions.

1. For reconstitution, what type of diluent is needed? _____
2. How much diluent is needed? _____
3. What is this vial's total strength? _____
4. How soon must this medication be used? _____

LABEL 2:

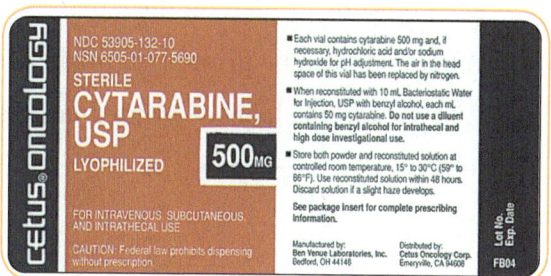

Cytarabine 500 mg.
Used with permission from Bedford Laboratories, A Division of Ben Venue Laboratories. A Boehringer-Ingelheim Company.

Using the Cytarabine label, answer the following questions.

1. What is this vial's total dosage strength? _____
2. What volume of diluent is needed? _____
3. What kind of diluent is needed? _____
4. What is the reconstituted dosage strength per mL? _____
5. How long will this medication be potent? _____

LABEL 3:

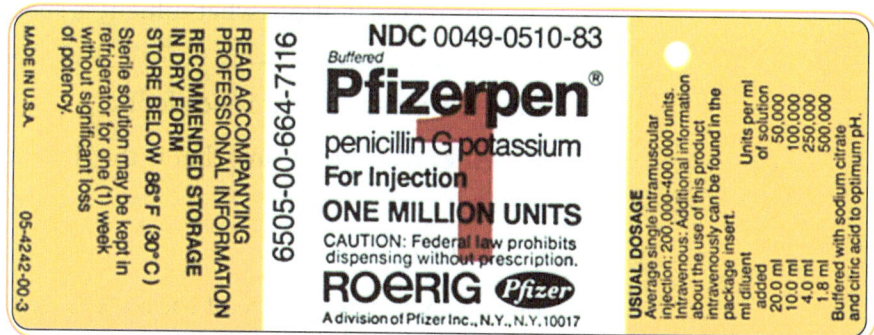

Pfizerpen 1 million units.
Used with permission from Pfizer, Inc.

Using the Pfizerpen label, answer the following questions.

1. What is this vial's total dosage strength? _____
2. To prepare a 100,000 units/mL strength, how much diluent is needed? _____
3. To prepare a 500,000 units/mL strength, how much diluent is needed? _____
4. To prepare a 50,000 units/mL strength, how much diluent is needed? _____
5. Where can the information on the type of diluent for this medication be found? _____
6. How must this medication be stored? _____

7. If this medication is reconstituted at 1:10 a.m. on Dec. 18, what must be printed on the label? _____

8. What else must be printed on the label? _____

9. Why should the label be printed and not handwritten? _____

LABEL 4:

Zithromax 500 mg.
Used with permission from Pfizer, Inc.

Using the Zithromax label, answer the following questions.

1. What is the generic name for Zithromax? _____
2. What is this vial's total strength? _____
3. For reconstitution, what diluent is specified? _____
4. How much diluent is needed? _____
5. After reconstitution, what is the final suspension strength? _____

Critical Thinking

A pharmacy has only three of the 3 g Unasyn® powder-for-injection vials on hand due to a back order. They receive a physician order for 32 mL of Unasyn® injection at a concentration of 375 mg/mL. According to the package insert, they are to dilute every 1.5 g of the powder with 3.2 mL of sterile water.

1. Do they have enough vials on hand to prepare this order? *Note that after dilution, they can withdraw up to 8 mL of Unasyn from each vial.* _____

2. How many vials will they need to fulfill this order? _____

3. If the dose ordered was for 1600 mg of Unasyn® instead, how many milliliters of the diluted solution will be dispensed? _____

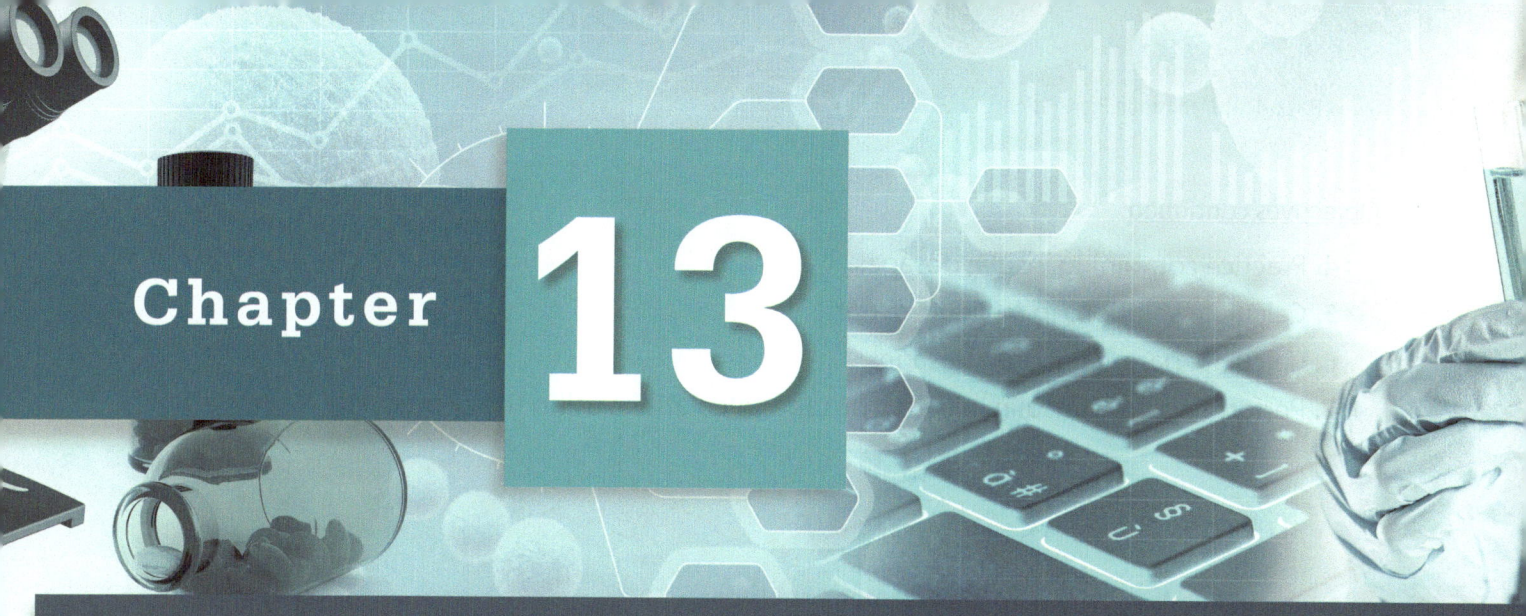

Chapter 13

Parenteral Medication Labels and Dosage Calculation

Outline

Overview
Reading Metric Solution Labels
Percent and Ratio Solution Labels
Solutions Measured in International Units
    Insulin Injections
    Types of Insulin
    Insulin Labels
    Mixing Insulins
    Measuring Insulin in an Insulin Syringe
    Combination Insulin Dosage
Solutions Measured as Milliequivalents
Calculating Parenteral Drug Dosages

Objectives

Upon completion of this chapter, you should be able to:

1. Given a metric solution label, identify information including dosage, brand name, and action time.
2. Given the prescription ordered and on-hand medication, calculate the amount to prepare one dose.
3. Demonstrate how to measure insulin in an insulin syringe.

Objectives continued

4. Practice combining insulin dosages.
5. Calculate solutions in milliequivalents.
6. Calculate parenteral drug dosages.
7. Perform accurate insulin injection dosage calculations using the appropriate-sized syringe.

Key Terms

international units
parenteral
percentage solutions
units

Overview

Parenteral forms of medication are selected when a rapid response time to medication is desired or if the patient is not able to take the medication orally. Injectable drug forms may be available as a solution or a powder. Some vitamins, a few antibiotics, and biologics such as vaccines are expressed in terms of **units**. The U.S. Food & Drug Administration (FDA) approved the measures of potency for these substances, as set forth in the *United States Pharmacopeia (USP)*. They also conform to international standards (**international units**).

Reading Metric Solution Labels

It is important for the pharmacy technician to be able to read and interpret metric solution labels. The most common units of measurement seen on medication labels are metric units, including milligrams, grams, milliliters, and so forth.

■ **Example 1:**

See the label for Vistaril in **Figure 13-1**. Note that the generic name of the drug is hydroxyzine hydrochloride and its trade name is Vistaril. Its dosage strength is 50 mg per mL and the total contents of the vial are 10 mL. Most intramuscular and subcutaneous dosages consist of one-half to double the average dosage strength. For this IM Vistaril, this is 50 mg per mL. Therefore, the following applies:

- For 25 mg, 0.5 mL would be administered.
- For 50 mg, 1 mL would be administered.
- For 75 mg, 1.5 mL would be administered.
- For 100 mg, 2 mL would be administered.

These dosages are within the common 0.5 to 3 mL IM volume.

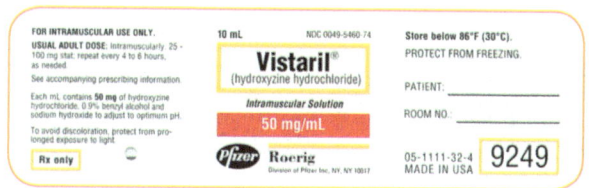

Figure 13-1 Vistaril 50 mg/mL.
Label reproduced with permission of Pfizer, Inc.

■ Example 2:

Figure 13-2 shows a Robinul (glycopyrrolate) label, with a dosage strength of 0.2 mg/mL. Therefore, the following applies:

- If the dosage was 0.1 mg, 0.5 mL would be administered.
- If the dosage was 100 mcg, 0.5 mL would be administered.
- If the dosage was 0.2 mg, 1 mL would be administered.
- If the dosage was 200 mcg, 1 mL would be administered.
- If the dosage was 0.4 mg, 2 mL would be administered.
- If the dosage was 400 mcg, 2 mL would be administered.

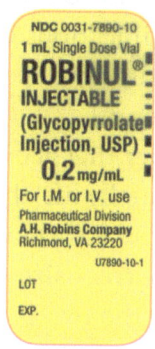

Figure 13-2 Robinul 0.2 mg/mL.
Courtesy of ESI Lederle, Philadelphia, PA.

Percent and Ratio Solution Labels

Percent and ratio solution labels are used for drugs labeled as **percentage solutions**. These solutions often express the dosage strength in metric measures as well as in percentage strength. **Figure 13-3** shows a label for lidocaine that is available as a 2% solution. Notice that below this information is listed 20 mg/mL. Lidocaine hydrochloride is usually ordered in milligrams, but when used as a local anesthetic, it may be used as a percentage strength solution.

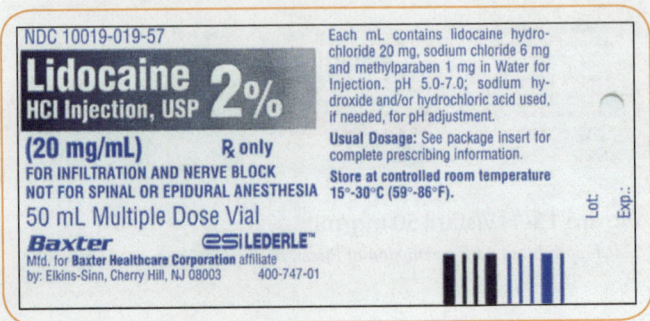

Figure 13-3 Lidocaine 2%.
© Baxter Healthcare Corporation

Solutions Measured in International Units

Many medications are measured in international units, including insulin, penicillin, heparin, and others. These medications are usually expressed in units per milliliter.

Insulin Injections

Insulin is a hormone released from the pancreas. It is essential for glucose, proteins, and fat metabolism. Patients who suffer from insulin-dependent diabetes are required to receive insulin injections each day. Insulin is measured in units and the most frequent supply dosage is 100 units per mL. U-100 is the abbreviation of 100 units per mL.

Pharmacy technicians must remember that accuracy in insulin preparation and administration is critical. Potentially life-threatening situations may result from inaccurate measurement. The information on the insulin label must be correctly interpreted and the correct size syringe must be selected for administration of insulin. These are the two most important factors for the pharmacy technician to understand regarding insulin injections.

Types of Insulin

There are several sources of insulin, which include:

- Human insulin (the most common type)
  - Biosynthetic—bacteria genetically altered to create human insulin
  - Semisynthetic—pork insulin chemically altered to produce human insulin
- Beef insulin—from the pancreas of a cow (no longer commonly used)
- Pork insulin—from the pancreas of a pig (no longer commonly used)
- Beef–pork mixture—a combination of beef and pork insulin (no longer commonly used)

Timing of Action

Insulins are classified by the timing of their action. **Figures 13-4a** through **e** illustrate various insulin labels arranged by the three action times:

- Rapid-acting (regular, lispro)
- Intermediate-acting (NPH, or neutral protamine hagedorn)
- Long-acting (Lantus, Levemir)

The two most common types of insulin used are regular and NPH insulin. You can see the uppercase, bold letters on each insulin label as follows: R for regular insulin; and N for NPH insulin. These letters are important visual identifiers when selecting the insulin type.

Insulin Labels

Insulin labels are identified by the manufacturer, brand and generic names, storage information, supply dosage or concentration, and expiration date (**Figure 13-5**).

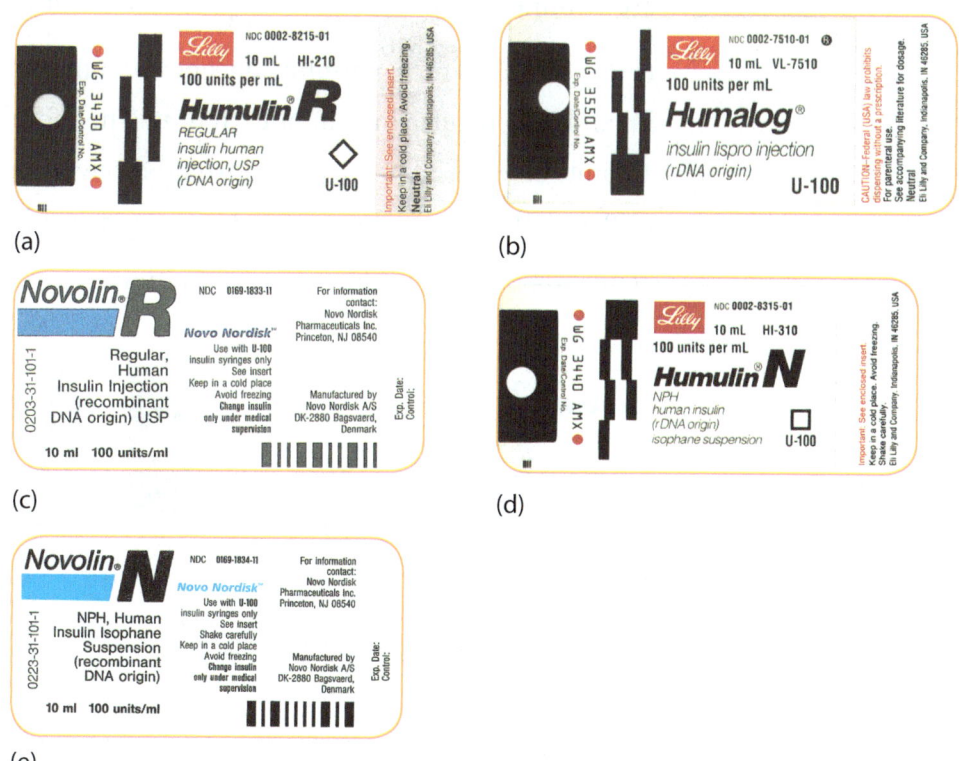

Figure 13-4 (a) Humulin R 10 mL, (b) Humalog 10 mL, (c) Novolin R, (d) Humulin N 10 mL, (e) Novolin N 10 mL.

(a), (b), and (d) Copyright Eli Lilly and Company. Used with permission. (c) and (e) Courtesy of Novo Nordisk Pharmaceuticals, Inc.

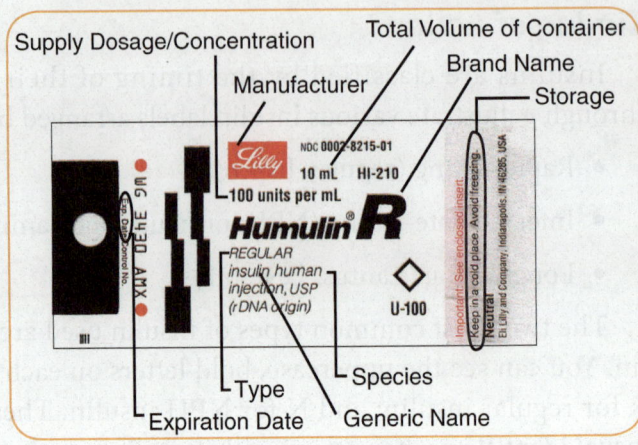

Figure 13-5 Humulin R.
© Eli Lilly and Company. Used with permission

Mixing Insulins

Premixed insulin combinations, including Humalog mixtures, that are commercially available are $\frac{70}{30}$ U-100 insulin and $\frac{50}{50}$ U-100 insulin (**Figure 13-6**). The $\frac{70}{30}$ insulin concentration means there is 70% NPH insulin and 30% regular insulin in each unit. Therefore, if the prescriber orders 10 units of $\frac{70}{30}$ insulin, the patient would receive 7 units of NPH insulin (70% or 0.7 × 10 units = 7 units) and 3 units of regular insulin (30% or 0.3 × 10 units = 3 units) in the $\frac{70}{30}$ concentration.

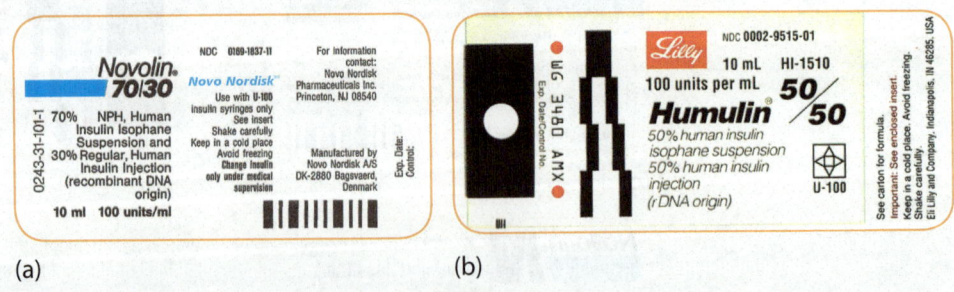

(a) (b)

Figure 13-6 (a) Novolin $\frac{70}{30}$, (b) Humulin $\frac{50}{50}$.
(a) Courtesy of Novo Nordisk Pharmaceuticals, Inc., (b) Copyright Eli Lilly and Company. Used with permission

The $\frac{50}{50}$ insulin concentration means each unit has 50% NPH insulin and 50% regular insulin. Therefore, if the physician orders 16 units of $\frac{50}{50}$ insulin, the patient would receive 8 units of NPH insulin (50% or 0.5 × 12 units = 8 units) and 8 units of regular insulin (50% or 0.5 × 16 units = 8 units).

Measuring Insulin in an Insulin Syringe

Measuring insulin with an insulin syringe is quite simple. The insulin syringe obtains a correct dosage without mathematical calculation. The syringes are the *standard* (100-unit) capacity and the *lo-dose* (50-unit and 30-unit) capacities.

Standard U-100 Insulin Syringe

The standard U-100 insulin syringe is a dual-scale syringe with 100 units/mL capacity. It is calibrated on one side in even-numbered, 2-unit increments (2, 4, 6 . . .) with every 10 units labeled (10, 20, 30 . . .). It is calibrated on the reverse side in odd-numbered, 2-unit increments (1, 3, 5 . . .) with every 10 units labeled (5, 15, 25 . . .). The measurement of 73 units of U-100 insulin is shown in **Figure 13-7**.

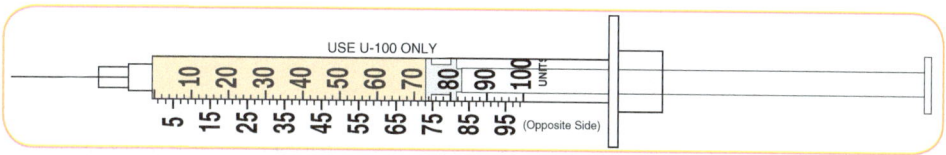

Figure 13-7 Standard U-100 insulin syringe measuring 73 units.
© Cengage Learning 2013

Lo-Dose U-100 Insulin Syringes

The lo-dose U-100 insulin syringe is a single-scale syringe with 50 units/0.5 mL capacity. It is calibrated in 1-unit increments with every 5 units (5, 10, 15 . . .) labeled up to 50 units. The enlarged 50-unit calibration of this syringe makes it easy to read 32 units. To measure 32 units, withdraw 100 units of insulin to the 32-unit mark (**Figure 13-8**).

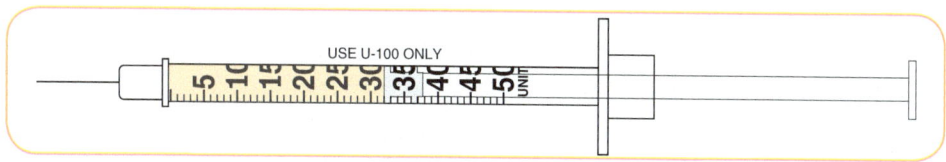

Figure 13-8 50 Unit Lo-Dose U-100 insulin syringe measuring 32 units.
© Cengage Learning 2013

The lo-dose U-100 insulin syringe is another single-scale syringe with 30 units/0.3 mL capacity. It is calibrated in 1-unit increments with every 5 units (5, 10, 15 . . .) labeled up to 30 units. The enlarged 30-unit calibration accurately measures very small amounts of insulin, such as for children. To measure 12 units, withdraw 100 units of insulin to the 12-unit mark (**Figure 13-9**).

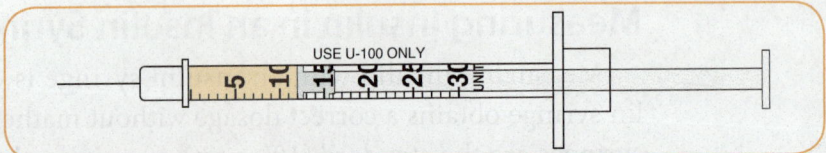

Figure 13-9 30 Unit Lo-Dose U-100 insulin syringe measuring 12 units.
© Cengage Learning 2013

Combination Insulin Dosage

Some patients may use two types of insulin that have been ordered to be administered at the same time. To avoid injecting the patient twice, it is common practice to draw up both insulins in the same syringe.

■ **Example 1:**

> Ordered: *Novolin R regular U-100 insulin 12 units with Novolin N NPH U-100 insulin 40 units SC with breakfast*

To accurately draw up both insulins into the same syringe, the pharmacy technician must know the total units of both insulins: 12 + 40 = 52 units. Withdraw 12 units of the Regular U-100 insulin (clear) and then withdraw 40 more units of the NPH U-100 insulin (cloudy) up to the 52-unit mark (**Figure 13-10**). In this case, the smallest capacity syringe that can be used is the Standard U-100 insulin syringe. It is important to remember that regular insulin must always be withdrawn from the vial into the syringe *first*. This prevents contaminating the vial of regular (clear) insulin with the NPH (cloudy) insulin, since if contaminated, it can affect the action of the insulin.

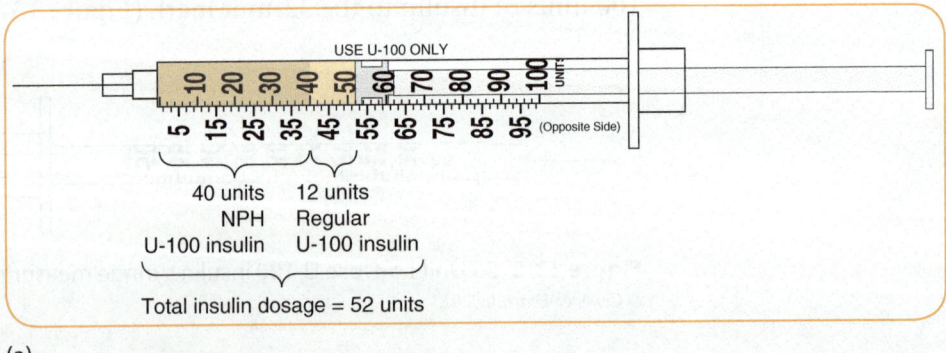

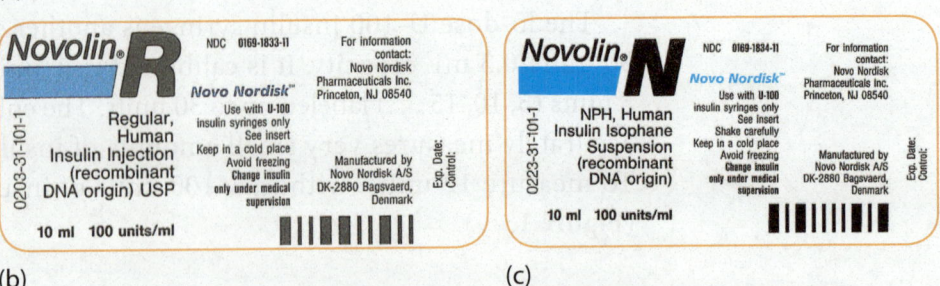

Figure 13-10 (a) Combination insulin dosage, (b) Novolin R, (c) Novolin N 10 mL.
(a) Copyright Cengage Learning 2013, (b) and (c) Courtesy of Novo Nordisk Pharmaceuticals, Inc.

The second example gives step-by-step directions for this procedure. Look closely at **Figures 13-11** and **13-12** to see the procedure as you study Example 2. Notice that to withdraw regular insulin (clear) first and then NPH insulin (cloudy), you must inject the dose amount of air into the NPH insulin vial before you inject the dose amount of air into the Regular insulin vial.

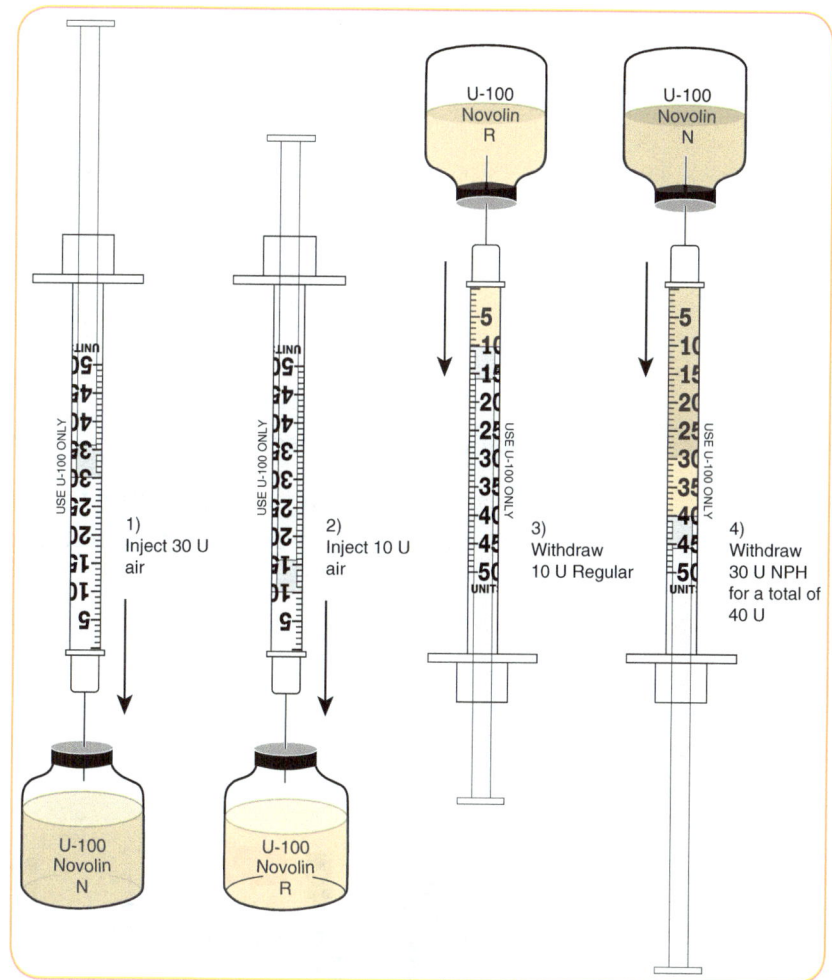

Figure 13-11 Procedure for drawing up combination insulin dosage: 10 Units Regular U-100 insulin with 30 Units NPH U-100 insulin.
© Cengage Learning 2013

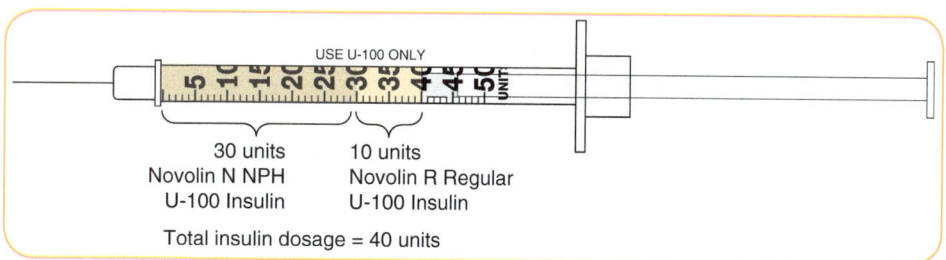

Figure 13-12 Combination insulin dosage.
© Cengage Learning 2013

Example 2:

A prescriber orders Novolin R regular U-100 insulin 10 units with Novolin N NPH U-100 insulin 30 USC $\frac{1}{2}$ hour before dinner.

1. Draw back and inject 30 units of air into the NPH insulin vial (cloudy liquid). Remove the needle.

2. Draw back and inject 10 units of air into the regular insulin (clear liquid) and leave the needle in the vial.

3. Turn the vial of regular insulin upside down, and draw out the insulin to the 10-unit mark on the syringe. Make sure all air bubbles are removed.

4. Roll the vial of the NPH insulin in your hands to mix; do not shake it. Insert the needle into the NPH insulin vial; turn the vial upside down; and slowly draw back to the 40-unit mark, being careful not to exceed the 40 unit calibration. 10 units of regular + 30 units of NPH = 40 units of insulin total.

Stop and Review
Calculating Insulin Doses

1. Read the following labels. Identify the insulin brand name and its action time (rapid-acting, intermediate-acting, or long-acting).

a. Insulin brand name _____

Action time _____

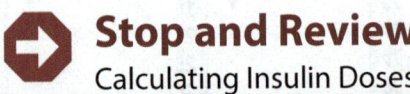

Humulin R.
© Copyright Eli Lilly and Company. Used with permission.

b. Insulin brand name _____

Action time _____

Novolin N 10 mL.
Courtesy of Novo Nordisk

c. Insulin brand name _____

Action time _____

Humulin U.
© *Eli Lilly and Company. Used with permission.*

d. Insulin brand name _____

Action time _____

Humalog 10 mL.
© *Eli Lilly and Company. Used with permission.*

e. Insulin brand name _____

Action time _____

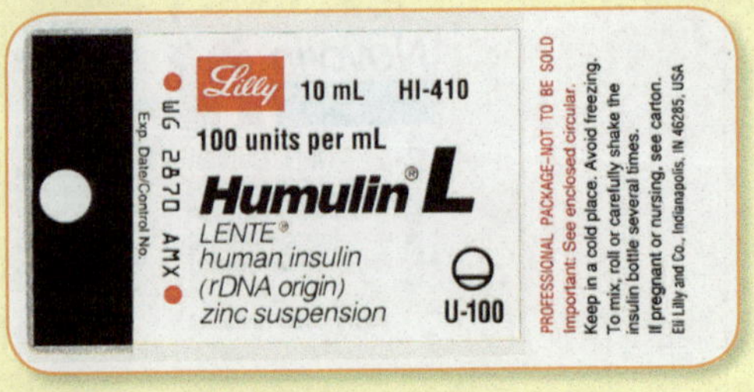

Humulin L 10 mL.
© Eli Lilly and Company. Used with permission.

f. Describe the three syringes available to measure U-100 insulin.
_____

g. What would be your preferred syringe choice to measure 24 units of U-100 insulin?
_____

h. What would be your preferred syringe choice to measure 35 units of U-100 insulin?
_____

i. There are 60 units of U-100 insulin per _____ mL.

j. There are 25 units of U-100 insulin per _____ mL.

k. 65 units of U-100 insulin should be measured in a(n) _____ syringe.

l. True or false? The 50-unit lo-dose U-100 insulin syringe is intended to measure U-50 insulin only. _____

2. Identify the U-100 insulin dosage indicated by the colored area of the syringe.

a. _____ units

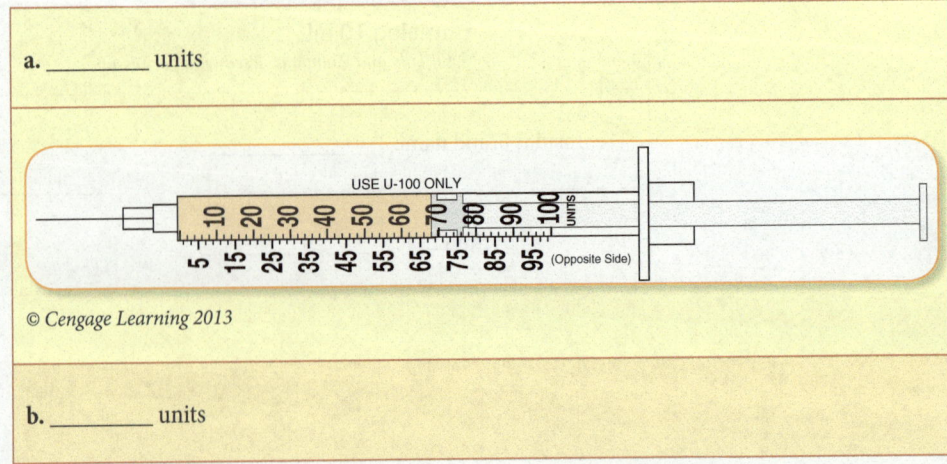

© Cengage Learning 2013

b. _____ units

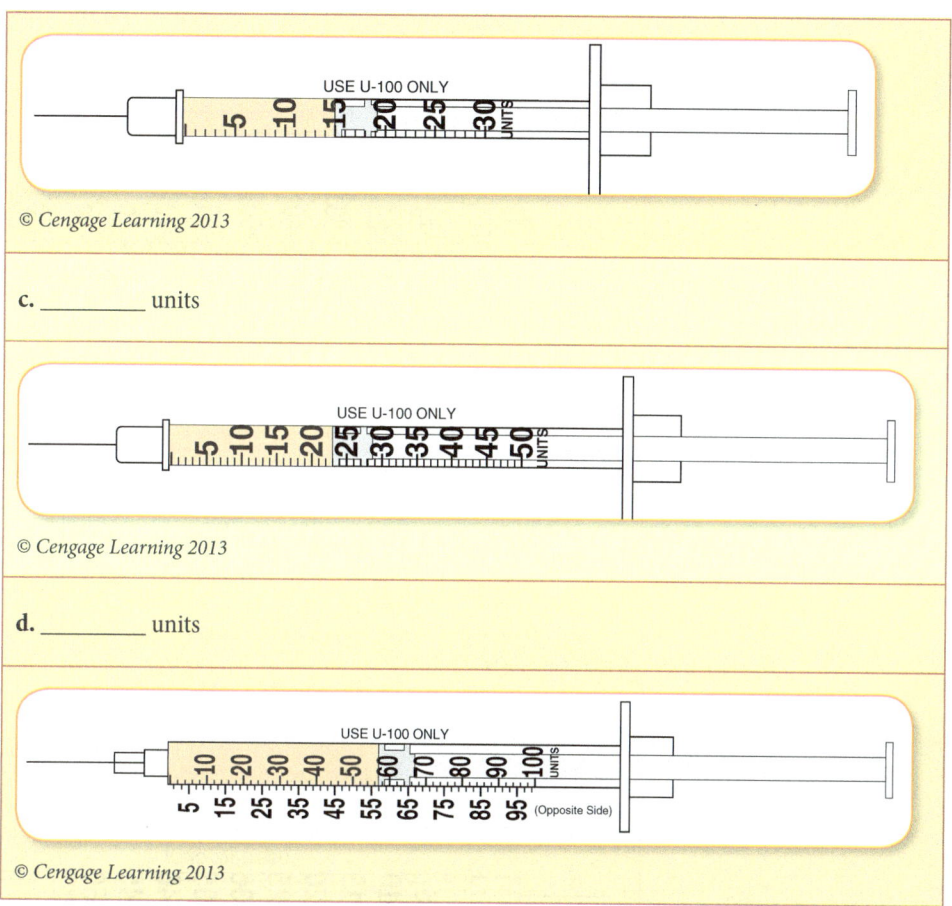

c. _____ units

d. _____ units

3. Draw an arrow on the syringe to identify the given dosages.

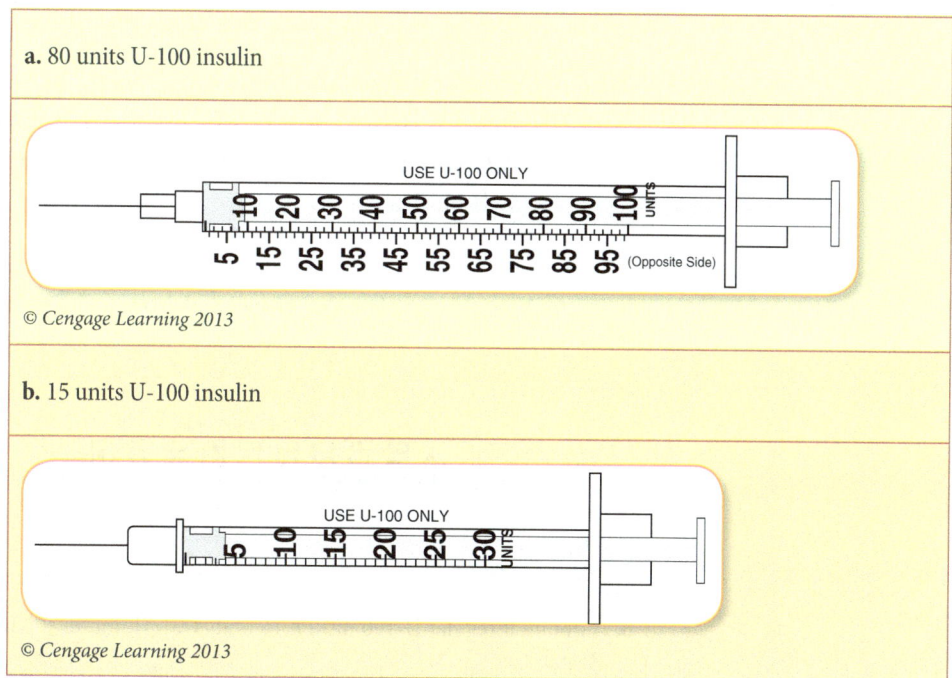

a. 80 units U-100 insulin

b. 15 units U-100 insulin

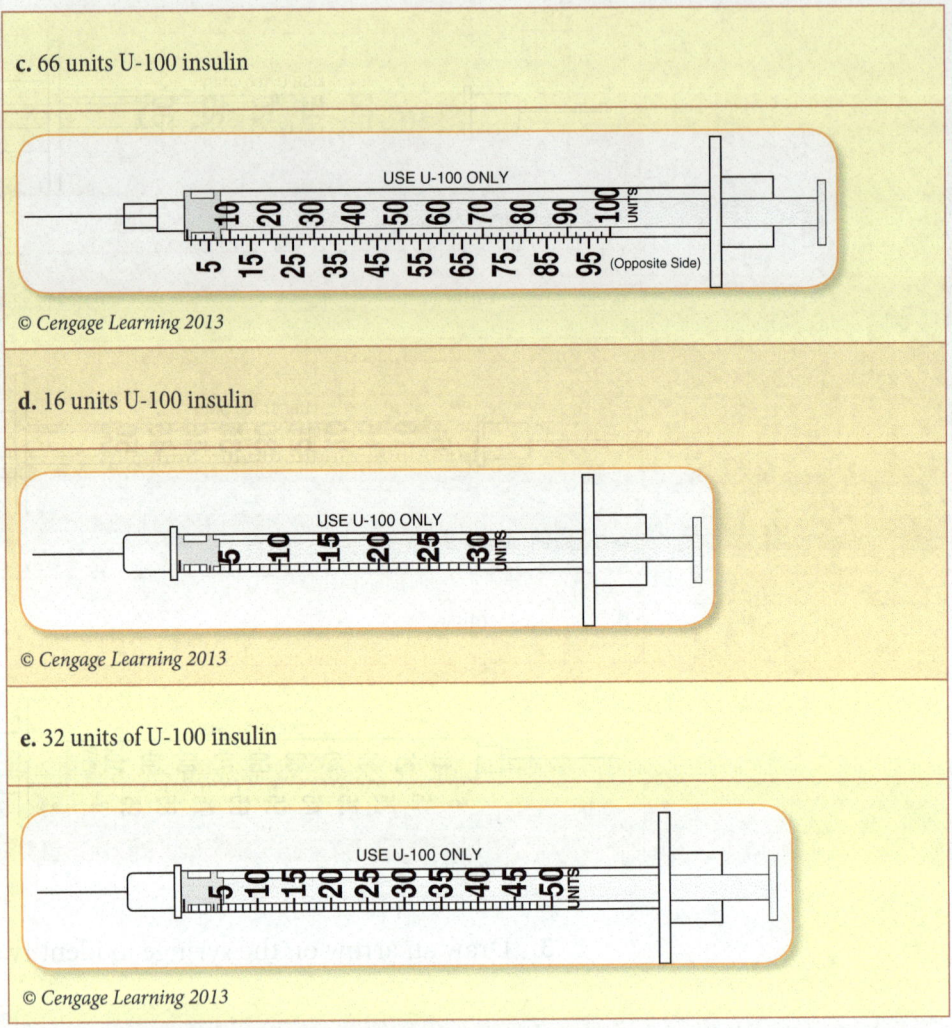

c. 66 units U-100 insulin

d. 16 units U-100 insulin

e. 32 units of U-100 insulin

4. Draw arrows and label the dosage for each of the combination insulin orders to be measured in the same syringe. Label and measure the insulins in the correct order, indicating which insulin will be drawn up first.

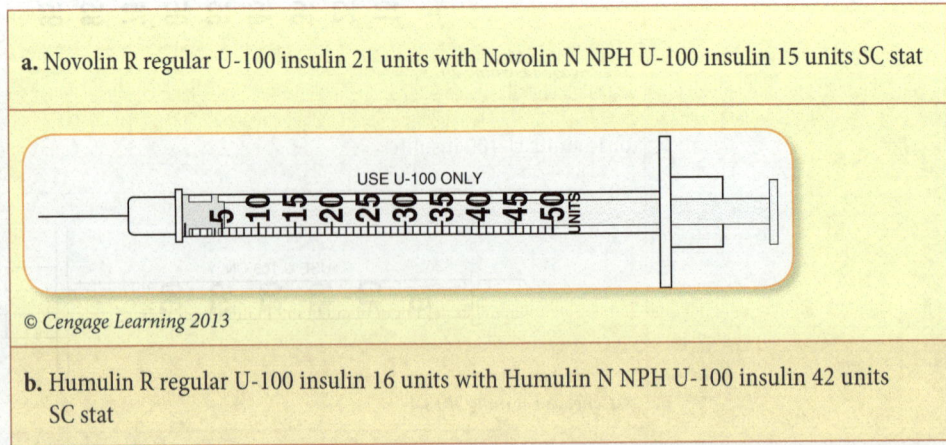

a. Novolin R regular U-100 insulin 21 units with Novolin N NPH U-100 insulin 15 units SC stat

b. Humulin R regular U-100 insulin 16 units with Humulin N NPH U-100 insulin 42 units SC stat

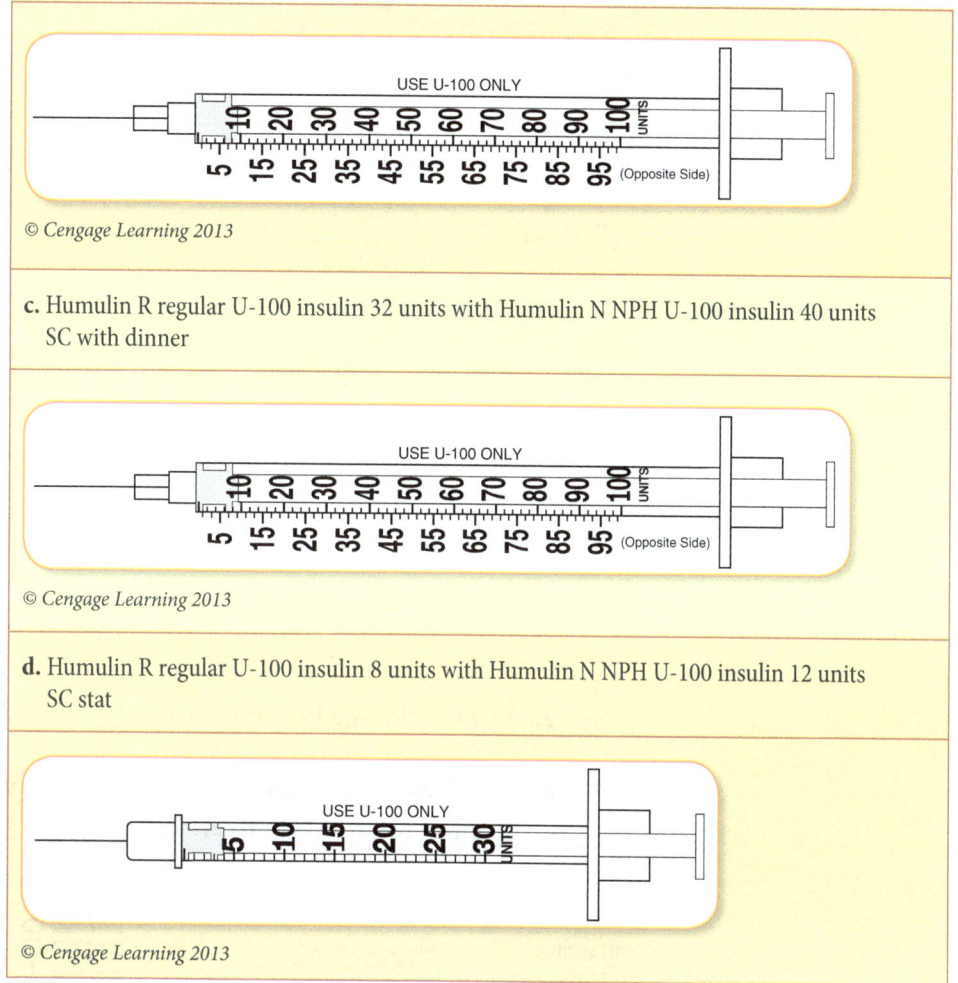

c. Humulin R regular U-100 insulin 32 units with Humulin N NPH U-100 insulin 40 units SC with dinner

d. Humulin R regular U-100 insulin 8 units with Humulin N NPH U-100 insulin 12 units SC stat

Solutions Measured as Milliequivalents

Other medications are measured as milliequivalents (mEq). An example of a medication measured in mEq is calcium gluconate (see **Figure 13-13**). This medication has a 10% strength, and the vial contains a dosage of 0.465 mEq/mL.

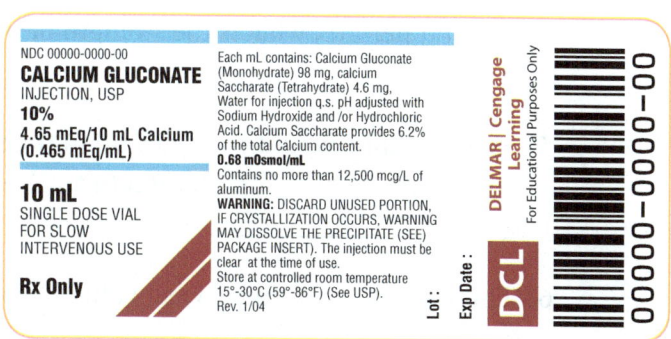

Figure 13-13 Calcium Gluconate 10 mL.
© Cengage Learning 2013

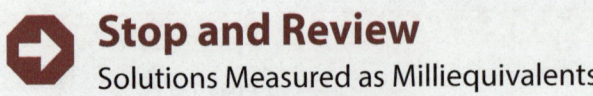

Stop and Review
Solutions Measured as Milliequivalents

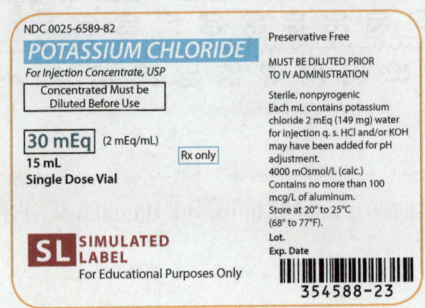

Potassium Chloride label.
© Cengage Learning 2013

Use the preceding label to answer the following questions.

1. For this vial, what are the total dosage and volume?
   _____

2. List the dosage in mEq per mL. _____

3. What volume would be drawn up if you were asked to prepare 15 mEq for addition to an IV? _____

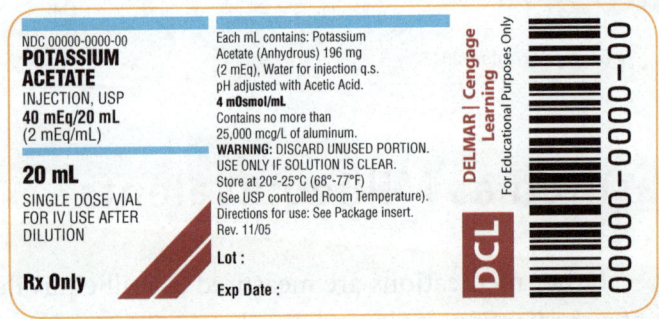

Potassium Acetate.
© Cengage Learning 2013

Use the preceding label to answer the following questions.

4. In mEq per mL, what is the strength of this solution?
   _____

5. What volume would you draw up in the syringe if you were asked to prepare 40 mEq for addition to an IV solution?
   _____

6. For a dosage of 20 mEq, what volume would you need?
   _____

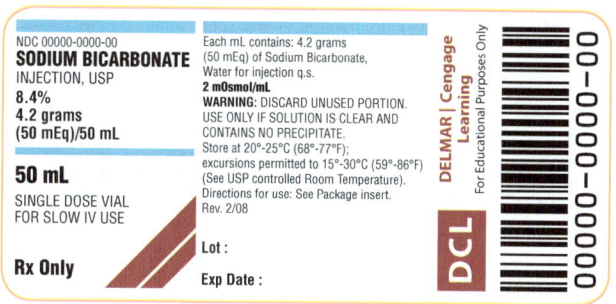

Sodium Bicarbonate.
© Cengage Learning 2013

Use the preceding label to answer the following questions.

7. In mEq/mL, what is the dosage strength? _____

8. What is this vial's total volume, and how many mEq does it contain? _____

9. What is the strength per mL in grams? _____

10. What volume would you draw up in a syringe if you were asked to prepare 10 mL of an 8.4% sodium bicarbonate solution? _____

Calculating Parenteral Drug Dosages

Parenteral medications are measured in proper syringes. The amount of solution delivered is called the desired dose of drug. The dosage strength on an injectable drug's label represents the amount of medication contained within a volume of solution. For example, xylocaine 1% (label drug) can be interpreted as 100 mL contains 1g of xylocaine. Another example is Compazine 5 mg/mL, which means 1 mL contains 5 mg of Compazine.

When the dosage ordered and the dose on hand have different units, the dosage ordered must be converted to the desired dose. Use this formula to calculate the amount of an injectable drug by the formula method:

$$\frac{D \text{ (desired)}}{H \text{ (have)}} \times Q \text{ (quantity)} = X \text{ (amount)}$$

■ Example 1:

Measure 0.33 mL in a 1 mL syringe.

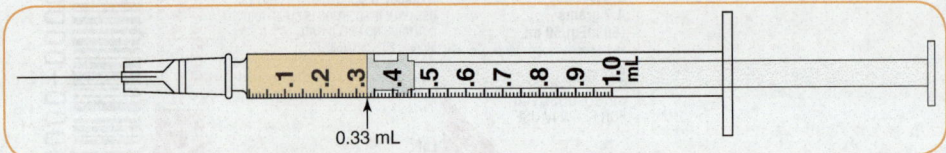

■ Example 2:

Round 1.33 mL to 1.3 mL, and measure in a 3 mL syringe.

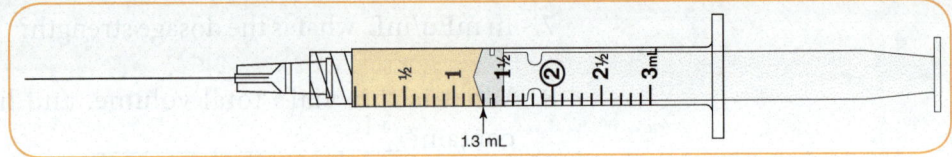

■ Example 3:

Measure 0.6 mL in either a 1 mL or 3 mL syringe.

(Notice that the amount is measured in tenths, but the 1 mL syringe would be preferable.)

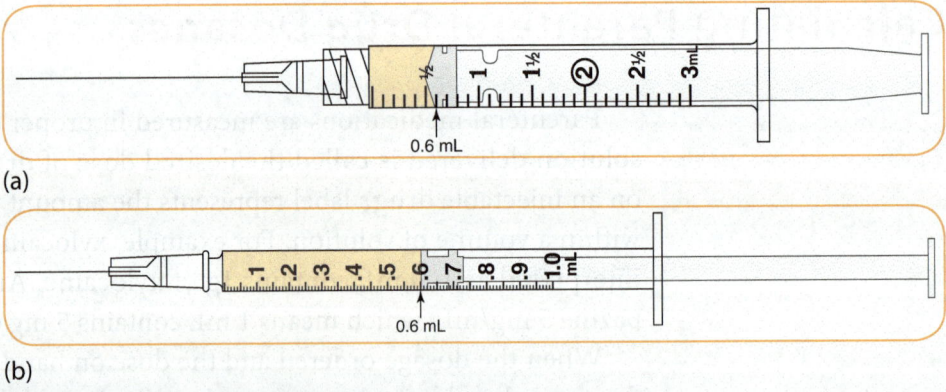

(a)

(b)

(a) and (b) Copyright Cengage Learning 2013

■ Example 4:

Measure 0.65 mL in a 1 mL syringe. (Notice that the amount is measured in hundredths and is less than 1 mL.)

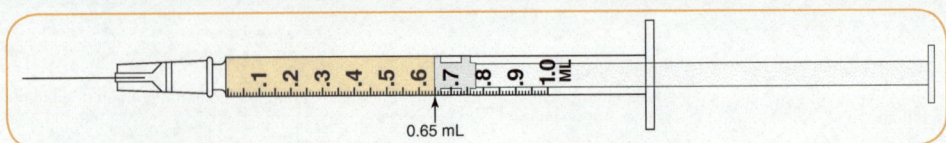

An amber color has been added to selected syringe drawings throughout the text to represent a specific amount of medication, as indicated in the example or problem. Because the color used may not correspond to the actual color of the medication named, it must not be used as a reference for identifying medications.

The following are some examples of parenteral dosage calculations.

■ Example 5:

Ordered: *Vistaril 100 mg IM stat*

On hand: Vistaril IM solution 50 mg/mL in a 10 mL multiple-dose vial

The amount that should be administered to the patient follows:

$$\frac{D}{H} \times Q = \frac{100 \text{ mg}}{50 \text{ mg}} \times 1 \text{ mL} = 2 \text{ mL}$$

Give intramuscularly immediately.

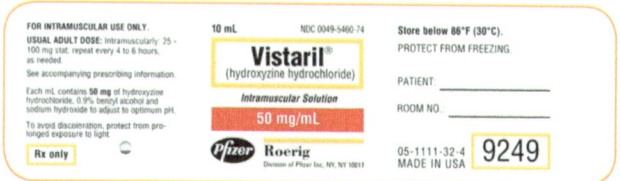

Vistaril 50 mg/mL.
Label reproduced with permission of Pfizer, Inc.

Select a 3 mL syringe and measure 2 mL of Vistaril 50 mg/mL. Look carefully at the illustration to clearly identify the part of the black rubber stopper that measures the exact dosage.

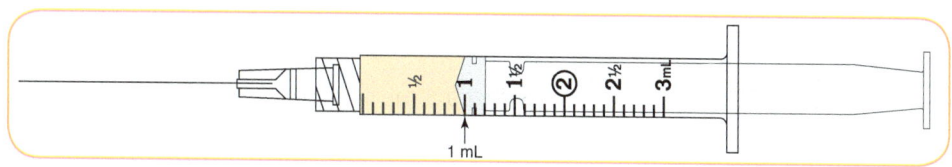

© Cengage Learning 2013

■ Example 6:

Ordered: *heparin 8000 units SC b.i.d.*

On hand: A vial of heparin sodium injection 10,000 units/1 mL

$$\frac{D}{H} \times Q = \frac{8000 \text{ U}}{10,000 \text{ U}} \times 1 \text{ mL} = \frac{8}{10} \text{ mL} = 0.8 \text{ mL}$$

Give subcutaneously twice daily.

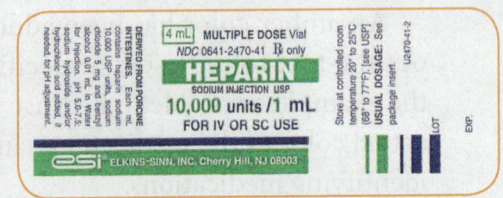

Heparin 1 mL.
Courtesy of ESI Lederle, a Business Unit of Wyeth Pharmaceuticals, Philadelphia, PA

Select a 1 mL or a 3 mL syringe and measure 0.8 mL of heparin 10,000 units/mL. Heparin is a very potent anticoagulant drug. It is safest to measure it in a 1 mL syringe.

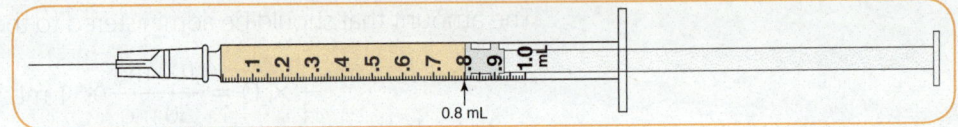

© Cengage Learning 2013

■ Example 7:

Ordered: *Cleocin Phosphate 150 mg IM q12h*

On hand: Cleocin Phosphate (clindamycin injection) 300 mg/2 mL

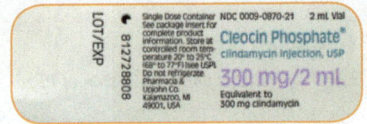

Cleocin Phosphate 300 mg.
Label reproduced with permission of Pfizer, Inc.

$$\frac{D}{H} \times Q = \frac{150 \text{ mg}}{300 \text{ mg}} \times 2 \text{ mL} = \frac{2}{2} = 1 \text{ mL}$$

Give intramuscularly every 12 hours.

Select a 3 mL syringe, and measure 1 mL of Cleocin 300 mg/2 mL.

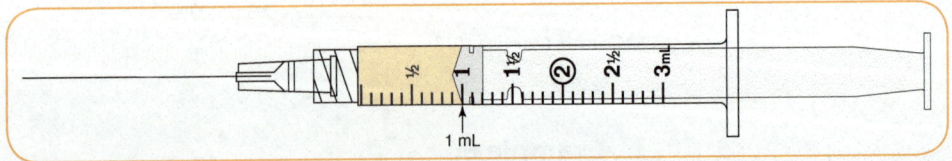

© Cengage Learning 2013

■ Example 8:

Ordered: *Robinul 150 mcg IM stat*

On hand: Robinul 0.2 mg/mL

$$0.2 \times 1000 = 0.200\text{.} = 200 \text{ mcg}$$

Equivalent: 1 mg = 1000 mcg

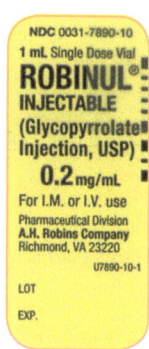

Robinul 0.2 mg/mL.
Courtesy of ESI Lederle, Philadelphia, PA

$$\frac{D}{H} \times Q = \frac{150 \text{ mcg}}{200 \text{ mcg}} \times 1 \text{ mL} = \frac{3}{4} = 0.75 \text{ mL}$$

Give intramuscularly immediately.

Select a 1 mL syringe, and measure 0.75 mL of Robinul 0.2 mg/mL.

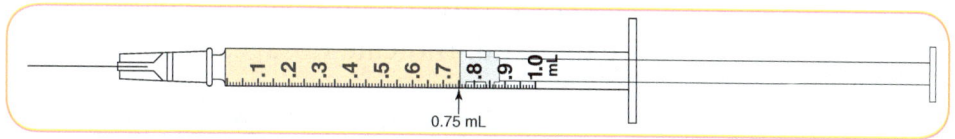

© Cengage Learning 2013

Example 9:

Ordered: *morphine sulfate gr $\frac{1}{6}$ IM q3-4h p.r.n.*

The label on the dosette vial states morphine sulfate 10 mg/mL.

On hand: morphine sulfate 10 mg/mL

Equivalent: gr i = 60 mg

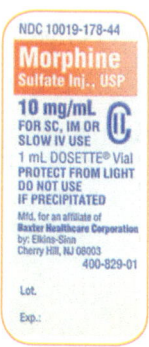

Morphine 10 mg/mL.
Courtesy of Baxter Healthcare Corporation

$$\text{gr}\frac{1}{6} \times \frac{60}{1} = 10 \text{ mg}$$

$$\frac{D}{H} \times Q = \frac{10 \text{ mg}}{10 \text{ mg}} \times 1 \text{ mL} = 1 \text{ mL}$$

Give intramuscularly every 3 to 4 hours as needed for pain.

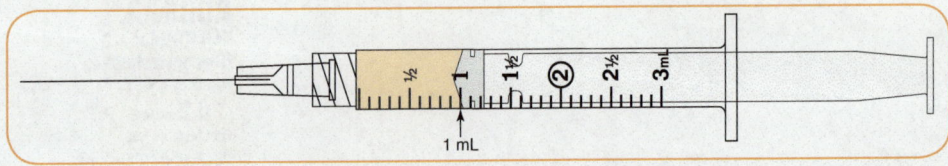

© Cengage Learning 2013

Test Your Knowledge

Calculate one dose of each of the drug orders numbered 1 through 12. Draw an arrow on the syringe, indicating the calibration line that corresponds to the dose to be administered. The labels provided following these questions are the drugs that are on hand. Indicate dosages that must be administered.

1. Haldol 1.5 mg IM q8h

   Give: _____ mL

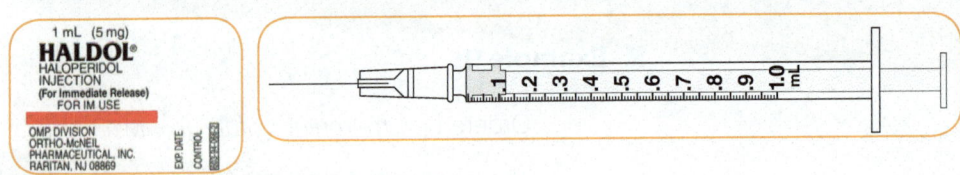

Haldol 1 mL.
Courtesy of Ortho-McNeil Pharmaceuticals

2. Thorazine 40 mg IM q6h

   Give: _____ mL

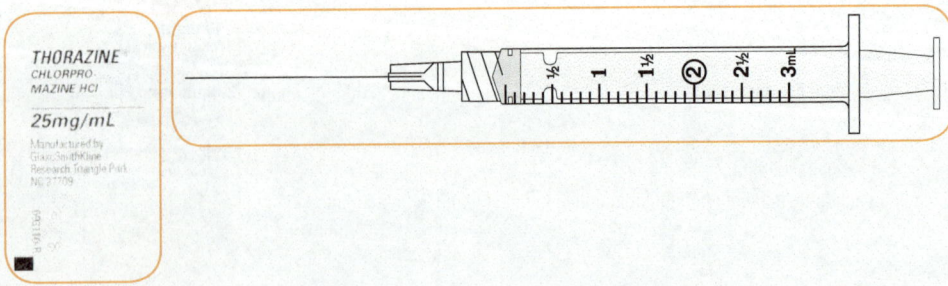

Thorazine 25 mg/mL.
Reprinted with permission from GlaxoSmithKline

3. Inapsine 1 mg IV stat.

   Give: _____ mL

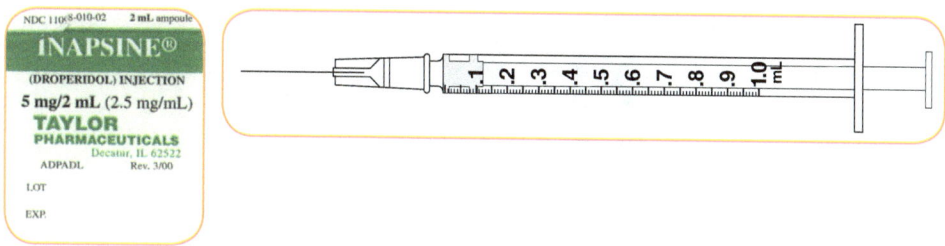

Inapsine 5 mg/2 mL.
Courtesy of Akorn Inc.

4. Nebcin 100 mg IM q8h.

   Give: _____ mL

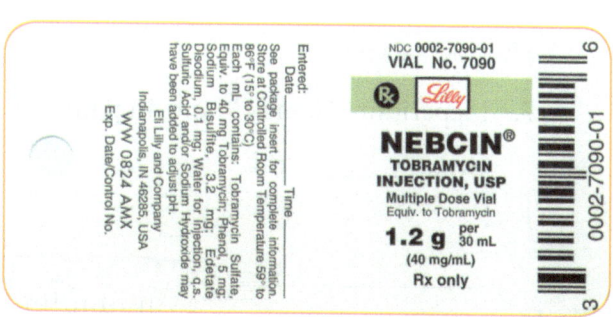

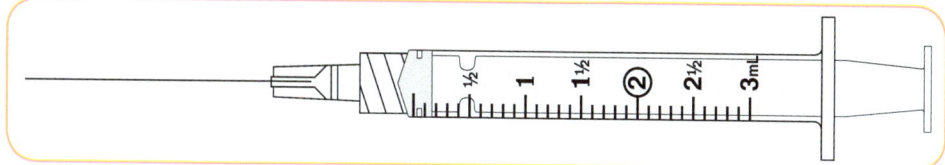

Nebcin 1.2 g per 30 mL.
© *Eli Lilly and Company. Used with permission.*

5. Epoetin alpha 12,000 units SC q.d. × 10 days

   Give: _____ mL

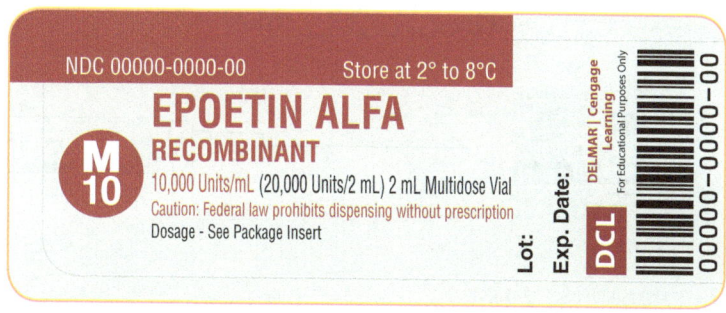

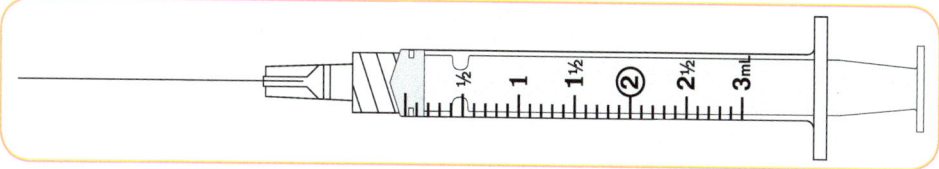

Epoetin alfa recombinant M10, 20,000 Units/2 mL.
© *Cengage Learning 2013*

6. Humulin regular U-100 insulin 22 units SC stat

    Give: _____ units

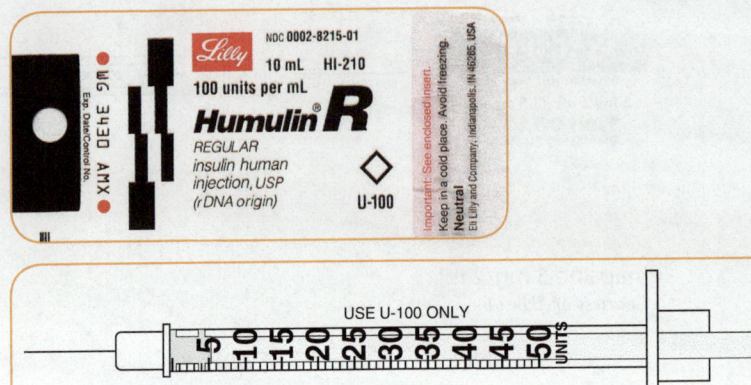

Humulin R.
© Eli Lilly and Company. Used with permission.

7. Meperidine 60 mg IM q3–4h p.r.n., pain

    Give: _____ mL

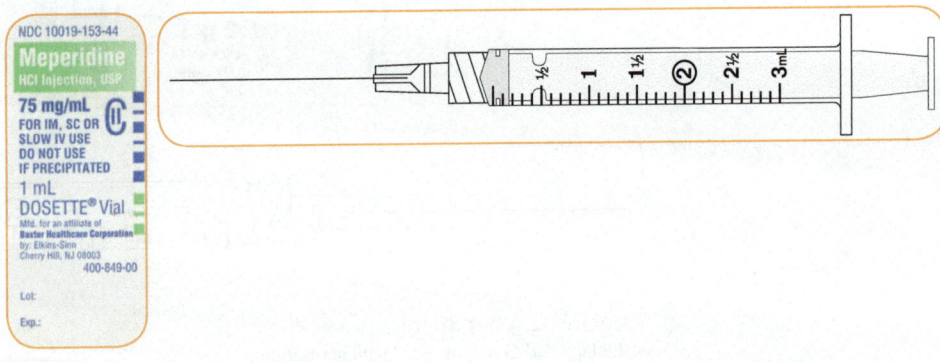

Meperidine 75 mg/mL.
Courtesy of Baxter Healthcare Corporation

8. Phenergan 15 mg IM q3–4h p.r.n., nausea and vomiting

    Give: _____ mL

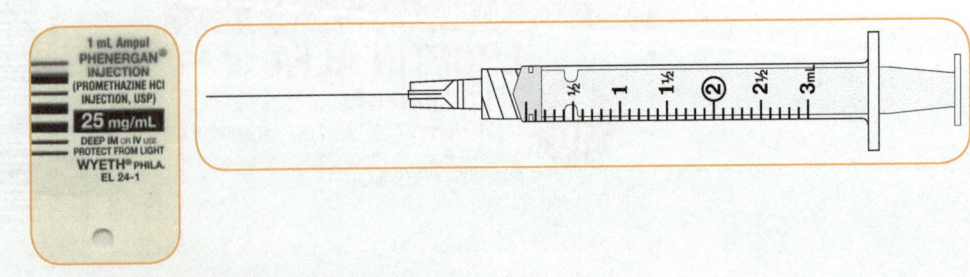

Phenergan 25 mg/mL.
Courtesy of Wyeth Pharmaceuticals, Philadelphia, PA

9. Reglan 7 mg IM stat

   Give: _____ mL

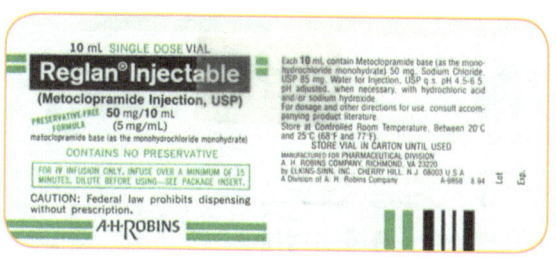
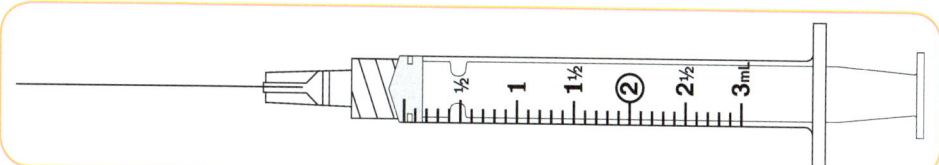

Reglan Injectable, 50 mg/10 mL.
Courtesy of ESI Lederle, Philadelphia, PA

10. Filgrastim 225 mcg SC q.d. × 2 weeks

    Give: _____ mL

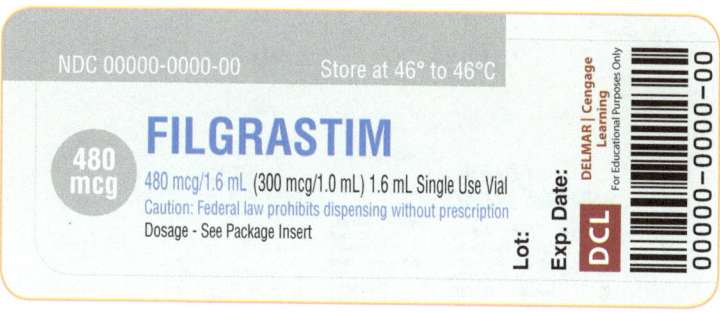
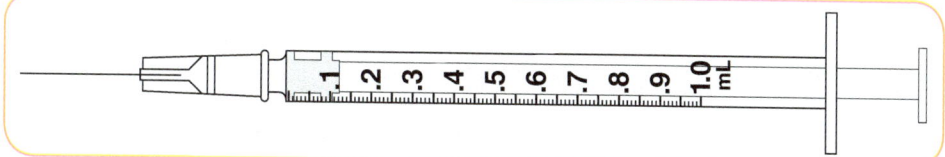

Filgrastim 480 mcg/1.6 mL (300 mcg/1.0 mL).
© *Cengage Learning 2013*

11. Novolin R Regular U-100 insulin 32 units with Novolin N NPH U-100 insulin 54 units SC with breakfast.

    Give: _____ units

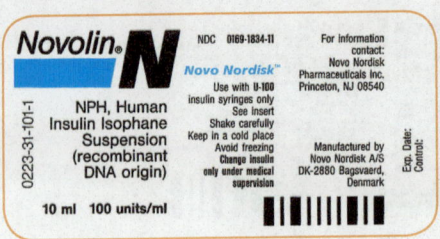
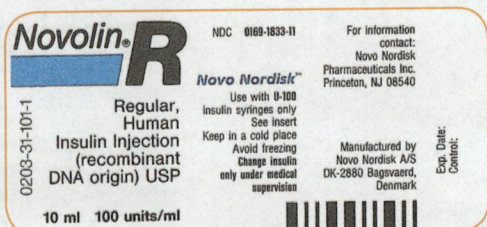

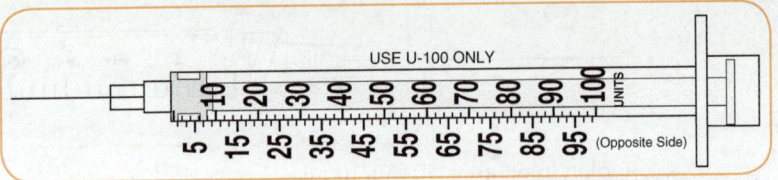

Novolin N 10 mL (100 units/mL) and Novolin R 10 mL (100 units/mL).
Courtesy Novo Nordisk

12. Novolin $\frac{70}{30}$ U-100 insulin 46 units SC with dinner.

    Give: _____ units

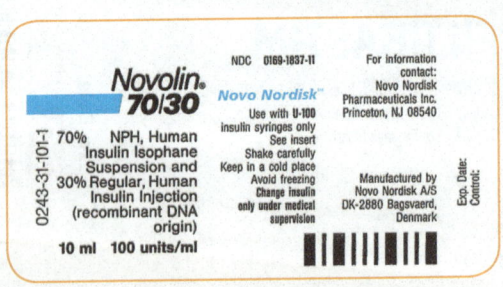

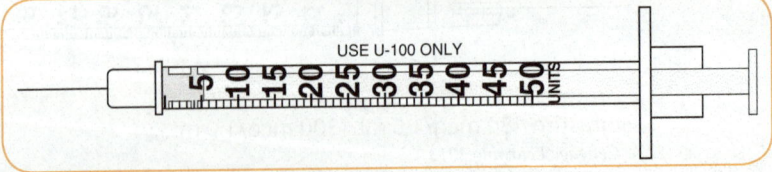

Novolin $\frac{70}{30}$, 10 mL (100 units/mL).
Courtesy Novo Nordisk

Calculate the amount you will prepare for one dose. Indicate the syringe you will select to measure the medication.

13. Ordered: *Demerol 35 mg IM q4h p.r.n., pain*

    On hand: *Demerol 50 mg/1 mL*

    Give: _____ mL   Select: _____ syringe

14. Ordered: *Atarax 40 mg IM q4–6h p.r.n., agitation*
    On hand: Atarax 50 mg/mL
    Give: _____ mL   Select: _____ syringe

15. Ordered: *Garamycin 40 mg IM q8h*
    On hand: Garamycin 80 mg/2 mL
    Give: _____ mL   Select: _____ syringe

16. Ordered: *heparin 3500 units SC q12*
    On hand: heparin 5000 units/mL
    Give: _____ mL   Select: _____ syringe

17. Ordered: *Lasix 60 mg IV stat*
    On hand: Lasix 20 mg per 2 mL ampule
    Give: _____ mL   Select: _____ syringe

18. Ordered: *Phenergan 35 mg IM q4h p.r.n., nausea and vomiting*
    On hand: Phenergan 50 mg/1 mL
    Give: _____ mL   Select: _____ syringe

19. Ordered: *vitamin B12 0.75 mg IM q.d.*
    On hand: vitamin B12 1000 mcg/mL
    Give: _____ mL   Select: _____ syringe

20. Ordered: *lidocaine 50 mg IV stat*
    On hand: lidocaine 2%
    Give: _____ mL   Select: _____ syringe

21. Ordered: *morphine sulfate gr $\frac{1}{4}$ IM stat*
    On hand: morphine sulfate 10 mg/mL
    Give: _____ mL   Select: _____ syringe

22. Ordered: *Cleocin 300 mg IM q.i.d.*
    On hand: Cleocin 0.6 g/4 mL
    Give: _____ mL   Select: _____ syringe

23. Ordered: *Dilantin 25 mg IV q8 h*
    On hand: Dilantin 100 mg/2 mL ampule
    Give: _____ mL   Select: _____ syringe

24. Ordered: *heparin 6000 units SC q12h*
    On hand: heparin 10,000 units/mL vial
    Give: _____ mL   Select: _____ syringe

25. Ordered: atropine gr $\frac{1}{150}$ IM on call to O.R.

    On hand: atropine 0.4 mg/mL

    Give: _____ mL   Select: _____ syringe

26. Ordered: Thorazine 10 mg deep IM q.i.d.

    On hand: Thorazine 25 mg/mL

    Give: _____ mL   Select: _____ syringe

27. Ordered: Epogen 1400 units SC tiw

    On hand: Epogen 2000 units/mL

    Give: _____ mL   Select: _____ syringe

28. Ordered: Adrenalin 0.2 mg SC stat

    On hand: Adrenalin 1:2000 solution

    Give: _____ mL   Select: _____ syringe

29. Ordered: Brethine 0.25 mg SC stat

    On hand: Brethine 1 mg/mL

    Give: _____ mL   Select: _____ syringe

30. Ordered: magnesium sulfate 250 mg IM q.d.

    On hand: magnesium sulfate 10% solution

    Give: _____ mL   Select: _____ syringe

31. Ordered: Calciferol 24,000 IU IM q.d.

    On hand: Calciferol 500,000 IU/5 mL

    Give: _____ mL   Select: _____ syringe

32. Ordered: Robinul 0.15 mg IM stat

    On hand: Robinul 0.2 mg/mL

    Give: _____ mL   Select: _____ syringe

Critical Thinking

Describe how to prevent a medication error in the following example.

A patient presents with nausea, and a physician orders oral Compazine liquid. Due to the patient's difficulty in taking the medication normally, the physician has instructed that a needleless syringe be supplied along with the medication, which the patient can use to self-administer the medication. The pharmacy technician processing the order accidentally packages it with needles so that the medication may be self-injected, along with appropriate self-injection instructions.

1. If the patient followed these instructions and did self-inject the medication, how would the medication be absorbed?

2. What could possibly develop at the site of the injection as a result of the self-injection?

A 56-year-old patient was hospitalized. The physician ordered Novolin R regular unit-100 insulin, 12 units, with Novolin N NPH unit-100 insulin, 40 units subcutaneously, with breakfast.

3. For this administration of combined insulins, what is the smallest capacity syringe that can be used?

4. Which of the insulins must always be withdrawn from the vial into the syringe first, and why?

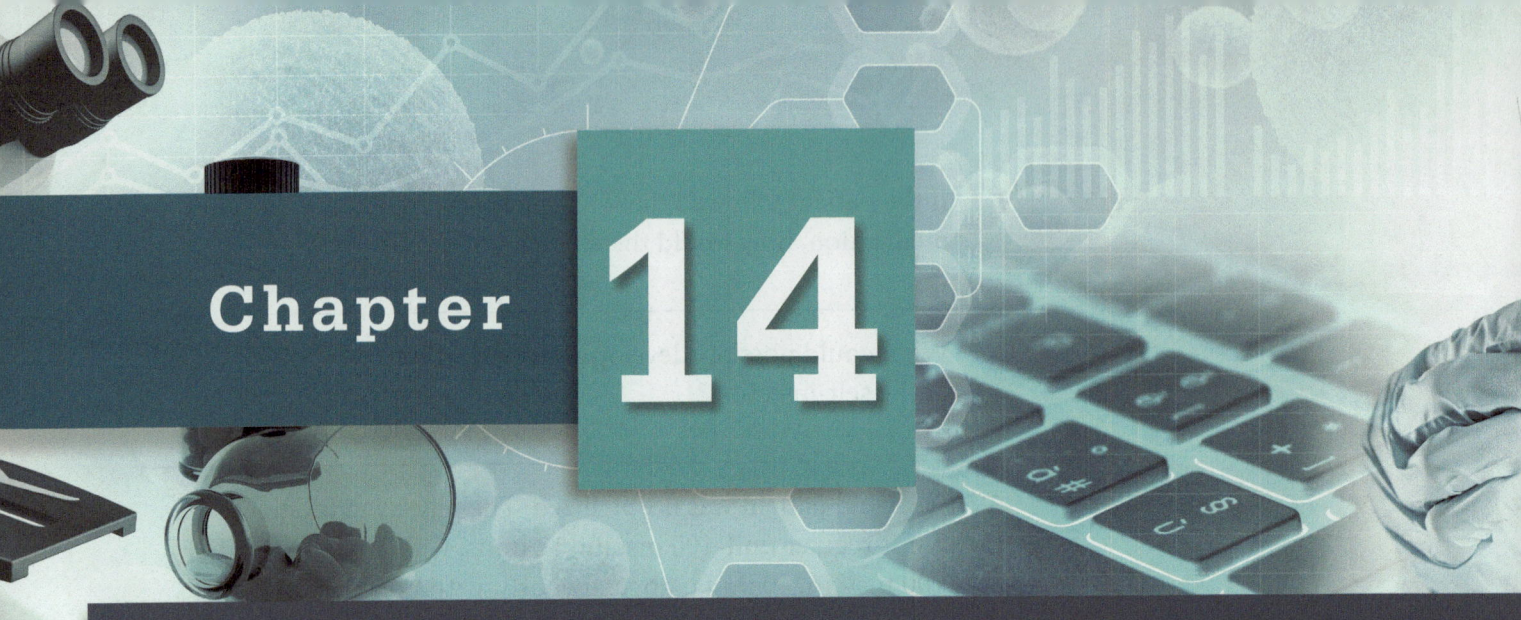

Chapter 14

Intravenous Flow Rate Calculations

Outline

Overview

IV Push

Continuous Intravenous Infusions
  Solution Additives
  Percentage in IV Fluids
  Parenteral Nutrition

Calculating IV Components as Percentages
  Calculating IV Flow Rates
  Calculating Flow Rates Using Ratio and Proportion
  Calculating Flow Rates Using Dimensional Analysis
  Calculating Flow Rates Using the Formula Method
  Calculating Flow Rates Using the Shortcut Method
  Adjusting IV Flow Rates
  Flow Rates for Electronic Regulation

Heparin Intravenous Calculations
  Calculating IV Flow Rate from Units per Hour Ordered
  Calculating Units per Hour Infusing from IV Flow Rate

Intermittent Intravenous Injections
  IV Piggybacks (IVPB)

Objectives

Upon completion of this chapter, you should be able to:

1. Calculate IV flow rates for manual regulation.
2. Calculate flow rates in drops per minute and milliliters per hour by using the formula method.
3. Calculate IV flow rates for electronic regulation.
4. Calculate IV flow rates from units per hour ordered and vice versa.
5. Calculate infusion times.
6. Calculate IVs as percentages.
7. Calculate drops per minute (gtt/min) flow rates using dimensional analysis.
8. Calculate IV flow rates using the shortcut method.
9. Given an image of IV tubing, identify the drop factor calibration shown.

Key Terms

continuous IV infusions
controllers
D_5W
heparin lock
infusion pumps
intermittent intravenous infusion
intermittent peripheral infusion device
IV bolus
IV push
saline lock
syringe pump

Overview

Intravenous (IV) fluids and drugs may be administered for many different reasons. Intravenous therapy is prescribed to persons requiring electrolyte replacement, fluid, calories, vitamins, or other nutritional substances. It may also be prescribed for administration of medications, chemotherapy, or for transfusion of blood products. There are about 200 different manufactured IV fluids. Approximately 90 percent of all hospitalized patients, and some in outpatient settings, receive IV therapy. Regulation of IV fluids is normally not a responsibility of pharmacy technicians. Pharmacists and technicians are involved with compounding IV fluids. This chapter explains the basic concepts of IV therapy and flow rate calculations.

Calculation errors can have serious, even fatal, consequences. Drug information inserts must be read carefully, and attention must be paid to the amount of drug that can be given per minute. If the drug is administered into the blood circulation at a rate faster than that specified in the drug literature, adverse reactions to the medication are likely to occur.

Heparin is an anticoagulant that inhibits new blood clot formation, and it keeps already-existing clots from becoming larger. It is often mixed in IV solutions for postoperative administration to prevent clot formation from venous stasis. Heparin dosages are based on body weight (in kilograms) or on a patient's clotting time, which is checked frequently during administration. Pharmacy technicians may be involved with heparin intravenous calculations in sterile compounding.

IV Push

Drugs that are administered by the IV injection route are often referred to as **IV push**. This route has a rapid onset of action, and calculation errors can have serious or even fatal consequences. Calculating the amount of drug needed to infuse by direct IV infusion can be determined by using the ratio and proportion method.

■ Example 1:

Ordered: *Dilantin 200 mg IV stat*

On hand: Dilantin 250 mg/5 mL; IV infusion not to exceed 50 mg/min

Give: $\dfrac{D}{H} \times V = \dfrac{200}{250} \times 5 = 4 \text{ mL}$

or

$$H : V :: D : X$$

$$250 \text{ mg} : 5 \text{ mL} :: 200 \text{ mg} : X \text{ mL}$$

$$250X = 5 \times 200 = 1000$$

$$X = \dfrac{1000}{250}$$

$$X = 4 \text{ mL}$$

Minutes :: desired drug : desired minutes

50 mg : 1 minute :: 200 mg : x minutes

$$50X = 200$$

$$X = 4 \text{ minutes}$$

■ Example 2:

Ordered: *furosemide 120 mg IV stat*

On hand: furosemide 10 mg/mL; IV infusion not to exceed 40 mg/min

a. $H : V :: D : X$

10 mg : 1 mL :: 120 mg : X

$$10X = 120$$

$$X = 12 \text{ mL of Lasix}$$

or

$$\frac{D}{H} \times V = \frac{1 \text{ mL} \times 120 \text{ mg}}{10 \text{ mg} \times 1} = 12 \text{ mL of Lasix}$$

b. On hand : minutes :: desired drug : desired minutes

$$40 \text{ mg} : 1 \text{ min} :: 120 \text{ mg} : X$$

$$40X = 120$$

$$X = 3 \text{ min}$$

■ Example 3:

Ordered: *Ativan 3 mg IV push 20 min preoperatively*

On hand: Ativan 4 mg/mL with drug literature guidelines of "IV infusion not to exceed 2 mg/min"

How much Ativan should you prepare? Use the formula:

$$\frac{D}{H} \times Q = \frac{3 \text{ mg}}{4 \text{ mg}} \times 1 \text{ mL} = 0.75 \text{ mL}$$

What is a safe infusion time?

$$\frac{D}{H} \times Q = \frac{3 \text{ mg}}{2 \text{ mg}} \times 1 \text{ min} = \frac{3}{2} = 1\frac{1}{2} \text{ min}$$

■ Example 4:

Ordered: *Cefizox 1500 mg IV push q8h*

On hand: Cefizox 2 g powder with directions: "For direct IV administration, reconstitute each 1 g in 10 mL sterile water and give slowly over 3–5 minutes"

How much Cefizox should you prepare?

$$2 \text{ g} = 2 \times 1000 = 2000 \text{ mg}$$

$$\frac{D}{H} \times Q = \frac{1500 \text{ mg}}{2000 \text{ mg}} \times 20 \text{ mL} = 15 \text{ mL}$$

What is a safe infusion time?

$$\frac{D}{H} \times Q = \frac{1500 \text{ mg}}{1000} \times 5 \text{ min} = \frac{15}{2} = 7.5 \text{ min}$$

Administer 15 mL over 7.5 min.

Stop and Review
Calculating IV Push Rates

1. Ordered:	*morphine sulfate 6 mg IV push q3h p.r.n., pain*
On hand:	*morphine sulfate 10 mg/mL with a written drug reference recommendation: "IV infusion not to exceed 2.5 mg/min"*
Given:	_____ mL/_____ min/_____ sec
2. Ordered:	*Oxacillin sodium 900 mg in 125 mL D_5W IV PB to be infused over 45 min*
Instructions:	Use an infusion pump.
Flow rate:	_____ mL/hr
3. Ordered:	*Versed 1.5 mg IV push stat*
On hand:	*Versed 1 mg/1 mL*
Instructions:	"Slowly titrate to the desired effect using no more than 1.5 mg initially given over 2-min period."
Prepare:	_____ mL Versed
Given:	_____ mL/15 sec
4. Ordered:	*Merrem 1 g in 100 mL D_5W IV PB to be infused over 50 min*
Instructions:	Use an infusion pump.
Flow rate:	_____ mL/hr
5. Ordered:	*Unasyn 1.5 g in 50 mL D_5W IV PB to be infused over 15 min*
Drop factor:	15 gtt/min
Flow rate:	_____ gtt/min
6. Ordered:	*Keflin 500 mg in 50 mL NS IV PB to be infused over 20 min*
Drop factor:	10 gtt/mL
Flow rate:	_____ gtt/min

7. Ordered:	*Ancef 1 g in 100 mL D_5W IV PB to be infused over 45 min*
Drop factor:	60 gtt/mL
Flow rate:	_____ gtt/min
8. Ordered:	*Zosyn 1.3 g in 100 mL D_5W IV PB to be infused over 30 min*
Drop factor:	60 gtt/mL
Flow rate:	_____ gtt/min
9. Ordered:	*Dilantin 150 mg IV push stat*
On hand:	Dilantin 250 mg/5 mL with drug insert, which states "IV infusion not to exceed 50 mg/min"
Given:	_____ mL/_____ min
10. Ordered:	*Cimetidine 300 mg IV push stat*
On hand:	Tagamet (cimetidine) 300 mg/2 mL
Instructions:	"For direct IV injection, dilute 300 mg in 0.9% NaCl to a total volume of 20 mL. Inject over at least 2 minutes."
Prepare:	_____ mL Tagamet
Dilute with:	_____ mL 0.9% NaCl for a total of 20 mL of solution
Administer:	_____ mL/15 sec

Continuous Intravenous Infusions

Continuous IV infusions replace or maintain fluids and electrolytes and serve as a vehicle for medication administration. IV fluids can be supplied in plastic solution bags or glass bottles with the volume of the IV fluid container typically varying from 50 mL to 1000 mL (**Figure 14-1**). Some IV bags may even contain more than 1000 mL. Solutions used for total parenteral nutrition usually contain 2000 mL or more in a single bag. The IV solution bag or bottle will be labeled with the exact components and amount of the IV solution. Pharmacy technicians often use abbreviations when

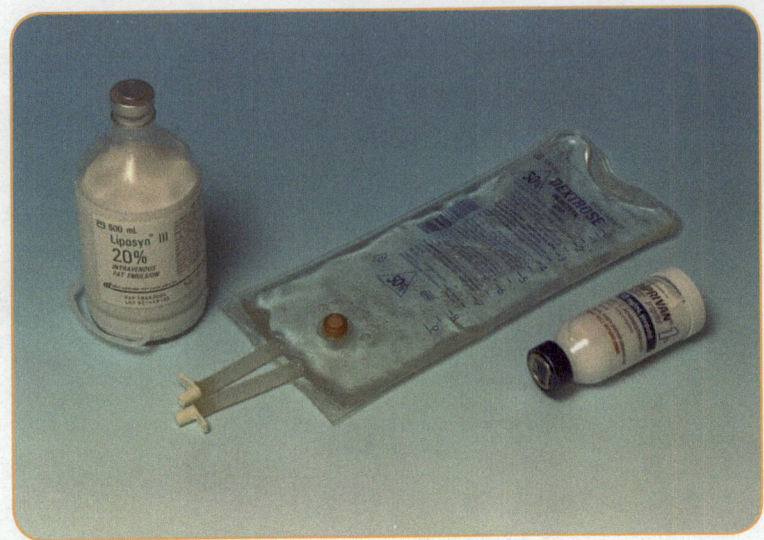

Figure 14-1 IV solutions come in various sizes.
© Cengage Learning 2013

communicating about the IV solution. Therefore, it is important for the technicians to know the common IV solution components and the solution concentration represented by such abbreviations (**Table 14–1**).

Table 14-1 Common IV Components and Solutions

Abbreviation	Solution	Component
D_5W	Dextrose 5% in water	5% dextrose
D_5NS	Dextrose 5% in normal saline	5% dextrose in 0.9% sodium chloride
$D_5 \frac{1}{2} NS$	Dextrose 5% in 0.45% normal saline	5% dextrose in 0.45% sodium chloride
NS	Normal saline 0.9%	0.9% sodium chloride
½ NS	Normal saline 0.45%	0.45% sodium chloride
LR, RL, RLS	Lactated Ringer's solution, Ringer's lactated solution	Electrolytes

■ **Example 1:**

Suppose an order includes D_5W, which is dextrose 5% in water. and it is supplied as 5% dextrose injection (**Figure 14-2**). This means that the solution strength of the solute (dextrose) is 5%. The solvent is water. Read the IV bag label and notice that "each 100 mL contains 5 g dextrose . . ." For every 100 mL of solution, there are 5 g of dextrose.

Chapter 14 • Intravenous Flow Rate Calculations 245

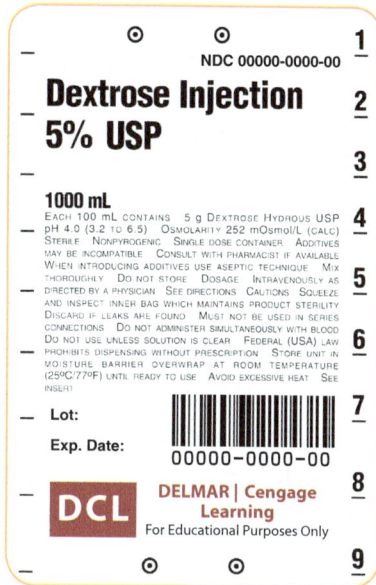

Figure 14-2 Dextrose Injection 5% USP.
© Cengage Learning 2013

■ **Example 2:**

Suppose a physician writes D₅LR on the prescription. This abbreviation means dextrose 5% in lactated Ringer's and is supplied as a lactated Ringer's and 5% dextrose injection, as shown in **Figure 14-3**.

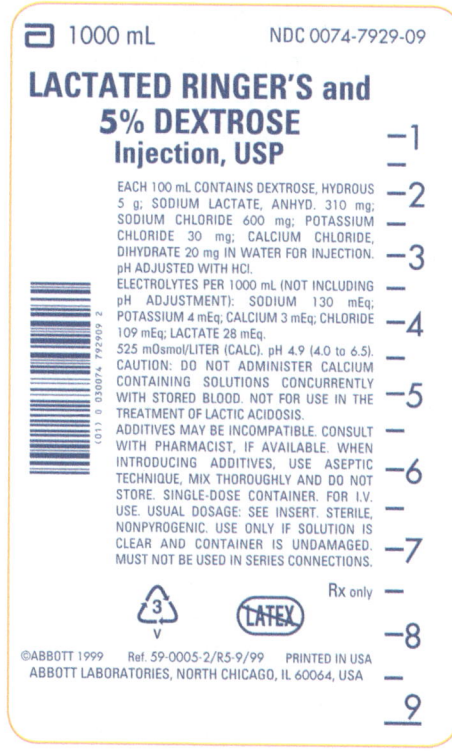

Figure 14-3 D₅LR.
Courtesy of Abbott Laboratories

Example 3:

A physician orders D₅NS 1000 mL IV q8h. This order is translated as "administer 1000 mL of 5% dextrose in normal saline intravenously every 8 hours." It is supplied as 5% dextrose and 0.9% sodium chloride. The common term for 0.9% sodium chloride is *normal saline* (also known as *physiologic saline*). In normal saline, the concentration of sodium chloride is 0.9 g (which is equal to 900 mg) per 100 mL of solution.

Solution Additives

In some cases, electrolytes, nutrients, and medications can be added and mixed with IV solutions. Antibiotics, potassium chloride, and water-soluble vitamins such as B and C are common additives. If additives are not prepackaged in the solution, the pharmacy technician needs to mix the additive and IV solution. The prescriber's order will explain how much additive is to be given, the amount and type of basic IV solution to use, and how long it should be infused.

Example 4:

The physician orders *D₅NS 20 mEq KCl/L*. This means to add 20 milliequivalents of potassium chloride per liter of 5% dextrose and 0.9% sodium chloride IV solution.

Stop and Review
Intravenous Solutions and Additives

1. For each of the following IV solutions labeled "a" through "h", specify the letter of the illustration corresponding to the fluid abbreviation, list the solute(s) of each solution and identify the strength (g/mL) of each solute, and identify the osmolarity (mOsm/L) of each solution.

	Letter of Matching Illustration	Components and Strength	Osmolarity (mOsm/L)
a. NS	_____	_____	_____
b. D₅W	_____	_____	_____
c. D₅NS	_____	_____	_____
d. D₅ $\frac{1}{2}$ NS	_____	_____	_____
e. D₅ $\frac{1}{4}$ NS	_____	_____	_____
f. D₅LR	_____	_____	_____
g. D₅ $\frac{1}{2}$ NS	_____	_____	_____
h. $\frac{1}{2}$ NS	_____	_____	_____

Chapter 14 • Intravenous Flow Rate Calculations   247

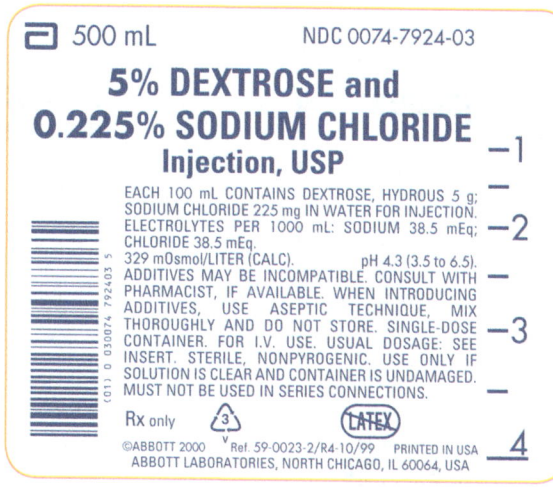

Label A

5% Dextrose and sodium chloride.
Courtesy of Abbott Laboratories

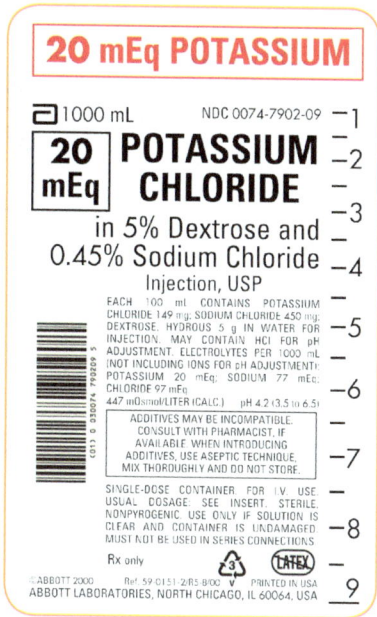

Label B

20 mEq Potassium Chloride.
Courtesy of Abbott Laboratories

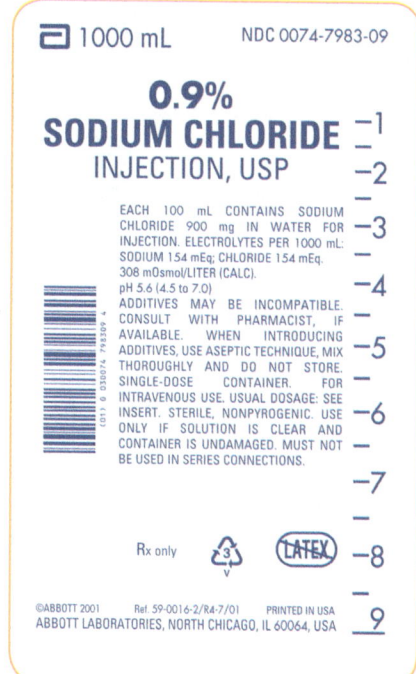

Label C

0.9% Sodium Chloride.
Courtesy of Abbott Laboratories

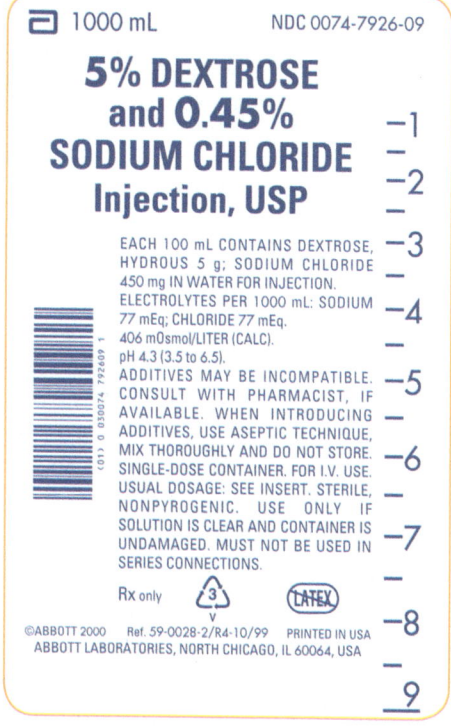

Label D

5% Dextrose and 0.45% Sodium Chloride.
Courtesy of Abbott Laboratories

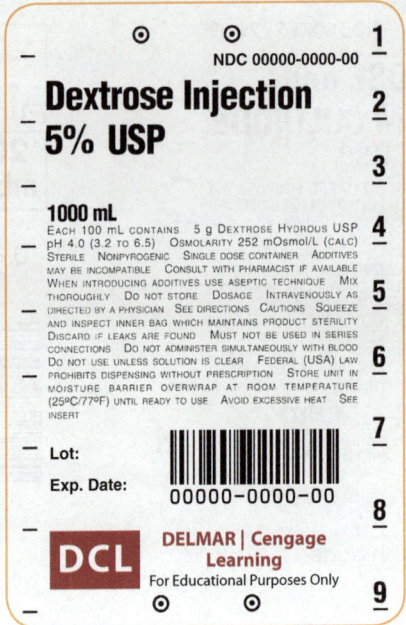

Label E

Dextrose Injection 5% USP.
© Cengage Learning 2013

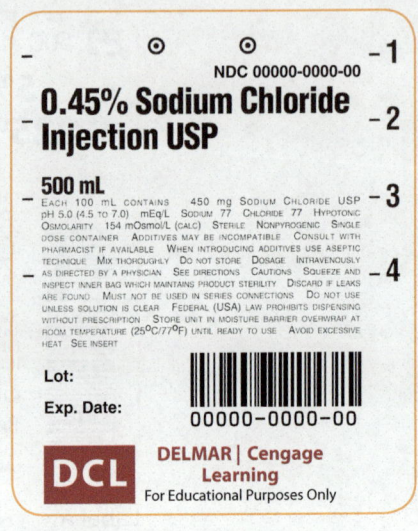

Label F

0.45% Sodium Chloride Injection.
© Cengage Learning 2013

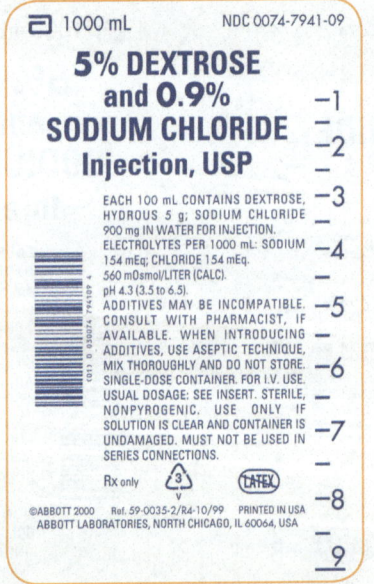

Label G

5% Dextrose and 0.9% Sodium Chloride.
Courtesy of Abbott Laboratories

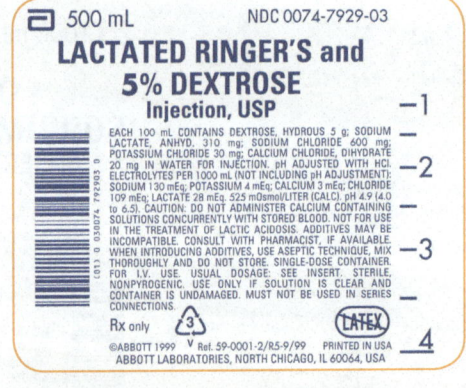

Label H

Lactated Ringer's and 5% Dextrose.
Courtesy of Abbott Laboratories

Percentage in IV Fluids

Because the term *percentage* means "grams of drug per 100 mL of fluid," a 5% dextrose solution has 5 grams of dextrose in each 100 mL of solution. Therefore, a 500 mL bag of a 5% solution contains 25 grams of dextrose. Likewise, a 500 mL bag of a 10% solution contains 50 grams of dextrose. All ingredients in any bag of solution are listed on the IV label. It is important to remember that percentages make IV fluids extremely different from each other. It is critical to read labels carefully and make sure that each IV is administered exactly as ordered.

Parenteral Nutrition

When a patient cannot eat normally, nutrients can be administered via a central vein. This is called *parenteral nutrition*. In general, parenteral nutrition solutions have high caloric content and various amounts of amino acids, glucose, and (sometimes) fat emulsions. Common types of parenteral nutrition include the following:

- Total parenteral nutrition (TPN)
- Partial parenteral nutrition (PPN)
- Hyperalimentation (nutrition that is in excess of maintenance needs)

Solutions that contain lipids appear opaque white and are usually infused slowly over a period of less than 24 hours. This is because they can become physically unstable and support bacterial growth if infused over 24 hours or longer. General intravenous administration precautions apply to parenteral nutrition, but greater care must be taken to prevent infection. These solutions are infused similarly to other IV solutions, with similar flow rates and infusion times.

Calculating IV Components as Percentages

The concept of calculating components of an IV solution by expressing them as a percentage is important because it helps in understanding that IV solutions provide much more than fluid. They also provide other components.

■ Example 1:

Ordered: D_5W 1000 mL

Calculate the amount of dextrose in 1000 mL D_5W. This can be calculated using ratio and proportion. Recall that % indicates g per 100 mL; therefore, 5% dextrose is 5 g dextrose per 100 mL of solution.

$$\frac{5 \text{ g}}{100 \text{ mL}} = \frac{X \text{ g}}{1000 \text{ mL}}$$

$$100X = 5000$$

$$X = \frac{5000}{100} = 50 \text{ g}$$

Example 2:

Ordered: $D_5\frac{1}{4}NS\ 500\ mL$

Calculate the amount of dextrose and sodium chloride in 500 mL.

$$\frac{5\ g}{100\ mL} = \frac{X\ g}{500\ mL}$$

$$100X = 2500$$

$$X = \frac{2500}{100} = 25\ g\ \text{dextrose}$$

$\frac{1}{4}$ NS = 0.225% NaCl = 0.225 g NaCl per 100 mL

Recall that NS, or normal saline, is 0.9% NaCl; therefore, $\frac{1}{2}$ NS is 0.45% NaCl, and $\frac{1}{4}$ NS is 0.225% NaCl.

$$\frac{0.225\ g}{100\ mL} = \frac{X\ g}{500\ mL}$$

$$100X = 112.5$$

$$X = 1.125\ g\ NaCl$$

500 mL $D_5\frac{1}{4}$ NS contains 25 g dextrose and 1.125 g sodium chloride.

Stop and Review
Calculating IVs as Percentages

1. Calculate the amount of dextrose and/or sodium chloride in each of the following IV solutions.

    a. 250 mL of NS

    sodium chloride _____ g

    b. 3 L of D_5NS

    dextrose _____ g

    sodium chloride _____ g

    c. 500 mL of D_5 0.33% NaCl

    dextrose _____ g

    sodium chloride _____ g

    d. 250 mL of $D_{10}W$

    dextrose _____ g

    e. 1000 mL of D_5NS

    dextrose _____ g

    sodium chloride _____ g

f. 750 mL of NS

sodium chloride _____ g

g. 0.75 L of 0.45% NaCl

sodium chloride _____ g

h. 300 mL of D_{12} 0.9% NaCl

dextrose _____ g

sodium chloride _____ g

i. 500 mL of $D_5 \frac{1}{2}$ NS

dextrose _____ g

sodium chloride _____ g

j. 0.5 L of $D_{10} \frac{1}{4}$ NS

dextrose _____ g

sodium chloride _____ g

Calculating IV Flow Rates

Intravenous fluids are administered via an intravenous infusion set. This primary line usually includes the sealed bottle or bag containing the fluids, a drip chamber connected to the bag or bottle by a small tube or spike, a roller clamp, and tubing that leads from the roller clamp down to and connecting with the needle or catheter at the site of insertion into the patient (**Figure 14-4**).

The nurse can regulate the rate either by using the roller clamp or by placing the tubing in an electronic infusion pump. Another type of IV tubing (the secondary intravenous tubing) is used when medications are administered by "piggybacking" into the primary line (**Figure 14-5**).

IV fluids are usually ordered for a certain volume to run for a stated period of time, such as *125 mL/h* or *1000 mL/8h*. The nurse may use electronic or manual regulating equipment to monitor the flow rate. The calculations performed to set the flow rate will depend on the equipment used to administer the IV solutions. It is important to note that in most settings, nurses will use IV pumps and not gravity-fed tubing.

The infusion of intravenous fluids is monitored in many different ways. Most times, for manual regulation, the bag containing the intravenous solution is hung 36 inches above the patient's heart so that gravity will draw the fluid into the patient. When the infusion is regulated, the roller clamp is used to adjust the rate of delivery. Therefore, the nurse manually regulates the IV rate. To calculate the ordered IV rate based on a certain number of drops

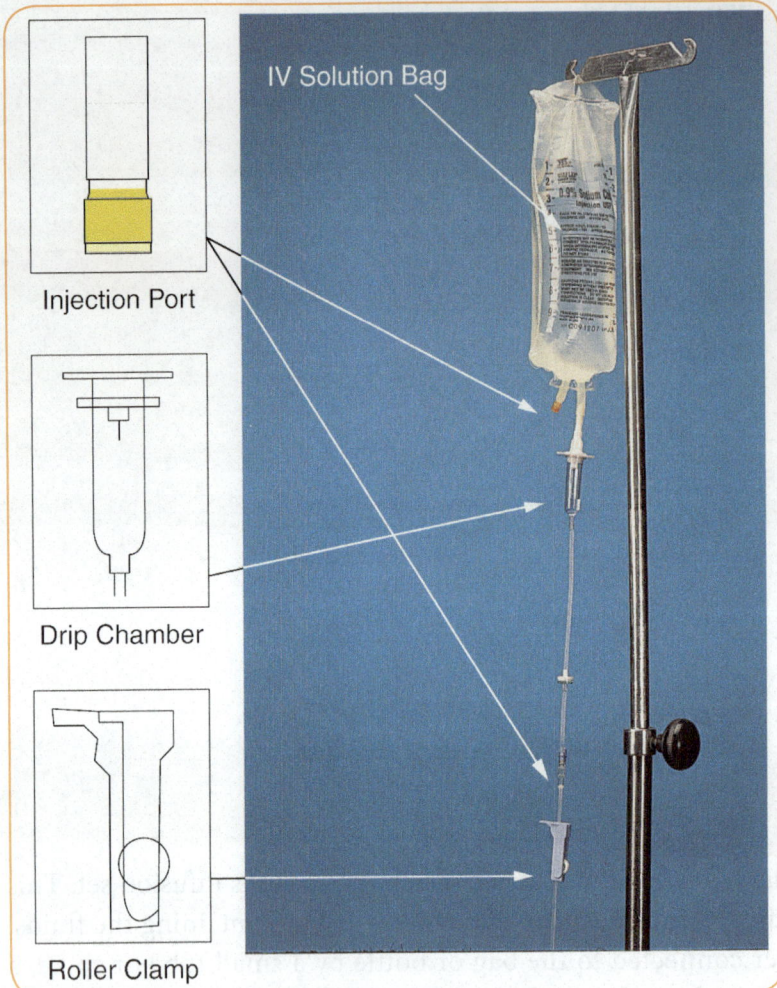

Figure 14-4 Standard IV set-up.
© Cengage Learning 2013

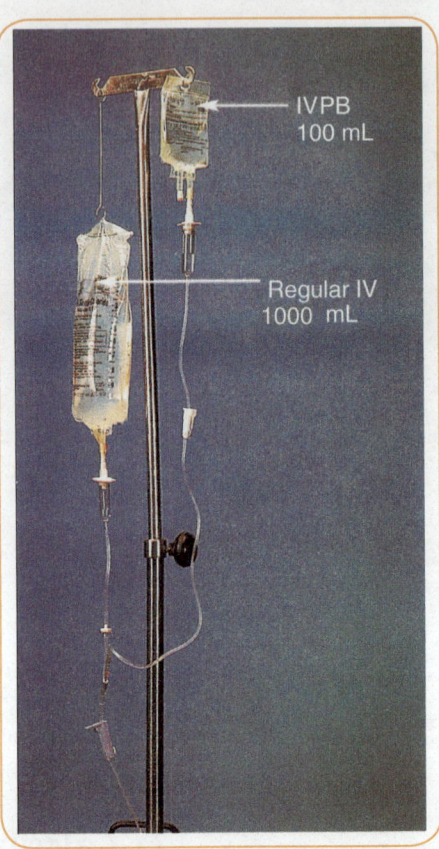

Figure 14-5 Piggyback IV set-up.
© Cengage Learning 2013

per minute (gtt/min), understand that this actually represents the ordered milliliters per hour. For calculating flow rate manually, you must count the number of drops falling into the drip chamber while holding a watch next to the drip chamber, to see how many drops fall in one minute (gtt/min). The number of drops dripping per minute into the IV drip chamber are controlled and counted by opening and closing the roller clamp. The drop factor is the number of drops per milliliter (gtt/mL) that a particular IV tubing set will deliver. It is written on the IV tubing package (**Figure 14-6**) and varies according to the manufacturer of the IV equipment. Standard or macrodrop IV tubing sets have a drop factor of 10, 15, or 20 gtt/mL. All microdrip IV tubing has a drop factor of 60 gtt/mL.

Figure 14-7 compares macrodrops and microdrops. **Figure 14-8** illustrates the size and number of drops in 1 mL for each drop factor. Notice that the fewer the number of drops per milliliter, the larger the actual drop size.

Chapter 14 • Intravenous Flow Rate Calculations 253

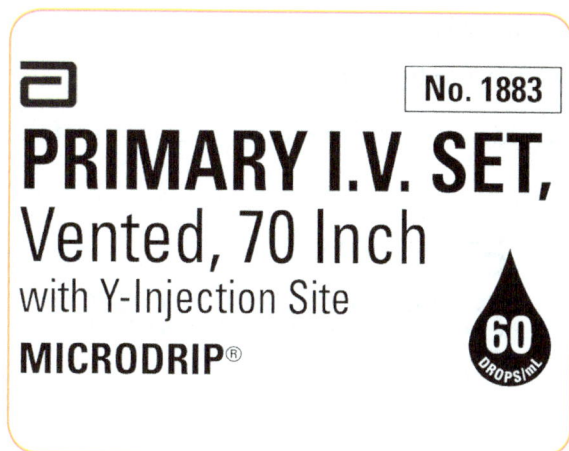

Figure 14-6 Primary intravenous infusion set.
Courtesy of Abbott Laboratories

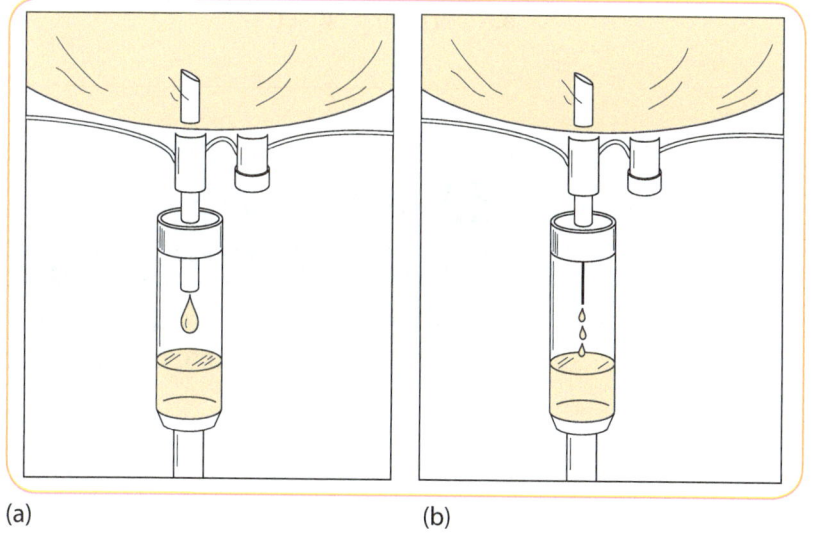

Figure 14-7 Intravenous drip chambers: (a) macrodrops; (b) microdrops.
© Cengage Learning 2013

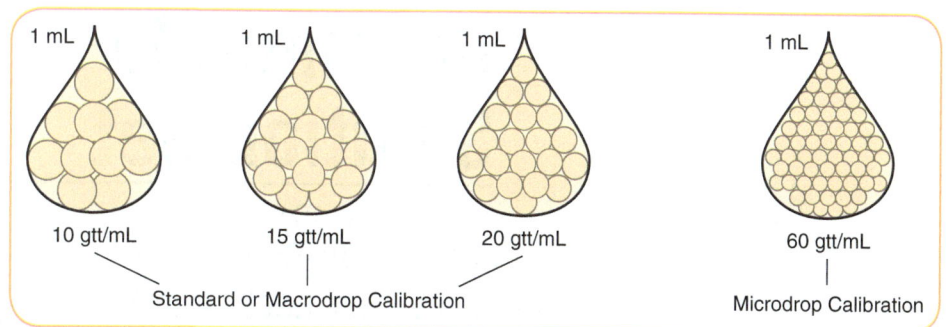

Figure 14-8 Comparison of calibrated drop factors.
© Cengage Learning 2013

Stop and Review
Calculating IV Flow Rates

1. Identify the drop factor calibration of the IV tubing pictured.

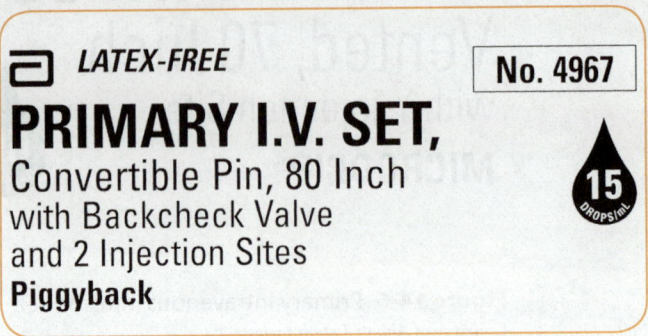

Courtesy of Abbott Laboratories

a. Primary IV set

_____

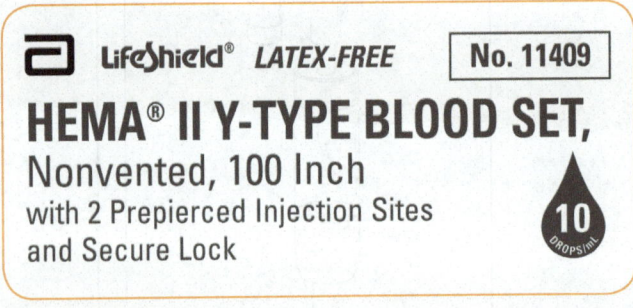

Courtesy of Abbott Laboratories

b. Hema II Y-type blood set

_____

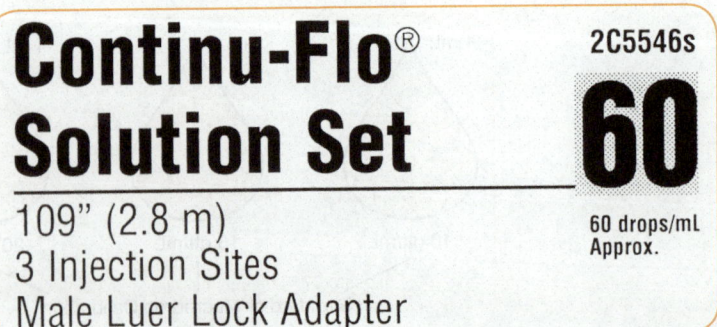

Courtesy of Abbott Laboratories

c. Continu-Flo

_____

Chapter 14 • Intravenous Flow Rate Calculations   255

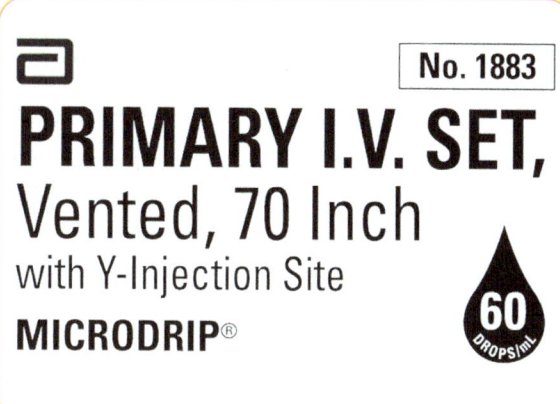

Courtesy of Abbott Laboratories

d. Primary IV set

Continu-Flo® Solution Set with DUO-VENT Spike
2C5541s
105" (2.7 m)
3 Injection Sites
Male Luer Lock Adapter
10
10 drops/mL
Approx.

Courtesy of Baxter Healthcare Corporation

e. Continu-Flo solution set

Calculating Flow Rates Using Ratio and Proportion

In this procedure, the flow rate is calculated in drops per minute (gtt/min) from the gtt/mL calibration of the required IV set. This is either 10, 15, 20, or 60 gtt/mL, with a specified order of milliliters per hour (mL/hr).

■ **Example 3:**

An IV is ordered to infuse at a rate of 125 mL/hr. The IV set is calibrated at 10 gtt/mL. What is the gtt/min flow rate?

First, convert the 125 mL/hr ordered to mL/min. This is done by dividing 125 mL by 60 minutes, which gives you approximately 2 mL/min.

Then calculate the gtt/min rate for 2 mL/min. Enter the 10 gtt/mL set calibration as the first ratio in this proportion. The X gtt in 2 mL is then entered:

$$\frac{10 \text{ gtt}}{1 \text{ mL}} = \frac{X \text{ gtt}}{2 \text{ mL}} = 20 \text{ gtt}$$

This is the same as the following:

$$10 \text{ gtt} : 1 \text{ mL} = X \text{ gtt} : 2 \text{ mL}$$

This also gives you the answer of X = 20 gtt.

Therefore, to infuse an IV at 125 mL/hr using a 10 gtt/mL calibrated set, you should set the drip rate at 20 gtt/min.

■ Example 4:

If an IV of 150 mL must be infused over 1 hour using an IV set calibrated at 15 gtt/mL, calculate the gtt/min flow rate.

First, convert the 150 mL/hr to mL/min. To do this, divide 150 mL by 60 minutes, which gives you 2.5 mL/min.

Then calculate the gtt/min rate for 2.5 mL/min as follows:

$$\frac{15 \text{ gtt}}{1 \text{ mL}} = \frac{X \text{ gtt}}{2.5 \text{ mL}} = 37.5 = 38 \text{ gtt}$$

This is the same as the following:

$$15 \text{ gtt} : 1 \text{ mL} = X \text{ gtt} : 2.5 \text{ mL}$$

The same answer is achieved:

$$X = 37.5 \text{ or } 38 \text{ gtt}$$

So, to infuse 150 mL/hr using a set calibrated at 15 gtt/mL, set the drip rate at 38 gtt/min.

■ Example 5:

An IV of 2500 mL must be infused over 24 hours using a 20 gtt/mL calibrated set. What is the gtt/min flow rate?

First, convert 2500 mL/24 hr to mL/hr:

$$2500 \text{ mL} \div 24 \text{ hr} = 104.1 = 104 \text{ mL/hr}$$

Convert 104 mL/hr to mL/min:

$$104 \text{ mL} \div 60 \text{ min} = 1.73 = 1.7 \text{ mL/min}$$

Calculate the gtt/min rate for 1.7 mL/min:

$$\frac{20 \text{ gtt}}{1 \text{ mL}} = \frac{X \text{ gtt}}{1.7 \text{ mL}} = 34 \text{ gtt}$$

Or:

$$20 \text{ gtt} : 1 \text{ mL} = X \text{ gtt} : 1.7 \text{ mL}$$

$$X = 34 \text{ gtt}$$

Therefore, to infuse an IV of 2500 mL in 24 hr using an IV set calibrated at 20 gtt/mL, set the flow rate at 34 gtt/min.

■ Example 6:

1000 mL must be infused IV over 5 hr using an IV set calibrated at 15 gtt/mL.

Convert 1000 mL/5 hr to mL/hr:

$$1000 \text{ mL} \div 5 \text{ hr} = 200 \text{ mL/hr}$$

Convert 200 mL/hr to mL/min:

$$200 \text{ mL} \div 60 \text{ min} = 3.3 \text{ mL/min}$$

Calculate the gtt/min rate for 3.3 mL/min:

$$\frac{15 \text{ gtt}}{1 \text{ mL}} = \frac{X \text{ gtt}}{3.3 \text{ mL}} = 49.5 \text{ (or 50) gtt}$$

Or:

$$15 \text{ gtt} : 1 \text{ mL} = X \text{ gtt} : 3.3 \text{ mL}$$

$$X = 49.5 = 50 \text{ gtt}$$

Therefore, to infuse 1000 mL in 5 hr using a set calibrated at 15 gtt/mL, set the rate at 50 gtt/min.

Stop and Review
Calculating gtt/min Flow Rates

1. A nurse starts to infuse an IV of 2000 mL in 12 hr using a 10 gtt/mL set.

   How many gtt/min should be given? _____

2. A physician orders an infusion of 500 mL in 3 hr using a 15 gtt/mL set.

   How many gtt/min should be given? _____

3. If an IV of 750 mL is ordered to infuse in 8 hr on a 10 gtt/mL set, how many gtt/min should be given? _____

4. A practitioner ordered 3000 mL volume to be infused in 24 hr on a set calibrated at 20 gtt/mL.

   How many gtt/min should be given? _____

5. A physician ordered 3500 mL to be infused in 24 hr using a set calibrated at 20 gtt/mL.

   How many gtt/min should be given? _____

6. 1500 mL must be infused in 5 hr using a 15 gtt/mL set.

   How many gtt/min should be given? _____

Calculating Flow Rates Using Dimensional Analysis

In dimensional analysis, calculations include two values: drops (gtt) and minutes (min), as follows.

■ **Example 7:**

Calculate a gtt/min flow rate for the infusion of 125 mL/hr using an IV set calibrated at 10 gtt/mL.

First, enter the gtt/min to be calculated as a common fraction:

$$\frac{gtt}{min}$$

Begin ratio entries as in calculating only the gtt numerator. Find the ratio containing gtt (the 10 gtt/mL set calibration). Enter 10 gtt as the numerator to match the gtt numerator being calculated. Therefore, 1 mL becomes the denominator:

$$\frac{gtt}{min} = \frac{10\ gtt}{1\ mL}$$

Match the mL denominator with the 125 mL (of the 125 mL/hr ordered). Therefore, 1 hr becomes the denominator:

$$\frac{gtt}{min} = \frac{10\ gtt}{1\ mL} \times \frac{125\ mL}{1\ hr}$$

A conversion ratio can then be entered, showing that 1 hr equals 60 minutes. The numerator will be 1 hr and the denominator will be 60 min. Notice that the minutes being calculated is easily placed as the final denominator of this equation:

$$\frac{gtt}{min} = \frac{10\ gtt}{1\ mL} \times \frac{125\ mL}{1\ hr} \times \frac{1\ hr}{60\ min}$$

Cross-multiply to cancel out the mL and hr in the equation. Do the math.

This results in 1250 divided by 60 = 20.8 or 21 gtt/min.

Therefore, to infuse 125 mL/hr using a 10 gtt/mL infusion set, the flow rate is 21 gtt/min.

■ **Example 8:**

To infuse 90 mL/hr, a 20 gtt/mL set is to be used. What is the gtt/min flow rate?

$$\frac{gtt}{min} = \frac{20\ gtt}{1\ mL}$$

$$\frac{gtt}{min} = \frac{20\ gtt}{1\ mL} \times \frac{90\ mL}{1\ hr}$$

$$\frac{gtt}{min} = \frac{20\ gtt}{1\ mL} \times \frac{90\ mL}{1\ hr} \times \frac{1\ hr}{60\ min}$$

After cancelling out the mL and hr, you find that:

1800 divided by 60 = 30 gtt/min

Therefore, to infuse 90 mL/hr using a 20 gtt/mL set, the rate is 30 gtt/min.

Stop and Review
Calculating gtt/min Flow Rates Using Dimensional Analysis

1. An order of 1250 mL must be infused in 12 hr using a 15 gtt/mL set.

   How many gtt/min should be given? _____

2. A physician ordered an IV of 2500 mL to be infused in 18 hr on a set calibrated at 10 gtt/mL.

   How many gtt/min should be given? _____

3. An order of 1000 mL must be infused in 6 hr using a 5 gtt/mL set.

   How many gtt/min should be given? _____

4. An order of 2750 mL must be infused in 22 hr on a 15 gtt/mL set.

   How many gtt/min should be given? _____

5. A physician ordered 500 mL in 3 hr using a 15 gtt/mL set.

   How many gtt/min should be given? _____

6. An IV of 1000 mL must be infused in 6 hr using a 10 gtt/mL set.

   How many gtt/min should be given? _____

Calculating Flow Rates Using the Formula Method

The formula method is used to determine the flow rate in drops per minute (gtt/min).

$$\frac{V}{T} \times C = R$$

$$\frac{\text{Volume (mL)}}{\text{Time (min)}} \times \text{Calibration or drop factor (gtt/mL)}$$

$$= \text{Rate (gtt/min)}$$

In this formula:
V = volume per hour to be infused in mL ordered by the prescriber
T = time converted to minutes ordered by the prescriber
C = calibration of tubing (drop factor) in gtt/mL
R = rate of the flow in gtt/min

■ **Example 9:**

The prescriber orders 1000 mL to be infused over 8 hours, with a drip factor of 30 gtt/mL. First, determine the mL/hour. 1000 mL/8 hours = 125 mL per hour. Then use this formula:

$$\frac{\text{mL/hour} \times \text{gtt/mL}}{60 \text{ minutes}}$$

Therefore,

$$\frac{125 \text{ mL/h} \times 30 \text{ gtt/mL}}{60 \text{ minutes}} = \frac{3750}{60}$$

$$= 62.5 \text{ gtt/min}$$

■ **Example 10:**

The physician orders 500 mL to be infused over 24 hours, with a drip factor of 60 gtt/mL.

$$\frac{500 \text{ mL}}{24 \text{ hours}} = 20.8 \text{ mL per hour}$$

$$\frac{20.8 \text{ mL/hr} \times 60 \text{ gtt/mL}}{60 \text{ minutes}} = \frac{1248}{60}$$

$$= 20.8 \text{ gtt/min}$$

(may be rounded to 21 drops per minute)

■ **Example 11:**

The physician orders 250 mL to be infused over 3 hours, with a drip factor of 15 gtt/mL. 250 mL/3 hours = 83.3 mL per hour

$$\frac{83.3 \text{ mL/hr} \times 15 \text{ gtt/mL}}{60 \text{ minutes}} = \frac{1249.5}{60}$$

= 20.8 gtt/min (rounded up to 21 gtt/min)

■ **Example 12:**

The prescriber orders 350 mL to be infused over 4 hours, with a drip factor of 8 gtt/mL. 350 mL/4 hours = 87.5 mL per hour

$$\frac{87.5 \text{ mL/hr} \times 8 \text{ gtt/mL}}{60 \text{ minutes}} = \frac{700}{60}$$

= 11.7 gtt/min (rounded to 12 gtt/min)

Stop and Review
Manually Calculating IV Flow Rates Using the Formula Method

1. Calculate the flow rate or watch count in gtt/min.

a. Ordered:	D_5NS IV at 150 mL/hr
Drop factor:	20 gtt/mL
Flow rate:	_____ gtt/min

b. Ordered:	3500 mL D$_5$LR IV to run at 160 mL/h
Drop factor:	15 gtt/mL
Flow rate:	_____ gtt/min
c. Ordered:	80 mL D$_5$W antibiotic solution IV to infuse in 60 min
Drop factor:	60 gtt/mL
Flow rate:	_____ gtt/min
d. Ordered:	250 mL LR IV at 50 mL/hr
Drop factor:	60 gtt/mL
Flow rate:	_____ gtt/min
e. Ordered:	480 mL packed red blood cells IV to infuse in 4 hours
Drop factor:	10 gtt/mL
Flow rate:	_____ gtt/min
f. Ordered:	2500 mL LR IV at 165 mL/hr
Drop factor:	20 gtt/mL
Flow rate:	_____ gtt/min
g. Ordered:	100 mL NS bolus IV to infuse in 60 min
Drop factor:	20 gtt/mL
Flow rate:	_____ gtt/min
h. Ordered:	Two 500 mL units of whole blood IV to be infused in 4 hours. Infusion set is calibrated to 20 drops per milliliter.
Flow rate:	_____ gtt/min

Calculating Flow Rates Using the Shortcut Method

This method is used when converting the volume and time in the formula method to mL/hr (or mL/60 min) to use as a shortcut for calculating flow rate.

■ Example 13:

Dr. Smith has ordered 125 mL/hr IV with a 20 gtt/mL infusion set. You can calculate this example using the following formula:

$$\frac{125 \text{ mL}}{60 \text{ min}} \times 20 \text{ gtt/mL} = \frac{125 \text{ gtt}}{3 \text{ min}}$$

$$= 41.7 \text{ gtt/min} = 42 \text{ gtt/min}$$

■ Example 14:

Ordered: *Normal saline 1000 mL IV at 125 mL/hr with a microdrop infusion set calibrated for 60 gtt/mL.*

Use the formula:

$$\frac{V}{T} \times C = R$$

$$\frac{125 \text{ mL}}{60 \text{ min}} \times 60 \text{ gtt/mL} = \frac{125 \text{ gtt}}{1 \text{ min}}$$

$$= 125 \text{ gtt/min}$$

Stop and Review

Manually Calculating IV Flow Rates Using the Shortcut Method

1. Calculate the IV flow rate in gtt/min using the shortcut method.

a. Ordered:	650 mL D_5 0.33% NaCl IV to infuse in 10 hr
Drop factor:	10 gtt/mL
Flow rate:	_____ gtt/min
b. Ordered:	500 mL D_5W 0.45% saline IV to infuse at 165 mL/hr
Drop factor:	10 gtt/mL
Flow rate:	_____ gtt/min
c. Ordered:	3 L NS IV to infuse at 125 mL/hr
Drop factor:	15 gtt/mL
Flow rate:	_____ gtt/min

d. Ordered:	400 mL D₅W IV to infuse at 50 mL/hr
Drop factor:	10 gtt/mL
Flow rate:	_____ gtt/min
e. Ordered:	0.5 L 0.45% NaCl IV to infuse in 20 hr
Drop factor:	60 gtt/mL
Flow rate:	_____ gtt/min
f. Ordered:	1000 mL D₅W IV to infuse at 200 mL/hr
Drop factor:	15 gtt/mL
Flow rate:	_____ gtt/min
g. Ordered:	2L NS IV to infuse at 60 mL/hr with microdrop infusion set of 60 gtt/mL
Flow rate:	_____ gtt/min
h. Ordered:	500 mL D₅LR to infuse in 6 hr
Drop factor:	20 gtt/mL
Flow rate:	_____ gtt/min

Adjusting IV Flow Rates

When medicines are added with IV fluids, the rate of flow must be carefully calculated, and close observation at regular intervals must be conducted. Various situations such as gravity, condition, and movement of the patient can alter the set flow rate of an IV, causing the IV to run ahead of or behind schedule. Therefore, the flow rate per minute may be adjusted by up to 25% more or less than the original rate, depending on the condition of the patient. In such cases, assess the patient. If the patient is stable, recalculate the flow rate to administer the total milliliters remaining over the number of hours remaining of the original order. If the patient is not stable, the physician must assess the rate of flow of IV fluids.

Use the following formula to recalculate the mL/hr and gtt/min for the time remaining and the percentage of variation.

First:
$$\text{Recalculated mL/hr} = \frac{\text{Remaining volume}}{\text{Remaining hours}}.$$

Then:
$$\frac{V}{T} \times C = \text{gtt/min}$$

Last:
$$\frac{\text{Adjusted gtt/min} - \text{ordered gtt/min}}{\text{Ordered gtt/min}} = \%\ \text{variation}$$

■ Example 15:

The prescriber has ordered 500 mL LR to run over 10 hr at 50 mL/hr. The drop factor is 60 gtt/mL and the IV is correctly infusing at 50 gtt/min. After $2\frac{1}{2}$ hours, you find 300 mL remaining. Almost half of the total volume has already been infused in about one-quarter the time. This IV infusion is ahead of schedule. You would compute a new flow rate for the 300 mL to complete the IV fluid order in the remaining $7\frac{1}{2}$ hours. The patient would require close assessment for fluid overload.

Step 1.
$$\frac{\text{Remaining volume}}{\text{Remaining hours}} = \text{Recalculate mL/hr}$$

$$\frac{300\ \text{mL}}{7.5} = 40\ \text{mL/hr}$$

Step 2.
$$\frac{V}{T} \times C = \frac{40\ \text{mL}}{60\ \text{min}} \times 60\ \text{gtt/mL} = 40\ \text{gtt/min}$$

(adjusted flow rate)

Step 3.
$$\frac{\text{Adjusted gtt/min} - \text{Ordered gtt/min}}{\text{Ordered gtt/min}}$$

$$= \%\ \text{of variation}$$

$$\frac{40 - 50}{50} = \frac{-10}{50} = -0.2 = -20\%$$

within the acceptable 25% of variation

Stop and Review
Adjusting Flow Rates

1. Compute the flow rate in drops per minute. Hospital policy permits recalculation of IVs when off schedule, with a maximum variation in rate of 25% for stable patients. Compute the % of variation.

a. Ordered:	*2000 mL NS IV for 16 hr at 125 mL/hr*
Drop factor:	15 gtt/mL
Original flow rate:	_____ gtt/min
After 6 hours, 650 mL of fluid have infused. Explain your next action.	
Solution remaining:	_____ mL
Time remaining:	_____ hr
Recalculated flow rate:	_____ mL/hr
Recalculated flow rate:	_____ gtt/min
Variation:	_____ %
Action:	_____
b. Ordered:	*1000 mL D$_5$W IV for 10 hr at 100 mL/hr*
Drop factor:	60 gtt/mL
Original flow rate:	_____ gtt/min
After 5 hours, 500 mL are remaining. Explain your next action.	
Time remaining:	_____ hr
Recalculated flow rate:	_____ mL/hr
Recalculated flow rate:	_____ gtt/min
Variation:	_____ %
Action:	_____

c. Ordered:	1000 mL NS IV for 8 hr at 125 mL/hr
Drop factor:	10 gtt/mL
Original flow rate:	_____ gtt/min
After 4 hours, 750 mL are remaining. Describe your next action.	
Time remaining:	_____ hr
Recalculated flow rate:	_____ mL/hr
Recalculated flow rate:	_____ gtt/min
Variation:	_____ %
Action:	_____
d. Ordered:	500 mL DNS IV for 5 hr at 100 mL/hr
Drop factor:	20 gtt/mL
Original flow rate:	_____ gtt/min
After 2 hours, 250 mL are remaining. Describe your next action.	
Time remaining:	_____ hr
Recalculated flow rate:	_____ mL/hr
Recalculated flow rate:	_____ gtt/min
Variation:	_____ %
Action:	_____
e. Ordered:	1500 mL lactated Ringer's IV for 12 hr at 125 mL/hr
Drop factor:	20 gtt/mL
Original flow rate:	_____ gtt/min

After 6 hours, 850 mL are remaining. Explain your next action.

Time remaining:	_____ hr
Recalculated flow rate:	_____ mL/hr
Recalculated flow rate:	_____ gtt/min
Variation:	_____ %
Action:	_____
f. Ordered:	*1000 mL D_5W IV for 8 hr at 125 mL/hr*
Drop factor:	20 gtt/mL
Original flow rate:	_____ gtt/min

After 4 hours, 800 mL are remaining. Explain your next action.

Time remaining:	_____ hr
Recalculated flow rate:	_____ mL/hr
Recalculated flow rate:	_____ gtt/min
Variation:	_____ %
Action:	_____
g. Ordered:	*1 L NS IV for 20 hr at 50 mL/hr*
Drop factor:	15 gtt/mL
Original flow rate:	_____ gtt/min

After 10 hours, 600 mL are remaining. Explain your next action.	
Time remaining:	_____ hr
Recalculated flow rate:	_____ mL/hr
Recalculated flow rate:	_____ gtt/min
Variation:	_____ %
Action:	_____
h. Ordered:	*1000 mL lactated Ringer's IV for 6 hr at 167 mL/hr*
Drop factor:	15 gtt/mL
Original flow rate:	_____ gtt/min
After 4 hours, 360 mL are remaining. Describe your next action.	
Time remaining:	_____ hr
Recalculated flow rate:	_____ mL/hr
Recalculated flow rate:	_____ gtt/min
Variation:	_____ %
Action:	_____

Flow Rates for Electronic Regulation

Intravenous fluids may be monitored electronically by an infusion device, which is known as a controller or pump. The indication for an electronic infusion device is determined by the need to strictly control the IV. Manufacturers provide special volumetric tubing that must be used with their infusion devices. This volumetric tubing ensures accurate, consistent IV infusions. Each device may be set for a specific flow rate and will set off an alarm if this rate is interrupted.

Controllers depend on gravity to maintain the desired flow rate by a compression and decompression mechanism that pinches the IV tubing, rather than forcing IV fluid into the system (**Figure 14-9**). They are often

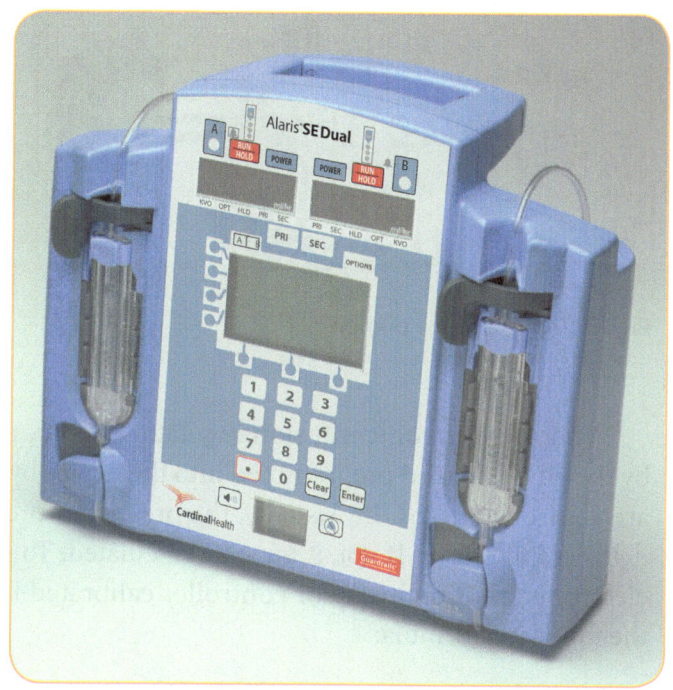

Figure 14-9 Alaris Dual Pump, a volumetric infusion Controller/Pump.
Photo courtesy of Cardinal Health, 2008. All rights reserved

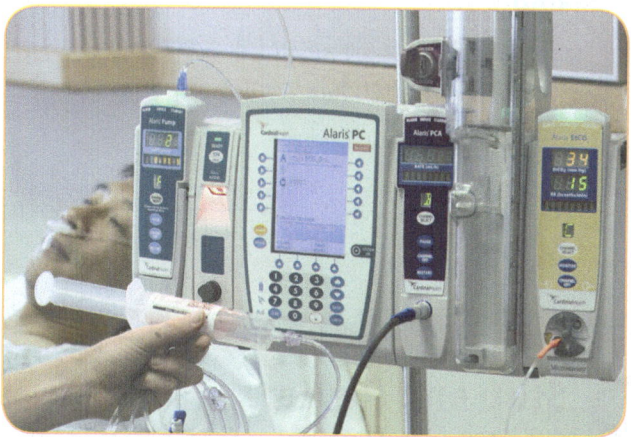

Figure 14-10 Infusion pump.
Photo courtesy of Cardinal Health, 2008. All rights reserved

referred to as electronic flow clamps because they control the selected rate of infusion by either drop counting (drops per minute) or volumetric delivery (milliliters per hour).

Infusion pumps do not rely on gravity but maintain the flow by displacing fluid at the ordered rate. Resistance to flow within the system causes positive pressure in relation to the flow rate (**Figure 14-10**).

A **syringe pump** is a kind of electronic infusion pump. It is used to infuse fluids or medications directly from a syringe. It is most often used in pediatric patients when small volumes of medication are administered at very low rates. It is also used in anesthesia, labor and delivery, and critical care when the drug cannot be mixed with other solutions or medications (**Figure 14-11**).

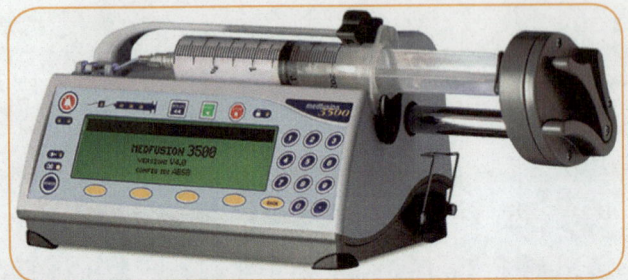

Figure 14-11 Syringe pump.
Courtesy of Smiths Medical

When an electronic infusion regulator is used, the IV volume is ordered by the physician and programmed into the device by the nurse. These devices are controlled in mL/hr. Usually, the prescriber orders the IV volume to be delivered in mL/hr. If not, it must be calculated. To regulate an IV volume by electronic infusion pump or controller calibrated in mL/hr, you should use the following formula:

$$\frac{\text{Total mL ordered}}{\text{Total hr ordered}} = \text{mL/hr}$$

■ Example 16:

Ordered: D_5W 250 mL IV over the next 2 hours by infusion pump

Use the formula:

$$\frac{\text{Total mL ordered}}{\text{Total hr ordered}} = \text{mL/hr}$$

$$\frac{250 \text{ mL}}{2 \text{ hr}} = 125 \text{ mL/1 hr}$$

Stop and Review
Calculating IV Flow Rates for Electronic Infusions

1. Calculate the flow rate that you will program the electronic infusion regulator for the following IV orders.

a. Ordered:	380 mL D_5 0.45% NaCl in 9 hr by infusion pump
Flow rate:	_____ mL/hr
b. Ordered:	150 mL antibiotic in D_5W IV in 2 hr by infusion pump
Flow rate:	_____ mL/hr

c. Ordered:	100 mL NS IV PB in 30 min by infusion pump	
Flow rate:	_____ mL/hr	
d. Ordered:	750 mL D_5W IV in 5 hr by infusion pump	
Flow rate:	_____ mL/hr	
e. Ordered:	3 L NS IV in 24 hr by controller	
Flow rate:	_____ mL/hr	
f. Ordered:	1800 mL Normal Saline IV to infuse in 15 hr by controller	
Flow rate:	_____ mL/hr	
g. Ordered:	1.5 L D_5NS IV in 12 hr by controller	
Flow rate:	_____ mL/hr	
h. Ordered:	2000 mL D_5W IV in 24 hr by controller	
Flow rate:	_____ mL/hr	

Heparin Intravenous Calculations

Heparin is commonly available in the 1000 unit (2 units per mL) strength shown in **Figure 14-12**, as well as other sizes. This label shows the drug name and its dosage strength clearly printed in red.

When a specific strength of heparin is not available, it must be prepared from a variety of available dosage strengths. The following examples refer to **Figure 14-13**, which shows four different heparin labels.

■ **Example 1:**

Using **Figure 14-13a**, determine how many mL are needed to add 20,000 units to an IV solution. Answer: _____

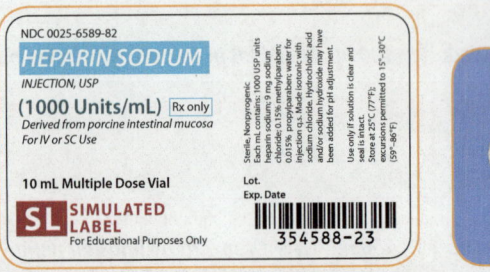
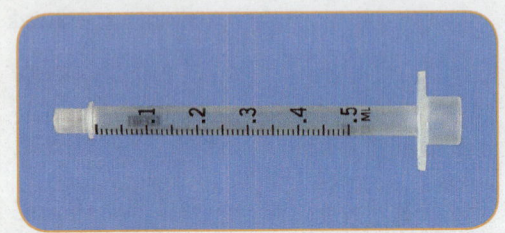

Figure 14-12 Heparin Sodium 1000 units.
© Cengage Learning 2013

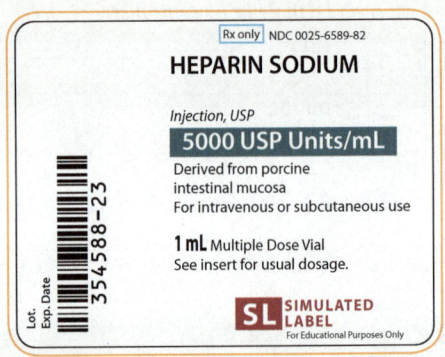
(a)

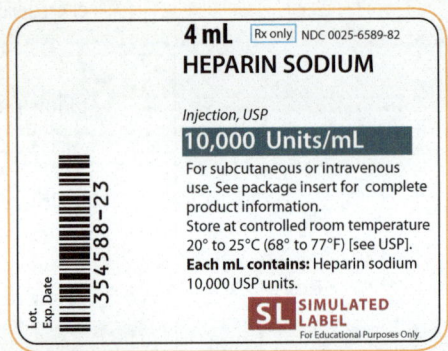
(b)

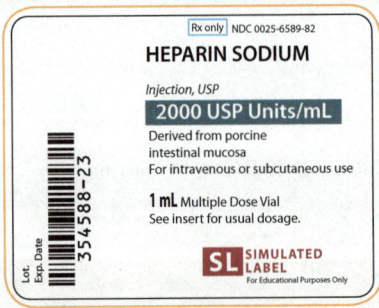
(c)

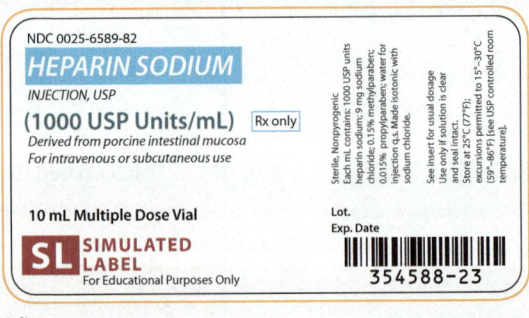
(d)

Figure 14-13 Untitled figure showing (a) Heparin Sodium 5000 USP Units/mL label, (b) Heparin Sodium 10,000 Units/mL label, (c) Heparin Sodium 2000 USP Units/mL label, and (d) Heparin Sodium 1000 USP Units/mL label. All four labels.
© Cengage Learning 2013

■ **Example 2:**

Using **Figure 14-13b**, determine how many mL are needed to add 20,000 units to an IV solution. Answer: _____

■ **Example 3:**

Using **Figure 14-13c**, determine how many mL are needed to add 12,000 units to an IV solution. Answer: _____

■ **Example 4:**

Using **Figure 14-13d**, determine how many mL are needed to add 10,000 units to an IV solution. Answer: _____

Calculating IV Flow Rate from Units per Hour Ordered

> **Remember**
>
> The mL/hr flow rate for an EID is identical to the gtt/min flow rate for a microdrip.

Heparin is usually ordered in units per hour to be administered via an electronic infusion device (EID). Therefore, calculating the flow rate in milliliters per hour (mL/hr) is usually required.

■ Example 5:

Heparin is ordered at 800 units/hr. It is on hand as 20,000 units in 1000 mL D_5W. What is the mL/hr flow rate?

$$\frac{mL}{hr} = \frac{1000\ mL}{20{,}000\ units}$$

Enter the next ratio, 800 units/hr, using units to match the denominator.

$$\frac{mL}{hr} = \frac{1000\ mL}{20{,}000\ units} \times \frac{800\ units}{1\ hr}$$

Cancel units to double-check and do the math.

$$\frac{mL}{hr} = \frac{1000\ mL}{20{,}000} \times \frac{800}{1\ hr} = 40\ mL/hr$$

A rate of 40 mL/hr is needed to infuse 800 units/hr from a solution strength of 20,000 units in 1000 mL.

■ Example 6:

Heparin is needed at 1100 units/hr from an available solution of 60,000 units in 1 L D_5W. What is the flow rate in mL/hr?

$$\frac{mL}{hr} = \frac{1000\ mL}{60{,}000\ units} \times \frac{1100\ units}{1\ hr}$$

$$\frac{mL}{hr} = \frac{1000\ mL}{60{,}000} \times \frac{1100}{1\ hr} = 18.33\ \text{(which is rounded to 18 mL/hr)}$$

Therefore, a rate of 18 mL/hr is needed to infuse 1100 units per hour from a 60,000 unit solution in 1 L solution.

■ Example 7:

Heparin must be infused at 1000 units/hr from a solution of 10,000 units in 250 mL D_5W. What is the flow rate in mL/hr?

Enter the mL/hr being calculated, and then locate the ratio containing mL (the 10,000 units/250 mL strength). This should be entered as the starting ratio with mL as the numerator, matching the mL numerator of units being calculated. Therefore, 10,000 units becomes the denominator.

$$\frac{mL}{hr} = \frac{250\ mL}{10{,}000\ units}$$

In the next numerator, the starting ratio denominator (units) must be matched. The rate ordered (1000 units/hr) is entered, with units as the numerator.

$$\frac{mL}{hr} = \frac{250\ mL}{10{,}000\ units} \times \frac{1000\ units}{1\ hr}$$

You then cancel alternate denominator/numerator units, leaving only the mL and hr. Do the math.

$$\frac{mL}{hr} = \frac{250\ mL}{10{,}000} \times \frac{1000}{1\ hr} = 25\ mL/hr$$

A rate of 25 mL/hr is needed to infuse 1000 units/hr from a solution strength of 10,000 units in 250 mL.

Stop and Review

Calculating IV Flow Rate from Units per Hour Ordered
Calculate the mL/hr flow rates.

1. The order is for 1500 units per hour of heparin from an available strength of 40,000 units in 1 L. _____

2. The order is for 50,000 units of heparin in 1 L D_5W to infuse at a rate of 2000 units per hour. _____

3. The order is for 800 units of heparin per hour from an available solution strength of 25,000 units in 500 mL NS.
_____

4. The order is for 1200 units per hour from a D_5W solution of 15,000 units in 1000 mL. _____

5. The order is for 2500 units per hour. The solution strength is 50,000 units in 1 L D_5W. _____

Calculating Units per Hour Infusing from IV Flow Rate

Another type of heparin calculation involves units/hr infusing from the mL/hr flow rate. You must use the units/mL solution strength and mL/hr rate of infusion.

■ **Example 8:**

A 500 mL IV containing 20,000 units of heparin is running at 30 mL/hr. How many units/hr are being infused?

$$\frac{units}{hr} = \frac{20{,}000\ units}{500\ mL} \times \frac{30\ mL}{1\ hr}$$

$$\frac{units}{hr} = \frac{20{,}000\ units}{500\ mL} \times \frac{30\ mL}{1\ hr} = 1200\ units/hr$$

Therefore, a 500 mL solution containing 20,000 units heparin running at 30 mL/hr is being infused at 1200 units/hr.

■ Example 9:

A 1 L solution of D_5W with 15,000 units of heparin is running at 60 mL/hr. How many units/hr are being infused?

$$\frac{\text{units}}{\text{hr}} = \frac{15,000 \text{ units}}{1000 \text{ mL}} \times \frac{60 \text{ mL}}{1 \text{ hr}}$$

$$\frac{\text{units}}{\text{hr}} = \frac{15,000 \text{ units}}{1000 \text{ mL}} \times \frac{60 \text{ mL}}{1 \text{ hr}} = 900 \text{ units/hr}$$

Therefore, a 1 L (1000 mL) solution containing 15,000 units heparin running at 60 mL/hr is being infused at 900 units/hr.

■ Example 10:

A 500 mL IV of D_5W containing 5000 units of heparin is running at 30 mL/hr. How many units/hr are being infused?

$$\frac{\text{units}}{\text{hr}} = \frac{5000 \text{ units}}{500 \text{ mL}} \times \frac{30 \text{ mL}}{1 \text{ hr}}$$

$$\frac{\text{units}}{\text{hr}} = \frac{5000 \text{ units}}{500 \text{ mL}} \times \frac{30 \text{ mL}}{1 \text{ hr}} = 300 \text{ units/hr}$$

Therefore, a 500 mL solution containing 5000 units heparin running at 30 mL/hr is being infused at 300 units/hr.

Stop and Review

Heparin Intravenous Calculations

Determine the units of heparin received per hour in the following examples.

1. A physician ordered an IV of 750 mL containing 30,000 units of heparin running at 25 mL/hr. _____

2. A physician ordered a solution of 20,000 units in 500 mL running at 30 mL/hr. _____

3. A 1 L DNS IV is needed, containing 30,000 units of heparin running at 40 mL/hr. _____

4. A 1 L DNS IV is needed, containing 20,000 units of heparin running at 30 mL/hr. _____

5. 25,000 units of heparin in a 500 mL solution must run at 30 mL/hr. _____

6. An IV containing 40,000 units of heparin in 1000 mL must run at 25 mL/hr. _____

7. A 1000 mL solution with 25,000 units heparin is running at 20 mL/hr. _____

8. A 1 L solution with 35,000 units heparin is running at 25 mL/hr. _____

9. An IV of 1 L DNS containing 20,000 units heparin is running at 20 mL/hr. _____

10. An IV of 1000 mL containing 40,000 units heparin is running at 35 mL/hr. _____

Intermittent Intravenous Injections

Intermittent intravenous infusions, such as IV piggyback and IV push, are used for IV administration of drugs and supplemental fluid. Intermittent peripheral infusion devices, also known as saline or heparin locks, are used to maintain venous access without continuous fluid infusion. In the case of a patient needing to get supplemental fluid therapy or IV medications, but not needing continuous replacement or maintenance IV fluid, intermittent IV infusion systems are generally used. These systems include IV piggyback, IV locks for IV push drugs, and volume control sets (such as Buretrol).

IV Piggybacks (IVPB)

A medication may be prescribed to be dissolved in a small amount of IV fluid, for example, 50 to 100 mL, and run "piggyback" to the regular IV fluids. Recall that the piggyback IV (or secondary IV) requires a secondary IV set.

■ **Example 1:**

Ordered: *Kefzol 500 mg in 100 mL D_5W IV PB to run over 30 min*

Drop factor: 20 gtt/mL

Determine the flow rate in gtt/min.

$$\frac{V}{T} \times C = \frac{100 \text{ mL}}{30 \text{ min}} \times 20 \text{ gtt/mL} = \frac{200 \text{ gtt}}{3}$$

$$= 66.7 \text{ gtt/min (which rounds up to 67 gtt/min)}$$

Saline and Heparin IV Locks for IV Push Drugs

IV locks are attached to the hub of the IV catheter that is situated in the vein. The lock is called a **saline lock**, meaning that saline is used to flush or maintain the IV catheter patency, or a **heparin lock** if heparin is used to maintain the IV catheter patency. These are used to ensure that the line remains open or unobstructed. Sometimes a more general term, such as **intermittent peripheral infusion device**, may be used. Medications can be given IV push, meaning that a syringe is attached to the lock and medication is pushed in. An **IV bolus**, usually a quantity of IV fluid, can be run in over a specified period of time through an IV setup that is attached to the lock.

In the majority of cases, it is easy to calculate mL/hr by dividing the total mL by the total hr. However, an IV with medication added or a piggyback IV may be prescribed to be injected in less than 1 hour by an electronic infusion device, but the pump or controller must still be set in mL/hr.

In this situation, the following formula can be used:

$$\frac{\text{Total mL ordered}}{\text{Total min ordered}} \times 60 \text{ min/hr} = \text{mL/hr}$$

■ Example 2:

Ordered: *Amoxicillin 500 mg IV in 50 mL $D_5\frac{1}{2}$NS in 30 min by controller.*

Use the following formula:

$$\frac{\text{Total mL ordered}}{\text{Total min ordered}} \times 60 \text{ min/hr} = \text{mL/hr}$$

$$\frac{50 \text{ mL}}{30 \text{ min}} \times \frac{60 \text{ min}}{1 \text{ hr}} = 100 \text{ mL/h}$$

📋 Test Your Knowledge

For the following questions, use the drop factor to calculate the flow rate in gtt/min.

Ordered:	*1000 mL 0.45% NaCl IV at 200 mL/hr*
1. Drop factor:	10 gtt/mL
Flow rate:	_____ gtt/min
2. Drop factor:	15 gtt/mL
Flow rate:	_____ gtt/min
3. Drop factor:	20 gtt/mL
Flow rate:	_____ gtt/min

Ordered:	540 mL D₅ 0.33% NaCl at 45 mL/hr
4. Drop factor:	10 gtt/mL
Flow rate:	_____ gtt/min
5. Drop factor:	15 gtt/mL
Flow rate:	_____ gtt/min
6. Drop factor:	20 gtt/mL
Flow rate:	_____ gtt/min
7. Drop factor:	60 gtt/mL
Flow rate:	_____ gtt/min
Ordered:	1 L hyperalimentation solution IV to infuse in 12 hr
8. Drop factor:	60 gtt/mL
Flow rate:	_____ gtt/min
9. Drop factor:	15 gtt/mL
Flow rate:	_____ gtt/min
10. Drop factor:	10 gtt/mL
Flow rate:	_____ gtt/min
11. Drop factor:	20 gtt/mL
Flow rate:	_____ gtt/min
Ordered:	2 L D₅NS IV to infuse in 20 hr
12. Drop factor:	20 gtt/mL
Flow rate:	_____ gtt/min

13. Drop factor:	60 gtt/mL
Flow rate:	_____ gtt/min
14. Drop factor:	10 gtt/mL
Flow rate:	_____ gtt/min
15. Drop factor:	15 gtt/mL
Flow rate:	_____ gtt/min

Complete the flow rate in drops per minute or milliliters per hour as requested. For these situations, hospital policy permits recalculating IVs when off schedule with a maximum variation in rate of 25%.

16. Ordered:	1L $D_{10}W$ IV to run from 1000 to 1800
Drop factor:	On electronic infusion pump
Flow rate:	_____ mL/hr
17. Ordered:	1000 mL D_5W IV per 24 hr
Drop factor:	60 gtt/mL
Flow rate:	_____ gtt/min
18. Ordered:	1000 mL D_5W IV for 6 hr
Drop factor:	15 gtt/mL
After 2 hours, 800 mL remain. Explain your next action. _____	
19. Ordered:	2.5 L NS IV to infuse at 125 mL/hr
Drop factor:	20 gtt/mL
Flow rate:	_____ gtt/min

20. Ordered:	*1500 mL D₅LR IV to run for 12 hr*
Drop factor:	*20 gtt/mL*
Flow rate:	_____ gtt/min

The IV tubing package in the following figure is the IV system available in your stock for manually regulated, straight gravity flow IV administration with macrodrop. The patient has an order for 500 mL D₅W IV q4h written at 1515, and you start the IV at 1530. Questions 21 through 30 refer to this situation.

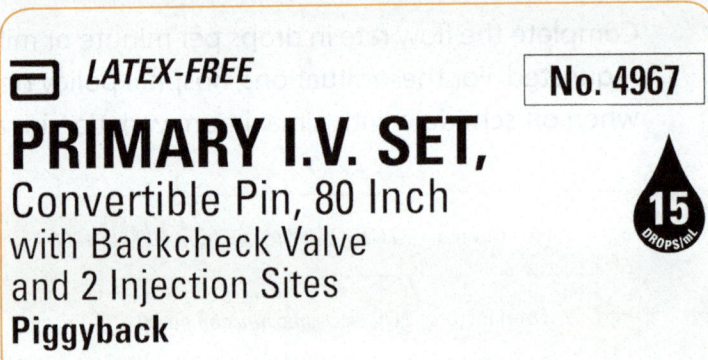

Primary I.V. Set.
Courtesy of Abbott Laboratories

21. How much IV fluid will the patient receive in 24 hours? _____

22. Who is the manufacturer of the IV infusion set tubing? _____

23. What is the drop factor calibration for the IV infusion set tubing? _____

24. What is the drop factor constant for the IV infusion set tubing? _____

25. Using the shortcut (drop factor constant) method, calculate the flow rate of the IV as ordered. Show your work.

    Shortcut method calculation: _____

    Flow rate: _____ gtt/min

26. Using the formula method, calculate the flow rate of the IV as ordered. Show your work.

    Formula method calculation: _____

    Flow rate: _____ gtt/min

27. At what time should you anticipate the first IV bag of 500 mL D$_5$W will be completely infused?

28. How much IV fluid should be infused by 1730? _____ mL

29. 100 mL of ampicillin is NS to run over 30 minutes. What is the flow rate?

30. 1600 mL of NS must be administered over 10 hours. How many mL/hour should be given?

31. 2 L of D$_5$W must be administered over 24 hours. The drop factor is 10 gtt/mL. How many drops per minute should be given?

32. 450 mL of fluid must run over 90 minutes using a tubing set to deliver 60 gtt/mL. How many drops per minute should be given?

33. 50 mL of an antibiotic must run over 30 minutes with tubing calibrated to deliver 45 gtt/mL. How many drops per minute should be given?

34. D$_5$ ½ NS is prescribed to run at 35 mL/hour with a drop factor of 60 gtt/mL. How many drops per minute should be given?

35. An IVPB of 500 mg ampicillin in 50 mL of fluid is prescribed to run at 50 gtt/minute. The drop factor is 60 gtt/mL. How long will the infusion take?

36. 2 L of D₅LR must infuse over 12 hours at 42 gtt/minute. After 6 hours, 850 mL of fluid remained. The drop factor is 30 gtt/mL. At what rate must the IV be set to complete the infusion in the original 12 hours?

37. A manually regulated IV is using a standard microdrop set (60 gtt/mL). How long will it take to infuse 150 mL of fluid to run at 30 gtt/minute?

38. 1 L of D₅W was ordered to infuse over 6 hours by infusion pump. What is the flow rate?

39. 1600 mL of D₅ ½ NS was ordered to infuse over 24 hours. What is the flow rate?

40. 1500 mL of D₅W was prescribed to be infused over 6 hours. With an IV set that delivers 10 gtt/mL, how many drops per minute should be infused?

41. 80 mL of an IVPB must run over 20 minutes with tubing calibrated to infuse 40 gtt/mL. How many drops per minute should be infused?

42. 600 mL of D₅W must be given to a patient, running at 30 gtt/minute. The drop factor of the tubing is 60 gtt/mL. How long will the infusion take?

43. Lidocaine (2 grams) was prescribed in 500 mL of fluid at 2 mg/minute, to be administered via an infusion pump. What is the flow rate?

44. A physician ordered a medication (40 mg) in 500 mL of fluid at 1 mg/minute. What is the flow rate in milliliters per hour?

45. A prescriber ordered Pentids 600,000 units in 100 mL. IVPB is to infuse over 1 hour by infusion pump, to deliver 15 gtt/mL. Calculate the flow rate in drops per minute.

46. 1 L of NS must infuse over 6 hours using tubing calibrated to deliver 20 gtt/mL. How many drops per minute should be infused?

47. A physician ordered 150 mL of an antibiotic to infuse over 30 minutes by an infusion pump. Calculate the flow rate.

48. D_5W must run at 150 mL/hour with a drop factor of 10 gtt/mL. Calculate how many drops per minute will be infused.

49. A 1000 mL solution containing 45,000 units of heparin must run at 25 mL/hr. Calculate the number of units of heparin per hour.

50. 25,000 units of heparin in a 1000 mL solution must run at 30 mL/hr. Calculate the number of units of heparin per hour.

51. A 1 L solution containing 35,000 units of heparin must run at 45 mL/hr. Calculate the number of units of heparin per hour.

52. A 500 mL solution containing 20,000 units of heparin must run at 20 mL/hr. Calculate the number of units of heparin per hour.

53. A solution of 1 L containing 25,000 units of heparin must run at 30 mL/hr. Calculate the number of units of heparin per hour.

54. A solution of 1 L of D_5W containing 30,000 units of heparin must run at 50 mL/hr. Calculate the number of units of heparin per hour.

55. Heparin 2000 units per hour is to be infused using a solution strength of 20,000 units in 500 mL. How many milliliters of heparin per hour should be infused?

56. A solution of 35,000 units of heparin in 1 L D_5W is to infuse via a volumetric pump at 1200 units/hour. How many milliliters of heparin per hour should be infused?

57. Calculate the IV flow rate for electronic regulation if the ordered medication was to be infused as 500 mL over 3 hours.

58. A 250 mL IV bag containing 25,000 of heparin is running at 18 mL/per hour. How many units per hour are being infused?

Critical Thinking

A 58-year-old hospitalized patient receives blood tests, which reveal that his potassium level is slightly decreased, at 3.1 mEq/L. The physician changes the patient's IV fluid to one liter of D_5 normal saline + 20 mEq of potassium chloride, at a rate of 75 mL/hr. The new IV fluid is prepared by the pharmacy technician for the hospital staff to use.

1. Using a drop factor of 20 gtt/mL, what is the rate in gtt/min?

2. If the physician instead ordered the same IV fluid at a rate of 100 mL/hr, what would the infusion time be?

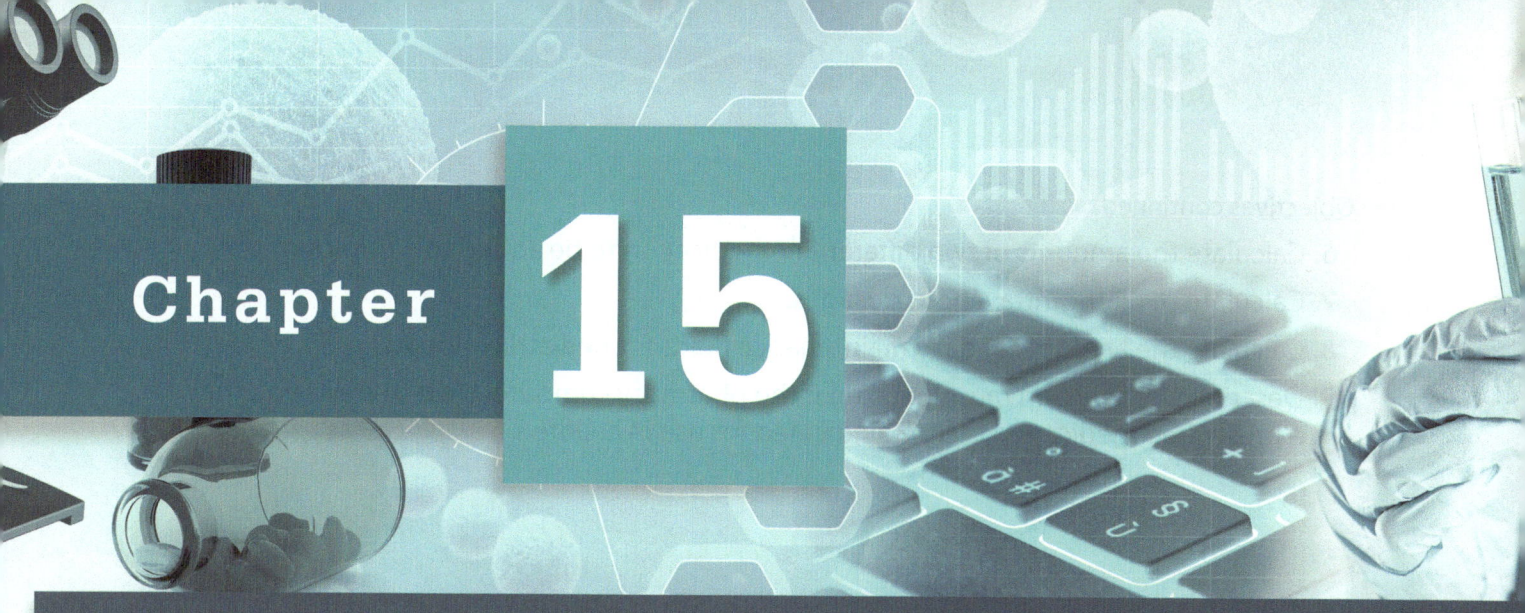

Chapter 15

Pediatric Drug Administration

Outline

Overview
Calculating Pediatric Dosages
    Body Weight Dosage Calculations
    Body Surface Area (BSA) Dosage Calculations
    Clark's Rule
    Young's Rule
    Fried's Rule
Intramuscular Drugs
Intravenous Drugs
    Intermittent IV Drug Infusion Using a Volume Control Set
Daily Maintenance Fluid Needs

Objectives

Upon completion of this chapter, you should be able to:

1. Use the two primary methods (body weight and body surface area) to calculate pediatric drug dosages.
2. Compare the ordered dosage with the recommended safe dosage.
3. Identify the steps in calculating body surface area from a pediatric nomogram.
4. Determine whether the ordered dosage is safe to administer.
5. Calculate an ordered IV medication to achieve an ordered concentration, given a specific on hand concentration.

Objectives continued

6. Calculate the amounts of two different IV medication to be added to a drip chamber.

7. Calculate pediatric intravenous dosages.

8. Calculate the amounts of daily maintenance fluids for pediatric patients.

9. Describe which action must be taken if the pharmacy computer system alerts you that a prescribed medication is contraindicated for use in children.

Key Terms

body surface area (BSA)
hypertonic solutions
nomogram
safe-dosage range

Overview

Administration of medications to children requires special attention and care because of their size and the way they metabolize drugs. Pharmacy technicians must understand calculations used for pediatric dosages. Accuracy is essential in all calculations. The calculations performed by the pharmacy technician must be supervised by a pharmacist. Pharmacists have ultimate legal responsibility for all pediatric dosages.

Children of different ages respond to medications differently. For example, many organ systems in newborns, infants, and toddlers are varied. Metabolism of medications in these groups compared with an adult dose will be completely different. Therefore, variations for children are so significant that no foolproof formula exists to determine the dosage of medications that a child should receive.

Calculating Pediatric Dosages

Pharmacists must be skillful in more advanced calculations for pediatric dosages. While pharmacy technicians must have an understanding of how this is done, pediatric dosing is actually regulated by law to pharmacists. The two main methods currently used for calculating safe pediatric dosages are body weight (such as mg/kg) and **body surface area (BSA)**. The first method uses a specific number of milligrams, micrograms, or units for each kilogram of body weight. Usually, drug data for pediatric dosage (mg/kg) are supplied by manufacturers in a drug information insert. BSA, measured in square meters (m^2), is considered a more accurate method than body weight. BSA takes into consideration the relationship between basal metabolic rate and surface area. BSA has primarily been used to calculate the dosage of antineoplastic agents (which are used in chemotherapy). Manufacturers are beginning to include BSA parameters (mg/m², mcg/m², units/m²) in drug information. Pharmacy computer systems used in prescribing alert pharmacy staff members when a drug prescribed for a pediatric patient is actually contraindicated for use in children. In such a case, a supervisor or the prescriber must be notified.

Body Weight Dosage Calculations

Standard adult dosages are determined by the drug manufacturer. Formulas must be provided for pediatric doses if the drug is intended to be given to children. Pediatric dose formulas are particularly important because dosage is usually recommended based on the requirements of an average-weight adult.

Dosages for newborns, infants, and children are based on their unique and changing body differences. Prescribers must consider the weight, height, body surface, age, and condition of the child as contributing factors to safe and effective drug dosages. The body weight method is more common in pediatric situations. Remember that both the body weight and BSA methods are also used for adults, especially in critical care situations, and the calculations are the same.

To calculate the amount of drug based on the child's body weight in kilograms, it is necessary to compare the child's ordered dosage to the recommended safe dosage from a reputable drug reference before administering the medication. During calculation and verification for safe pediatric dosages, follow these steps:

1. Convert the child's weight from pounds to kilograms.

2. Calculate the safe dosage in mg/kg or mcg/kg for a child of this weight, as recommended by a reputable drug reference: multiply mg/kg by the child's weight in kg (e.g., 1 kg = 2.2 lb or 1 g = 1000 mg).

3. Decide if the dosage is safe by comparing ordered and recommended dosages.

4. Calculate one dose.

5. Compare the prepared dosage to the ordered dosage and the recommended dosage, and have the pharmacist decide if the dosage is safe.

Note: The dosage per kg may be mg/kg, g/kg, mEq/kg, units/kg, milliunits/kg, and so forth.

■ Example 1:

The physician orders morphine sulfate 1.8 mg IM stat. The child weighs 79 lb. Is this dosage safe? First, convert pounds to kilograms:

$$79 \text{ lb} = 79 = 2.2 \div 35.90 \text{ kg} = 35.9 \text{ kg}$$

Next, calculate the milligrams per kilogram as recommend by a reputable drug source. A reputable drug source indicates that the usual IM/SC dosage may be initiated at 0.05 mg/kg/dose.

Decide if the dosage ordered is safe. For this child's weight, 1.8 mg is the recommended dosage, and 1.8 is the ordered dosage. This dosage is safe.

Calculate the dose.

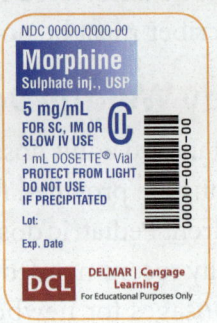

Morphine 5 mg/mL.
© Cengage Learning 2013

Ordered: *morphine sulfate 1.8 mg IM stat*

On hand: morphine sulfate 5 mg/mL

Administer:

$$\frac{D}{H} \times Q = \frac{1.8 \text{ mg}}{5 \text{ mg}} \times 1 \text{ mL} = 0.36 \text{ mL}$$

Or apply the ratio and proportion method:

5 mg : X mL :: 1.8 mg : 1 mL

$$\frac{5 \text{ mg}}{1 \text{ mL}} = \frac{1.8 \text{ mg}}{X \text{ mL}}$$

$$5X = 1.8$$

$$X = 0.36 \text{ mL}$$

This is a small child's dose. Measure 0.36 mL in a 1 mL syringe. The route is IM. The needle may need to be changed.

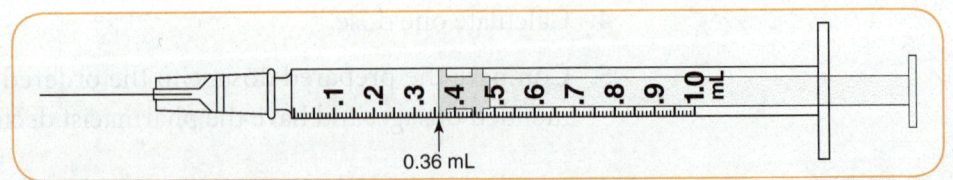

© Cengage Learning 2013

Single-Dosage Ranges

Single-dosage drugs are intended to be given once or prn. A dosage ordered by the body weight method is based on mg/kg/dose and is calculated by multiplying the recommended mg by the patient's kg weight for each dose. Some single-dosage medications indicate a minimum and maximum range, or a **safe-dosage range**.

■ Example 2:

The physician orders *Vistaril 20 mg IM q4–6h, p.r.n., nausea*. The child weighs 44 lb. Is this a safe dosage?

1. Convert lb to kg.

$$44 \text{ lb} = 44 \div 2.2 = 20 \text{ kg}$$

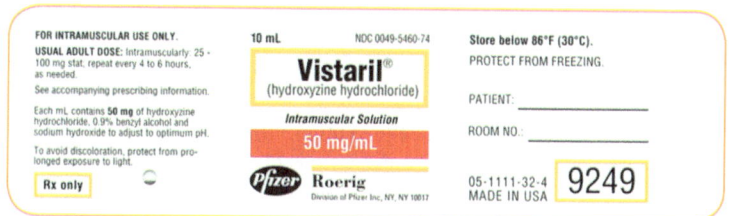

Vistaril 50 mg/mL.
Label reproduced with permission of Pfizer, Inc.

Calculate the recommended dosage. A reputable drug resource indicates that the usual IM dosage is 0.5 mg to 1 mg/kg/dose every 4 to 6 hours as needed.

Calculate the minimum and maximum safe dosage range.

Minimum per dose: 0.5 mg/kg/dose × 20 mg = 10 mg/dose

Maximum per dose: 1 mg/kg/dose × 20 kg = 20 mg/dose

2. Decide if the ordered dosage is safe. The recommended dosage is 10 mg to 20 mg, and the ordered dosage of 20 mg is within this range. Yes, the ordered dosage is safe.

3. Calculate one dose. Apply the three steps of dosage calculation.

Ordered: *Vistaril 20 mg IM q4–6h p.r.n., nausea*

On hand: Vistaril 50 mg/mL

$$\frac{D}{H} \times Q \frac{20 \text{ mg}}{50 \text{ mg}} \times 1 \text{ mL} = \frac{2}{5} \text{ML} = 0.4 \text{ mL}$$

Or apply the ratio and proportion method.

$$\frac{50 \text{ mg}}{1 \text{ mL}} = \frac{20 \text{ mg}}{X \text{ mL}}$$

$$50X = 20$$

$$\frac{50 X}{50} = \frac{20}{50}$$

$$X = 0.4 \text{ mL}$$

This is a small child's dose. Measure it in a 1 mL syringe. The route is IM. The needle may need to be changed.

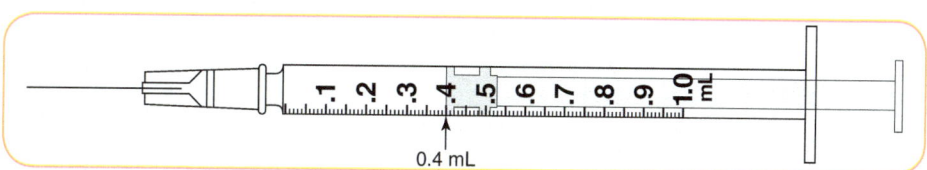

0.4 mL

Stop and Review
Calculating Pediatric Dosages by Body Weight
Calculate one safe pediatric dose.

1. Ordered:	*Keflex 125 mg p.o. q6h for a child who weighs 44 lb.* The recommended pediatric dosage of Keflex (cephalexin) is 25–50 mg/kg/day in 4 equally divided doses.
Child's weight:	_____ kg
Recommended minimum daily dosage for this child:	_____ mg/day
Recommended minimum single dosage for this child:	_____ mg/day
Recommended maximum daily dosage for this child:	_____ mg/day
Recommended maximum single dosage for this child:	_____ mg/day
Is the dosage in the recommended range for a healthy child?	_____
1a. Keflex is available in a suspension of 125 mg per 5 mL. If the dosage ordered in question 1 is safe, give _____ mL.	
2. Ordered:	*Chloromycetin 55 mg IV q12h for an 8-day-old newborn who weighs 2200 g.* The recommended dosage of Chloromycetin (chloramphenicol) for neonates less than 2 kg is 25 mg/kg once daily; and for neonates more than 2 kg and over 7 days of age, the recommended dosage is 50 mg/kg/day divided q12h.
Child's weight:	_____ kg
Recommended daily dosage for this child:	_____ mg/day
Recommended single dosage for this child:	_____ mg/dose
Is the ordered dosage safe?	_____

Chapter 15 • Pediatric Drug Administration 291

2a. Chloramphenicol is available as a solution for injection of 1 g per 10 mL. If the dosage ordered in question 2 is safe, how much should be given? _____ mg

3. Ordered:	*Suprax 120 mg p.o. q.d. for a child who weighs 33 lb.* The recommended dosage of Suprax (cefixime) for children under 50 kg is 8 mg/kg p.o. once daily or 4 mg/kg q12h.
Child's weight:	_____ kg
Recommended single dosage for this child:	_____ mg/dose
Is the ordered dosage safe?	_____

3a. Suprax is available as a suspension of 100 mg per 5 mL in a 50 mL bottle. If the dosage ordered in question 3 is safe, give _____ mL.

The labels provided represent the drugs available to answer questions 4 through 8. Verify safe dosage, indicate the amount to give, and draw an arrow on the accompanying measuring device. Explain unsafe dosages and describe the appropriate action to take.

4. Ordered:	*Nebcin 8 mg IM q6h for an infant who weighs 5000 g.* The recommended pediatric dosage of Nebcin (tobramycin) is 2–2.5 mg/kg q8h or 1.5–1.9 mg/kg q6h.
Infant's weight:	_____ kg
Recommended minimum single dosage for this infant:	_____ mg/dose
Recommended maximum single dosage for this infant:	_____ mg/dose
Is the dosage ordered safe?	_____

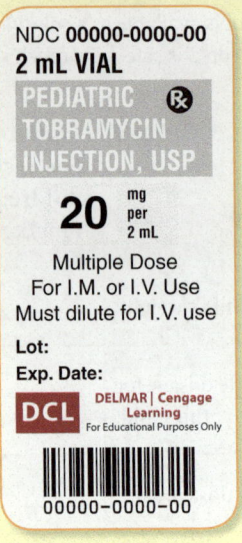

Nebcin Pediatric 20 mg per 2 mL.
© Cengage Learning 2013

4a. If the dosage ordered in question 4 is safe, give _____ mL.

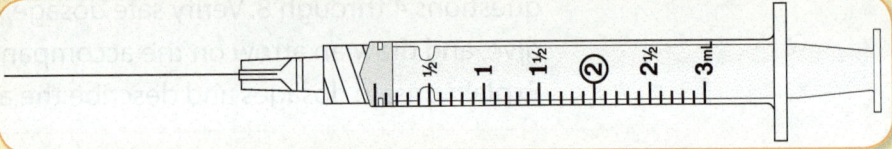

© Cengage Learning 2013

5. Ordered:	gentamicin 40 mg IV q8h for a premature neonate who is 5 days old and weighs 1800 g. The recommended dosage of gentamicin for children is 2–2.5 mg/kg q8h; for neonates, it is 2.5 mg/kg q8h; and for premature neonates less than 1 week of age, it is 2.5 mg/kg q12h.
Neonate's weight:	_____ kg
Recommended single dosage for this neonate:	_____ mg/dose
Is the dosage ordered safe?	_____

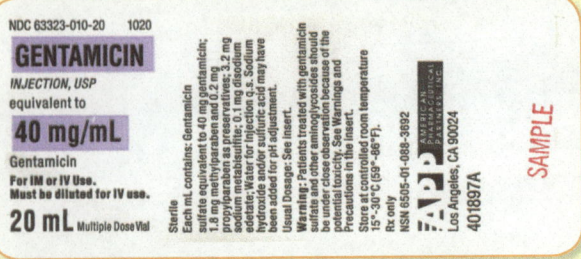

Gentamicin 40 mg/mL.
Courtesy of American Pharmaceutical Partners, Inc.

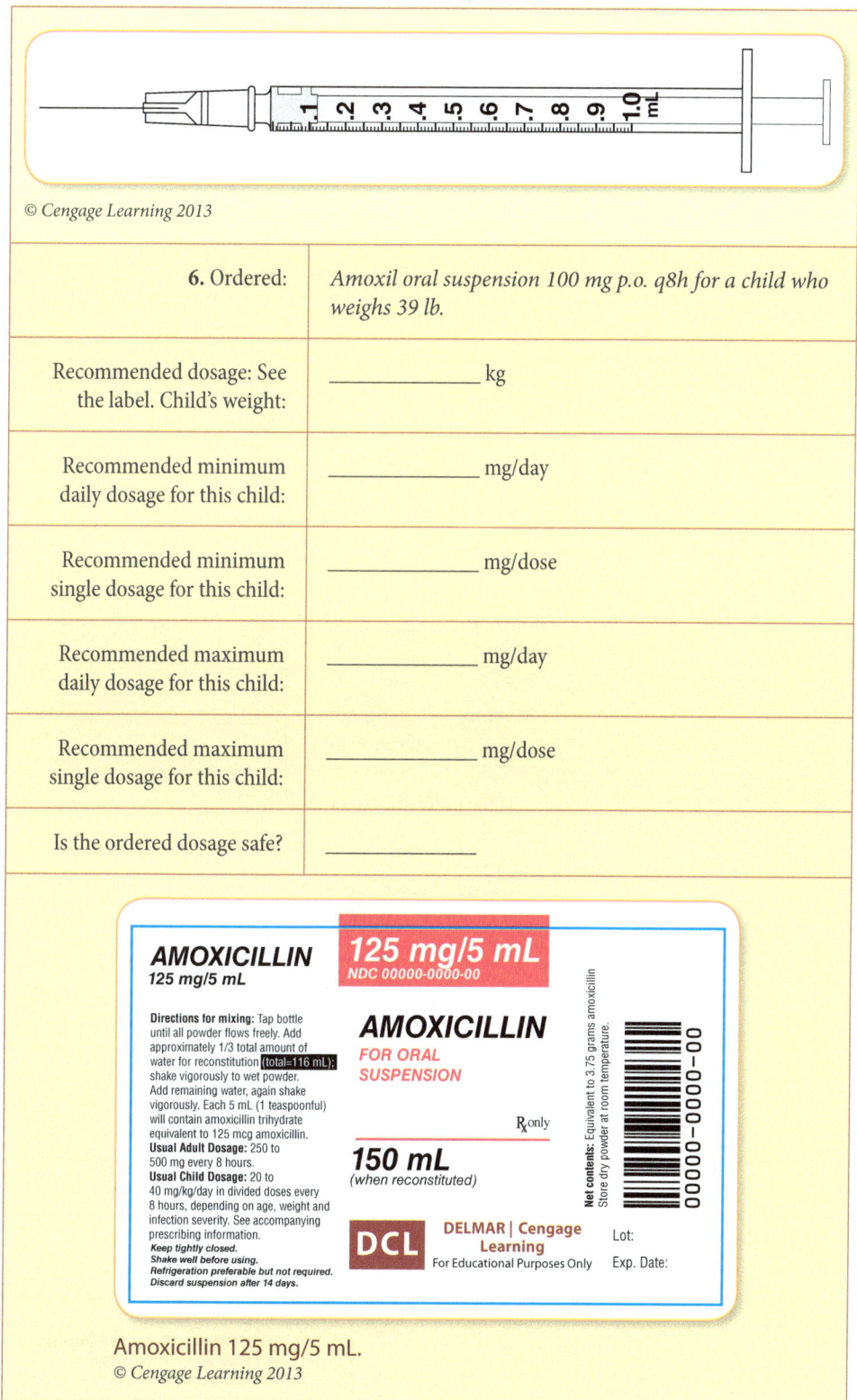

6. Ordered:	Amoxil oral suspension 100 mg p.o. q8h for a child who weighs 39 lb.
Recommended dosage: See the label. Child's weight:	_____ kg
Recommended minimum daily dosage for this child:	_____ mg/day
Recommended minimum single dosage for this child:	_____ mg/dose
Recommended maximum daily dosage for this child:	_____ mg/day
Recommended maximum single dosage for this child:	_____ mg/dose
Is the ordered dosage safe?	_____

Amoxicillin 125 mg/5 mL.
© Cengage Learning 2013

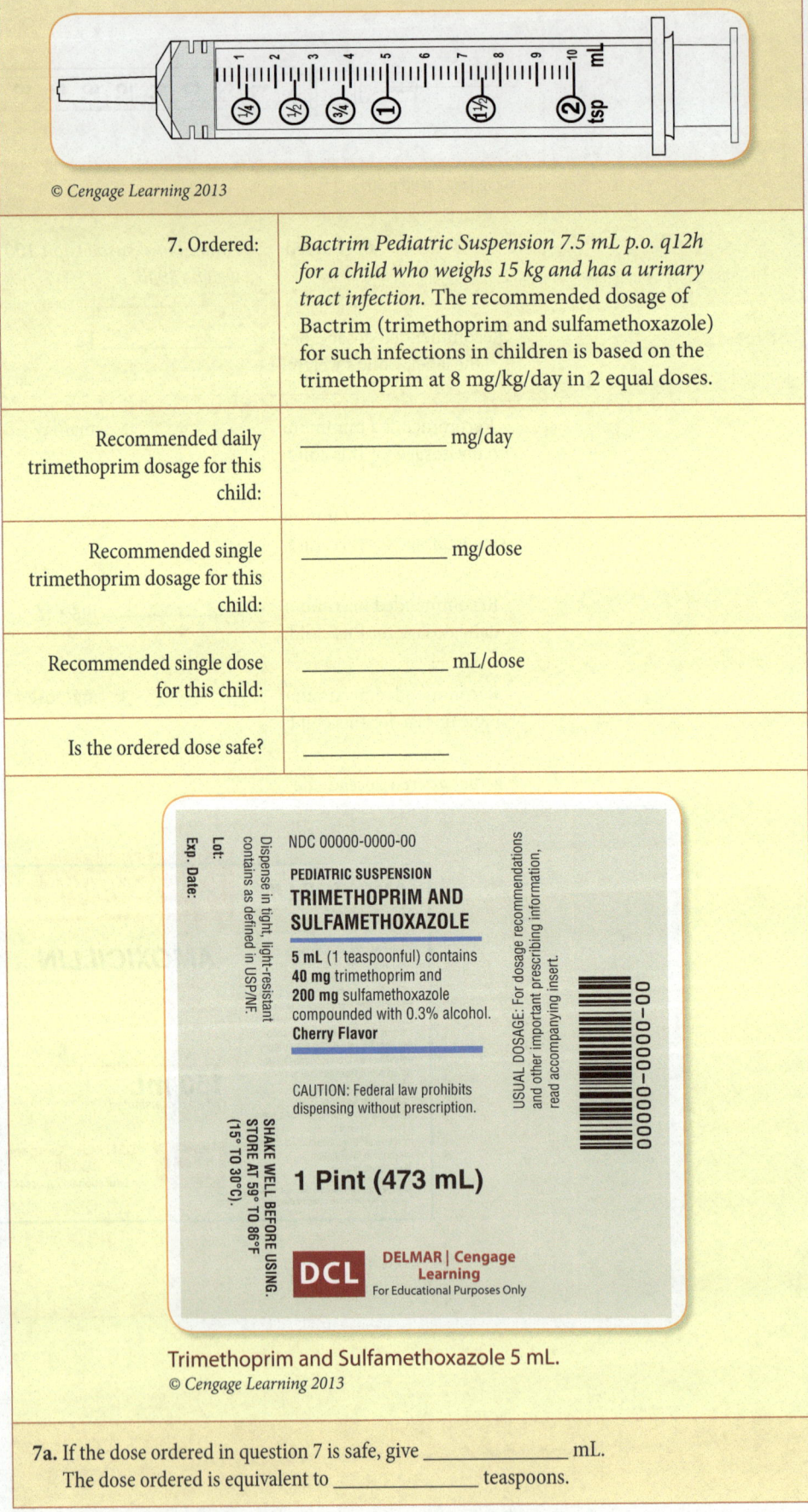

7. Ordered: *Bactrim Pediatric Suspension 7.5 mL p.o. q12h for a child who weighs 15 kg and has a urinary tract infection.* The recommended dosage of Bactrim (trimethoprim and sulfamethoxazole) for such infections in children is based on the trimethoprim at 8 mg/kg/day in 2 equal doses.

Recommended daily trimethoprim dosage for this child:	_____ mg/day
Recommended single trimethoprim dosage for this child:	_____ mg/dose
Recommended single dose for this child:	_____ mL/dose
Is the ordered dose safe?	_____

Trimethoprim and Sulfamethoxazole 5 mL.

7a. If the dose ordered in question 7 is safe, give _____ mL.
The dose ordered is equivalent to _____ teaspoons.

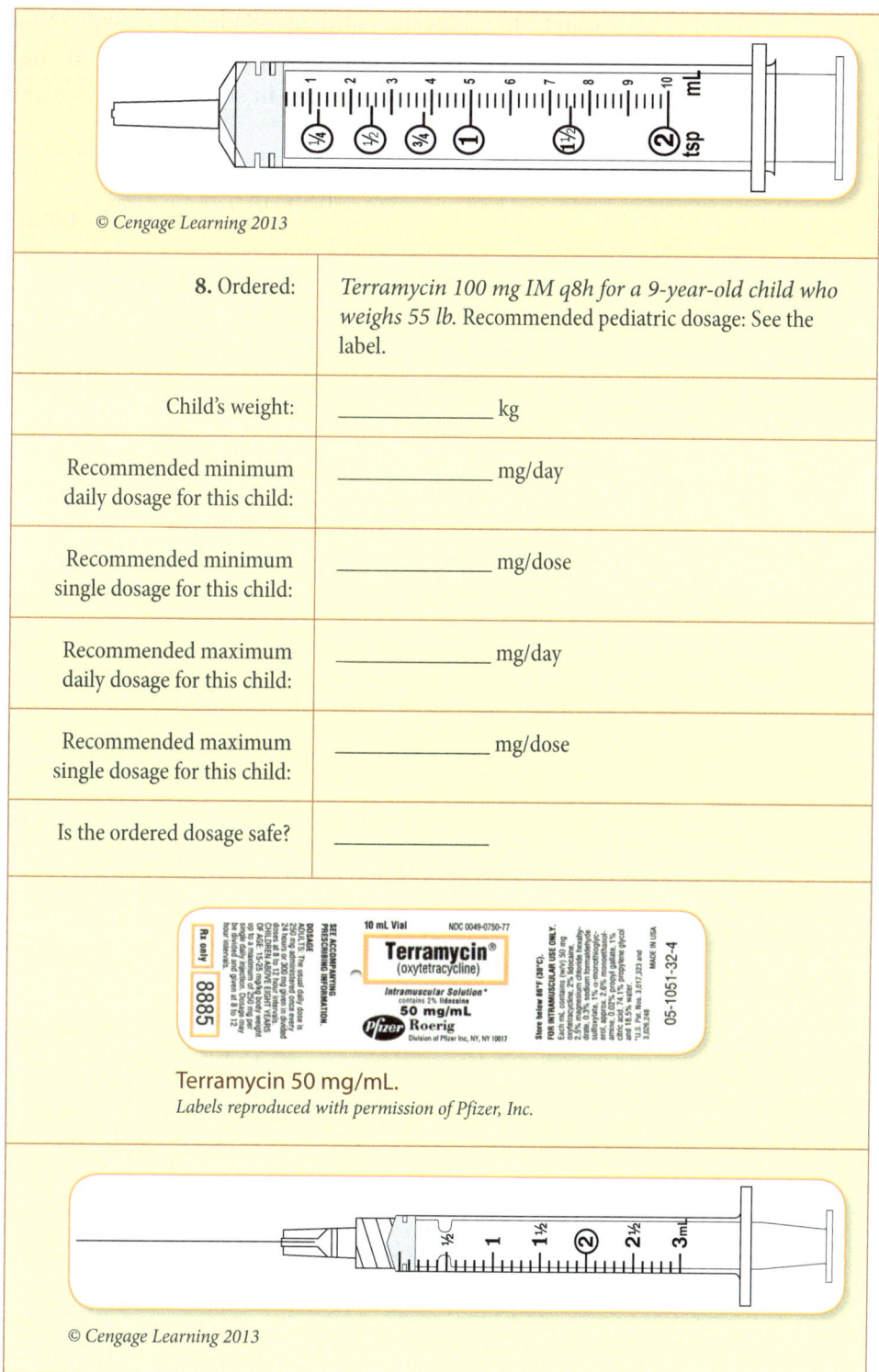

8. Ordered:	Terramycin 100 mg IM q8h for a 9-year-old child who weighs 55 lb. Recommended pediatric dosage: See the label.
Child's weight:	_____ kg
Recommended minimum daily dosage for this child:	_____ mg/day
Recommended minimum single dosage for this child:	_____ mg/dose
Recommended maximum daily dosage for this child:	_____ mg/day
Recommended maximum single dosage for this child:	_____ mg/dose
Is the ordered dosage safe?	_____

Terramycin 50 mg/mL.
Labels reproduced with permission of Pfizer, Inc.

Body Surface Area (BSA) Dosage Calculations

The BSA is used frequently in calculating dosages for infants and children. A patient's BSA is stated in square meters, or m^2. Pharmacy technicians can calculate the BSA by using a chart (**nomogram**) or formula calculation. Other information is needed for the calculation, such as the child's height, weight in kilograms, and age. Pediatric dosage in (square meters) is listed by the manufacturer or hospital pharmacy. The formula calculation is the most accurate. To determine BSA in square meters based on metric measurement of height and weight:

$$BSA\,(m^2) = \sqrt{\frac{ht\,(cm) \times wt\,(kg)}{3600}}$$

This formula may also be expressed as follows:

BSA = The square root of:

The patient's weight (in kilograms) multiplied by his or her height (in centimeters)
Divided by 3600

■ **Example 3:**

Use the metric formula to determine the BSA for a child whose height is 85 cm and weight is 13.9 kg (note that square meters is signified by m^2):

$$BSA = \sqrt{\frac{85 \times 13.9}{3600}}\,m^2$$

$$\sqrt{\frac{1181.5}{3600}}\,m^2$$

$$= 0.573\,m^2 = 0.57\,m^2$$

■ **Example 4:**

Calculate the BSA of a child who stands 98.4 cm and weighs 17.17 kg.

You need to find the square root of:

17.17 × 98.4, divided by 3600

Therefore,

The square root of 0.47 =

0.685 = 0.69 m^2 (rounded to hundredths)

To calculate BSA in m^2 based on household measurement of height and weight:

$$BSA\,(m^2) = \sqrt{\frac{ht\,(in.) \times wt\,(lb)}{3131}}$$

This formula may also be expressed as follows:

BSA = The square root of:

The patient's weight in pounds multiplied by his or her height in inches
Divided by 3131

■ Example 5:

Calculate the BSA for a baby whose height is 24 in. and weight is 12.2 lb.

$$BSA = \sqrt{\frac{24 \times 12.2}{3131}} m^2$$

$$\sqrt{\frac{292.8}{3131}} m^2 = 0.306 \ m^2 = 0.31 \ m^2$$

■ Example 6:

A child is 25 inches tall and weighs 35 pounds. What is his BSA?

You need to find the square root of:

$$35 \text{ pounds} \times 25 \text{ inches, divided by } 3131$$

Therefore,

The square root of $0.28 =$

$0.529 = 0.53 \ m^2$ (rounded to hundredths)

■ Example 7:

A child weighs 95 lb and stands 49 inches in height. What is her BSA?

You need to find the square root of:

$$95 \times 49, \text{ divided by } 3131$$

Therefore,

The square root of $1.49 =$

$1.220 = 1.22 \ m^2$ (rounded to hundredths)

Nomogram

When practitioners use a chart to estimate the BSA by plotting the height and weight and then connect the dots with a straight line, it is called a nomogram (**Figure 15-1**). Use a nomogram for determining the BSA for a child who has a normal height and weight. For a child who is underweight or overweight, the surface area is indicated by a straight line connecting the height and weight, intersecting the surface area (SA) column. This chart can be used for both children and adults for heights up to 240 cm (95 in.) and weights up to 80 kg (180 lb).

West's nomogram uses a calculation of the body surface area of infants and young children to determine the pediatric dose. The nomogram is used as a quick reference for pediatric doses. To use the nomogram, you need a straightedge ruler. Place one end of the ruler on the patient's height (either centimeters or inches) and the other edge on the weight (either kilograms or pounds). Draw a line to connect these two points; the meter-squared number is where the line intersects on the line labeled meters squared (m^2). Write this number down.

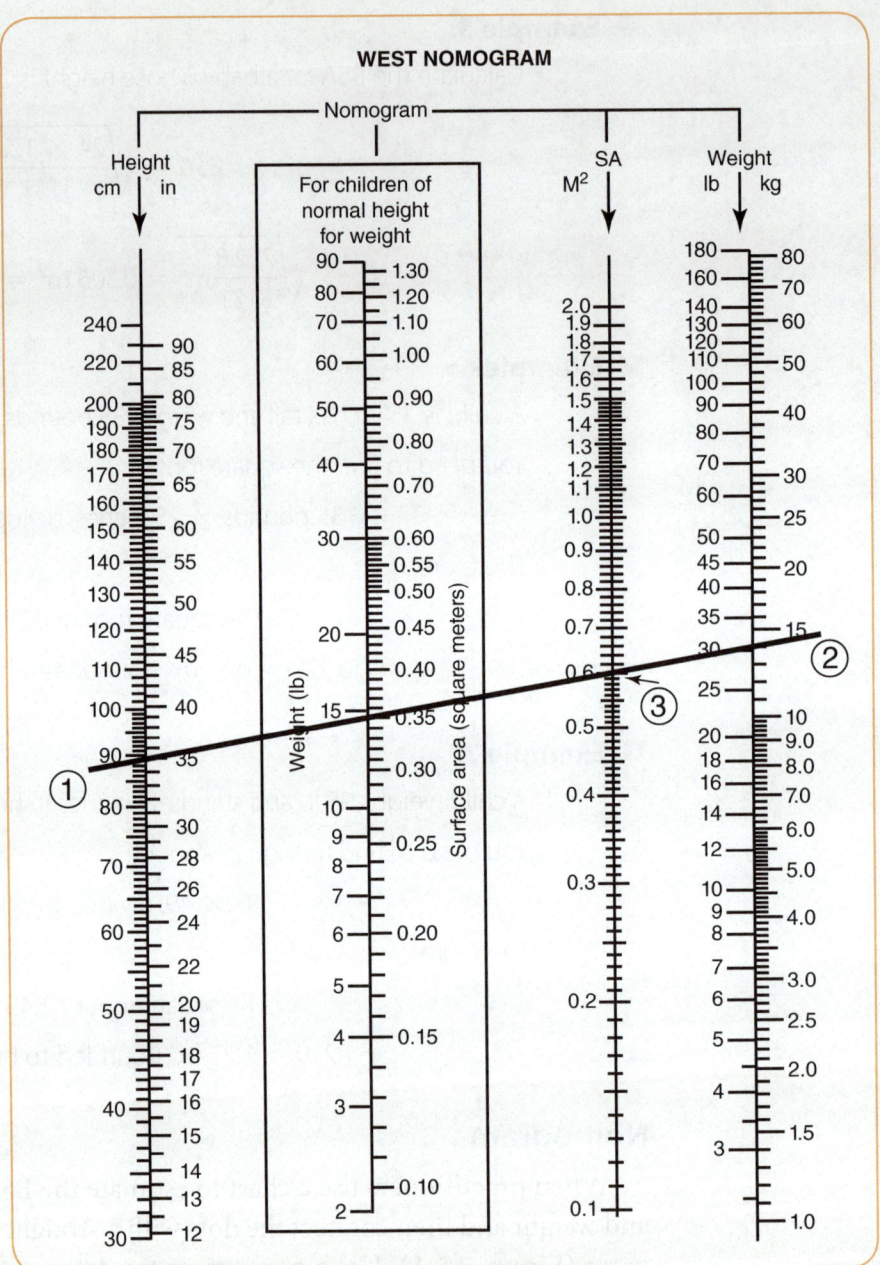

Figure 15-1 Nomogram for calculating body surface area.
From Nelson Textbook of Pediatrics *(16th ed.), by R.E. Behrman, R.M. Kliegman, and H.B. Jenson, 2000, Philadelphia: W.B. Saunders Company. Reprinted with permission.*

For pediatric doses, you can use the following formula:

$$\text{Pediatric dose} = \frac{\text{Body surface area (BSA) of child in m}^2}{1.7 \text{ m}^2 \text{ (average adult BSA)}} \times \text{Adult dose}$$

Stop and Review
Determining Pediatric Dosages by Body Surface Area
Use the appropriate formula to determine the BSA.

1. A child's height is 88 cm and her weight is 13.2 kg.
   _____

2. A child measures 94 cm in height and weighs 18 kg.
   _____

3. A child measures 26 in. tall and weighs 21 lb.
   _____

4. A child measures 65 cm tall and weighs 15 kg.
   _____

5. A child measures 92 cm tall and weighs 24 kg.
   _____

6. A teenager measures 135 cm tall and weighs 46 kg.
   _____

7. A child measures 43 in. tall and weighs 35 lb.
   _____

Find the BSA on the West nomogram (see **Figure 15-1**) for children with the following height and weight.

8. 21 in. and 81 lb: _____ m^2

9. 106 cm and 25 kg: _____ m^2

10. 41 in. and 32 lb: _____ m^2

11. 80 cm and 11 kg: _____ m^2

12. 140 cm and 30 kg: _____ m^2

13. 34 in. and 28 lb: _____ m^2

14. 122 cm and 32 kg: _____ m^2

15. 38 in. and 31 lb: _____ m^2

Clark's Rule

Using Clark's rule to calculate pediatric dosages is much more accurate than other pediatric methods. It is based on a child's weight and uses 150 lb (70 kg) as the average adult weight, while assuming that a child's dose is proportionately less. Calculate as follows:

$$\text{Pediatric dose} = \frac{\text{Child's weight in pounds}}{150 \text{ pounds}} \times \text{Adult dose}$$

■ **Example 8:**

Find the dose of cortisone for a 45 lb infant (adult dose = 100 mg).

$$\frac{45}{150} \times 100 \text{ mg} = 30 \text{ mg}$$

Note: **The use of Clark's rule, Young's rule, and Fried's rule has declined because of the use of nomograms and body surface area. However, it is still important for health professionals to understand the rules' concepts.**

Young's Rule

Young's rule is used for children who are between the ages of 1 and 12 years. Calculate as follows:

$$\text{Pediatric dose} = \frac{\text{Child's age in years}}{\text{Child's age in years} + 12} \times \text{Adult dose}$$

■ **Example 9:**

How much acetaminophen is the acceptable dosage for a 5-year-old child if the adult dose normally equals 1000 mg?

$$\text{Pediatric dose} = \frac{5 \text{ (years)}}{5 \text{ (years)} + 12} = 0.294 \times 1000 \text{ mg (adult dose)} = 294 \text{ mg}$$

Young's rule is not valid for children who are older than 12 years of age. If a child over 12 is still small enough in size to require a reduced dose, Clark's rule should be used to calculate the proper amount.

Fried's Rule

Fried's rule helps to estimate correct medication dosages for infants who are younger than 1 year of age. Calculate as follows:

$$\frac{\text{Age in months}}{150} \times \text{adult dose} = \text{child's dose}$$

Note: Young's and Fried's rules are the least accurate ways to measure doses for children.

> **》》》 Remember**
>
> Three steps are used to calculate pediatric drug dosages.
>
> **Step 1:** Convert pounds to kilograms, and then cross-multiply the ratio and round to the nearest whole number.
>
> **Step 2:** Calculate the drug dosage based on milligrams per kilogram of body weight and cross-multiply the ratio.
>
> **Step 3:** Calculate how much medication the patient would then receive based on the total amount allowed per day, divided into the proper amount of administrations per day.

■ Example 10:

Find the dose of phenobarbital for an 11-month-old infant if the adult dose = 400 mg.

$$\frac{11}{150} \times 400 \text{ mg} = 29 \text{ mg}$$

Intramuscular Drugs

The amount of medication to be administered in pediatric patients requires the pharmacy technician to consider the age and the size of the child. To be precise in calculating injection amounts, round the amount of the drug calculation to the nearest hundredth. When a pharmacy technician calculates dosages for pediatric injections, he or she uses the same method used for adults. The maximum volume of "intramuscular injections" for infants is 0.5–1 mL and for children more than 1 year old, it is 1 mL. For children older than 1 year, and up to 12 years, the amount is 1–1.5 mL.

■ Example 1:

Ordered: *Zinacef 50 mg/kg/day IM q6h*

On hand: *Zinacef 750 mg for injection*

Find the amount to administer.

According to the package insert, Zinacef may be administered to pediatric patients above 3 months of age at the rate of 50–100 mg/kg/day in divided doses every 6 to 8 hours.

$$1 \text{ kg} : 2.2 \text{ lb} :: ? \text{ kg} : 44 \text{ lb}$$

$$\frac{1 \text{ kg}}{2.2 \text{ lb}} = \frac{X \text{ kg}}{44 \text{ lb}}$$

$$44 = 2.2X$$

$$X = 20 \text{ kg}$$

Now, find the daily dosage.

$$\frac{50 \text{ mg}}{1 \text{ kg}} \times 20 \text{ kg} = \frac{50}{1} \times 20 = 1000 \text{ mg}$$

$$1000 \div 4 = 250 \text{ mg each dose}$$

After reconstitution, the Zinacef has a dosage strength of 220 mg/mL. To find the amount to administer for each dose:

$$250 \text{ mg} \times \frac{1 \text{ mL}}{220 \text{ mg}} = 250 \times \frac{1}{220} = 1.14 \text{ mL}$$

Intravenous Drugs

According to the size and age of children, the amount of medication to administer for intravenous drugs compared with adults is smaller. Volume control sets (**Figure 15-2**) are most commonly used to administer hourly fluids and intermittent IV medications to children. The fluid chamber will hold 100 mL to 150 mL of fluid to be infused in a specified time period as ordered, for example, for 60 minutes or less. The medication is added to the IV fluid in the chamber for a prescribed dilution volume. The IV bag acts only as a reservoir to hold future fluid infusions, and the nurse can fill the chamber for 1 to 2 hours. If more fluid infusions are needed, then the nurse can add to the amount. Only small, ordered quantities of fluid can be added, and the clamp above the chamber is fully closed.

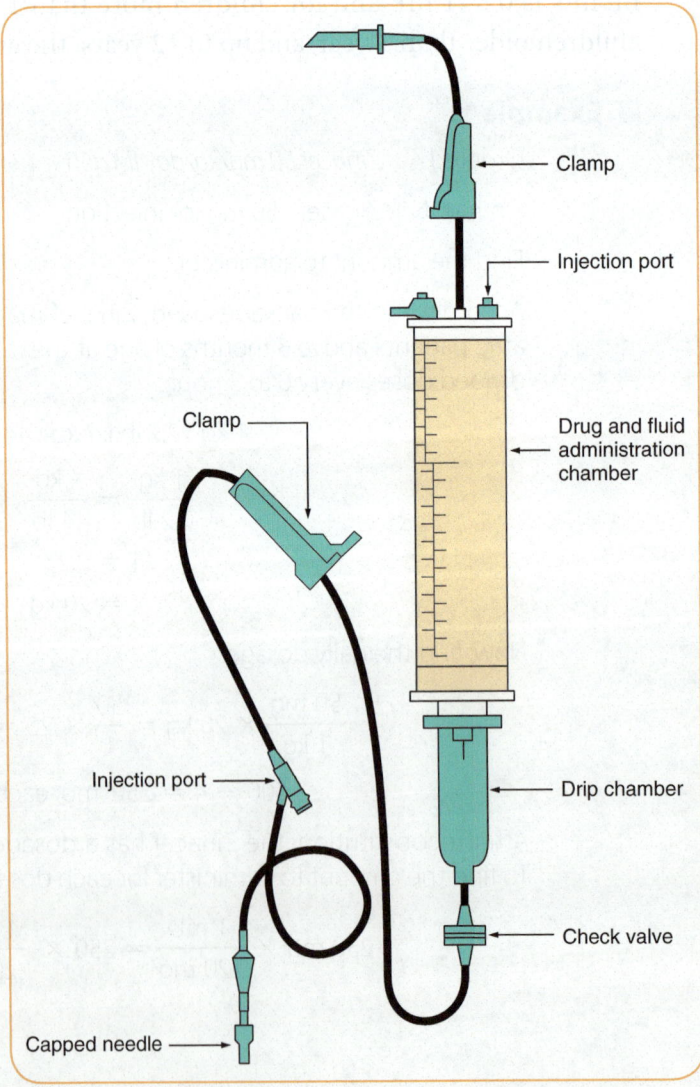

Figure 15-2 Volume control set.
© Cengage Learning 2013

Intermittent IV Drug Infusion Using a Volume Control Set

In place of a continuous IV infusion, children receiving IVs may receive them via means of a saline or heparin lock. Medication is injected into the volume control set chamber, and then an appropriate volume of IV fluid (to dilute the drug) is added. Then the IV tubing is attached to the child's IV lock to infuse over a specified amount of time. Once the chamber is empty and all the medication is infused, a flush of IV fluid is used to make sure that all the medication has cleared out of the tubing. Once the chamber empties, remember that some medication remains in the drip chamber, IV tubing, and IV lock (all above the height of the child's vein). Peripheral or central IV lines are not flushed with any standard amount of fluid. Manufacturers of IV tubing all have slight differences in their products, so the flush can vary from 15 mL to 50 mL, according to the tubing's overall length and any extra extensions added. It is necessary to verify hospital policy as to the correct volume to flush central and peripheral IV lines in children. For the examples in this text, 15 mL is used as the volume to flush a peripheral IV line unless otherwise specified.

In calculating the IV flow rate for the volume control set, consider the total fluid volume of the medication, the IV fluid used for diluting, and the volume of IV flush fluid. Volume control sets are microdrip sets that use a drop factor of 60 gtt/mL. Note that, usually, nurses are responsible for calculating flow rates and setting up equipment.

■ Example 1:

Ordered: *Claforan 250 mg IV q6h in 50 mL $D_5 \frac{1}{4} NS$ to infuse in 30 min followed by a 15 mL flush. Child has a saline lock.*

On hand: See the label.

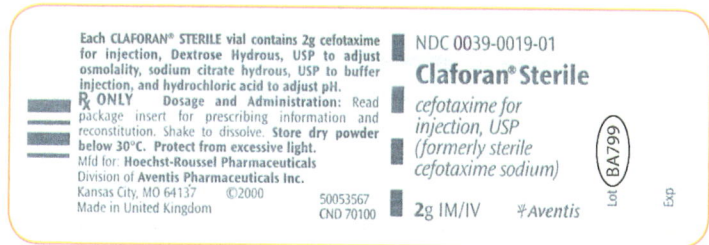

Claforan® Sterile.
Courtesy of Aventis Pharmaceuticals, Inc.

Instructions from the package insert for IV use are the following: Add 10 mL diluent for a total volume of 11 mL with a concentration of 180 mg/mL.

Step 1: Calculate the total volume of the intermittent IV flush: 50 mL + 15 mL = 65 mL.

Step 2: Calculate the flow rate of the IV medication and the IV flush. Remember: The drop factor is 60 gtt/mL.

$$\frac{V}{T} \times C = \frac{65 \text{ mL}}{30 \text{ min}} \times 60 \text{ gtt/mL}$$

$$= \frac{65 \text{ mL}}{1 \text{ min}} \times \frac{2 \text{ gtt}}{1 \text{ mL}} = 130 \text{ gtt/min}$$

Step 3: Calculate the volume of the medication to be administered:

$$\frac{D}{H} \times Q = \frac{250 \text{ mg}}{180 \text{ mg}} \times 1 \text{ mL} = 1.39 \text{ mL} = 1.4 \text{ mL}$$

Step 4: Add 1.4 mL Claforan 2 g to the chamber and fill with IV fluid to a volume of 50 mL. This provides the prescribed total volume of 50 mL in the chamber.

Step 5: Set the flow rate of the 50 mL of intermittent IV medication for 130 gtt/min. Follow with the 15 mL flush also set at 130 gtt/min. When complete, detach the IV tubing and follow the saline lock policy.

■ Example 2:

Ordered: *D$_5$NS IV at 30 mL/hr for continuous infusion and gentamicin 30 mg IV q8h over 30 min*

On hand: See the label.

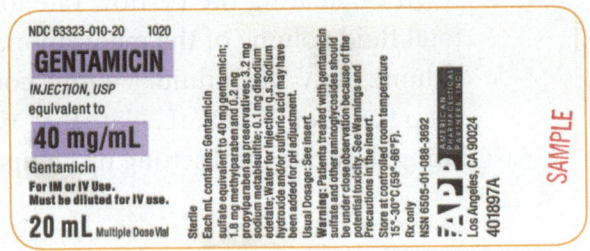

Gentamicin 40 mg/mL.
Courtesy of American Pharmaceutical Partners, Inc.

An infusion controller is in use with the volume control set.

Step 1: Calculate the dilution volume required to administer the gentamicin at the prescribed continuous flow rate of 30 mL/hr.

Calculate: Use ratio and proportion to verify your estimate.

$$\frac{30 \text{ mL}}{60 \text{ min}} = \frac{X \text{ mL}}{30 \text{ min}}$$

$$60X = 900$$

$$\frac{60X}{60} = \frac{900}{60}$$

$$X = 15 \text{ mL in 30 min}$$

Therefore, the IV fluid dilution volume required to administer 30 mg of gentamicin in 30 minutes is 15 mL to maintain the prescribed continuous infusion rate of 30 mL/hr.

Step 2: Determine the volume of gentamicin and IV fluid to add to the volume control chamber:

$$\frac{D}{H} \times Q = \frac{30 \text{ mg}}{40 \text{ mg}} \times 1 \text{ mL} = \frac{3}{4} \text{mL} = 0.75 \text{ mL}$$

Add 0.75 mL gentamicin and fill the chamber with D₅NS to the total volume of 15 mL.

Step 3: Set the controller to 30 mL/hr to deliver 15 mL of intermittent IV gentamicin solution in 30 minutes. Resume the regular IV, which will also flush out the tubing. The continuous flow rate will remain at 30 mL/hr.

Stop and Review

Calculating Pediatric Intravenous Drug Administrations

Calculate the amount of IV fluid to be added to the volume control chamber.

1. Ordered:	D₅ 0.33% NaCl IV at 66 mL/hr with Fortaz 720 mg IV q8h to be infused over 40 min by volume control set	
On hand:	Fortaz 1 g/10 mL	
Add _____ mL medication and _____ mL IV fluid to the chamber.		
2. Ordered:	D₅W at 30 mL/hr for continuous infusion with medication × 60 mg q6h to be infused over 20 min by volume control set	
On hand:	Medication × 60 mg/2 mL	
Add _____ mL medication and _____ mL IV fluid to the chamber.		
3. Ordered:	D₅ 0.45% NaCl IV at 48 mL/hr with Vibramycin 75 mg IV q12h to be infused over 2 hr volume control set	
On hand:	Vibramycin 100 mg/10 mL	
Add _____ mL medication and _____ mL IV fluid to the chamber.		
4. Ordered:	0.9% NaCl at 50 mL/hr for continuous infusion with Ancef 250 mg IV q8h to be infused over 30 min by volume control set	
On hand:	Ancef 125 mg/mL	
Add _____ mL medication and _____ mL IV fluid to the chamber.		

Calculate the IV flow rate to administer the following IV medications by using a volume control set, and determine the amount of IV fluid and medication to be added to the chamber. The ordered time includes the flush volume.

5. Ordered:	Antibiotic Z 15 mg IV b.i.d. in 25 mL 0.9% NaCl over 20 min. Flush with 15 mL.
On hand:	Antibiotic Z 15 mg 3 mL
Flow rate:	_____ gtt/min
Add _____ mL medication and _____ mL IV fluid to the chamber.	
6. Ordered:	Antibiotic Y 60 mg IV q8h in 50 mL $D_5 \frac{1}{3}$ NS over 45 min. Flush with 15 mL.
On hand:	Antibiotic Y 60 mg/2 mL
Flow rate:	_____ gtt/min
Add _____ mL medication and _____ mL IV fluid to the chamber.	
7. Ordered:	Ancef 0.6 g IV q12h in 50 mL D_5 NS over 60 min or an infusion pump. Flush with 30 mL.
On hand:	Ancef 1 g/10 mL
Flow rate:	_____ mL/hr
Add _____ mL medication and _____ mL IV fluid to the chamber.	
8. Ordered:	Medication X 75 mg IV q6h in 60 mL $D_5 \frac{1}{4}$ NS over 60 min. Flush with 15 mL.
On hand:	Medication X 75 mg/3 mL
Flow rate:	_____ gtt/min
Add _____ mL medication and _____ mL IV fluid to the chamber.	

Daily Maintenance Fluid Needs

Pharmacy technicians should also be familiar with calculating 24-hour maintenance IV fluids for pediatric patients. They must use the following formula for calculations:

- 100 mL/kg/day for the first 10 kg of body weight
- 50 mL/kg/day for the next 10 kg of body weight
- 20 mL/kg/day for each kg above 20 kg of body weight

This formula uses the child's weight in kilograms to estimate the 24-hour total fluid need, including oral intake.

These types of IV solutions usually contain a combination of saline, glucose, and potassium chloride and are known as **hypertonic solutions** (**Figure 15-3**).

Sodium chloride is usually concentrated between 0.225% and 0.9% ($\frac{1}{4}$ NS up to NS). Dextrose (glucose) for energy is usually concentrated between 5% and 12% for peripheral infusions. Plus, 20 mEq per liter of potassium chloride (20 mEq KCl/L) are added to continuous pediatric infusions.

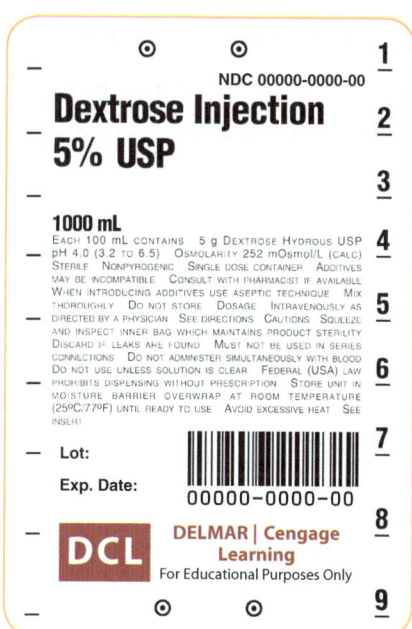

Figure 15-3 Dextrose Injection 5% USP.
© Cengage Learning 2013

■ Example 1:

Child who weighs 26 kg: 100 mL/kg/day × 10 kg = 1000 mL/day (for the first 10 kg)

50 mL/kg/day × 10 kg = 500 mL/day (for the next 10 kg)

20 mL/kg/day × 6 kg = 120 mL/day (for the next 6 kg)

Total: 1000 mL/day + 500 mL/day + 120 mL/day = 1620 mL/day, or per 24 hours

$$\frac{1620 \text{ mL}}{24 \text{ hr}} = 67.5 \text{ mL/hr} = 68 \text{ mL/hr}$$

■ **Example 2:**

Child who weighs 14 kg: 100 mL/kg/day × 10 kg = 1000 mL/day (for the first 10 kg)

50 mL/kg/day × 4 kg = 200 mL/day (for the remaining 4 kg)

Total: 1000 mL/day + 200 mL/day = 1200 mL/day, or per 24 hours

$$\frac{1200 \text{ mL}}{24 \text{ hr}} = 50 \text{ mL/hr}$$

■ **Example 3:**

Child who weighs 8 kg: 100 mL/kg/day × 8 kg = 800 mL/day or per 24 hours

$$\frac{800 \text{ mL}}{24 \text{ hr}} = 33.3 \text{ mL/hr} = 33 \text{ mL/hr}$$

Stop and Review
Calculating Daily Maintenance Fluids for Pediatric Patients

1. Calculate the total volume and hourly IV flow rate for a 3500 g infant receiving maintenance fluids. Infuse _____ mL at _____ mL/hr.

2. Calculate the total volume and hourly IV flow rate for a 13 kg child receiving maintenance IV fluids. Infuse _____ mL at _____ mL/hr.

3. Calculate the total volume and hourly IV flow rate for a 77 lb child receiving maintenance fluids. Infuse _____ mL at _____ mL/hr.

4. Calculate the total volume and hourly IV flow rate for a 25 kg child receiving maintenance IV fluids. Infuse _____ mL at _____ mL/hr.

5. Calculate the total volume and hourly IV flow rate for a 17.6 lb newborn receiving maintenance IV fluids. Infuse _____ mL at _____ mL/hr.

6. Calculate the total volume and hourly IV flow rate for an 8800 g child receiving maintenance IV fluids. Infuse _____ mL at _____ mL/hr.

7. Calculate the child's daily maintenance fluid needs for the following weights.

   a. 68.2 lb = _____ mL

   b. 13.3 lb = _____ mL

   c. 12 kg = _____ mL

   d. 43 kg = _____ mL

Test Your Knowledge

For Questions 1 through 7, verify the safety of the following pediatric dosages ordered. If the dosage is safe, calculate one dose and the IV volume to infuse one dose.

Ordered for a child weighing 15 kg:

D_5 0.45% NaCl IV at 53 mL/h with ampicillin 275 mg IV q4h infused over 40 min by volume control set

Recommended dosage: ampicillin 100–125 mg/kg/day in 6 divided doses

On hand: ampicillin 1 g/10 mL

1. Safe daily dosage range for this child: _____ mg/day to _____ mg/day.

   Safe single dosage range for this child: _____ mg/dose to _____ mg/dose. Is the ordered dosage safe? _____ If safe, give _____ mL/dose.

2. IV fluid volume to be infused in 40 min: _____ mL. Add _____ mL ampicillin and _____ mL D_5 0.45% NaCl to the chamber.

Ordered for a child who weighs 55 lb:

D_5 NS at 60 mL/hr with penicillin G potassium 525,000 units q4h to be infused over 20 min by control set

Recommended dosage: penicillin G potassium 100,000–250,000 units/kg/day in 6 divided doses q4hr.

On hand: penicillin G potassium 200,000 units/mL

3. Child's weight: _____ kg

   Safe daily dosage for this child: _____ units/day to _____ units/day

   Safe single dosage for this child: _____ units/dose to _____ units/dose

4. Is the ordered dosage safe? _____

5. IV fluid volume to be infused in 20 min: _____ mL. Add _____ mL penicillin G potassium and _____ mL D₅ NS to the chamber.

Ordered for a child who weighs 22 kg:

D₅ 0.225% NaCl IV at 50 mL/hr with Amikin 165 mg IV q8h to be infused over 30 min by volume control set

Recommended dosage: Amikin 15–22.5 mg/kg/day in 3 divided doses q 8 hr

On hand: Amikin 100 mg/2 mL

6. Safe daily dosage range for this child: _____ mg/day to _____ mg/day. Safe single dosage range for this child: _____ mg/dose to _____ mg/dose.

7. IV fluid volume to be infused in 30 min: _____ mL. Add _____ mL Amikin and _____ mL D₅ 0.225% NaCl to the chamber.

For questions 8 through 15, use the BSA formulas to calculate the BSA value.

8. Height: 4 ft; Weight: 80 lb; BSA: _____ m²
9. Height: 5 ft 6 in.; Weight: 136 lb BSA: _____ m²
10. Height: 68 in.; Weight: 170 lb BSA: _____ m²
11. Height: 64 in.; Weight: 63 kg BSA: _____ m²
12. Height: 164 cm; Weight: 58 kg BSA: _____ m²
13. Height: 100 cm; Weight: 17 kg BSA: _____ m²
14. Height: 60 cm; Weight: 6 kg BSA: _____ m²
15. Height: 85 cm; Weight: 11.5 kg BSA: _____ m²

For questions 16 through 18, calculate the ordered medication for each of the following IV bags to achieve the ordered concentration. On hand is KCl 2 mEq/mL.

16. Ordered: Add 30 mEq KCl per L of IV fluid.
    On hand: 360 mL IV solution
    Add: _____ mEq; _____ mL

17. Ordered: Add 20 mEq KCl per L of IV fluid.
    On hand: 700 mL IV solution
    Add: _____ mEq; _____ mL

18. Ordered: *Add 15 mEq KCl per L of IV fluid.*

    On hand: 250 mL IV solution

    Add: _____ mEq; _____ mL

To calculate the daily volume of pediatric maintenance IV fluids to answer questions 19 through 22, allow the following:

100 mL/kg/day for the first 10 kg of body weight

50 mL/kg/day for the next 10 kg of body weight

20 mL/kg/day for each kg of body weight above 20 kg

19. Calculate the total volume and hourly IV flow rate for a 78 lb child receiving maintenance fluids.

    Infuse _____ mL at _____ mL/hr

20. Calculate the total volume IV flow rate for a 21 kg child receiving maintenance fluids.

    Infuse _____ mL at _____ mL/hr

21. Calculate the total volume and hourly IV flow rate for a 2400 g infant receiving maintenance fluids.

    Infuse _____ mL at _____ mL/hr

22. Calculate the total volume and hourly IV flow rate for a 33 lb child receiving maintenance fluids.

    Infuse _____ mL at _____ mL/hr

Calculate the volume for one dose of safe dosages. Refer to the BSA formulas or the West nomogram, as needed, to answer questions 23 through 32.

23. A child is 140 cm tall and weighs 43.5 kg. The recommended IV dosage of Adriamycin is 20 mg/m^2. Use the BSA formula to calculate the safe IV dosage of Adriamycin for this child.
    BSA: _____ m^2

    Safe dosage: _____ mg

24. Calculate the dose amount of Adriamycin for the child in Question 23.

    On hand: Adriamycin 2 mg/mL

    Give: _____ mL

25. Use the BSA nomogram to determine the safe IM dosage of Oncaspar for a child who is 42 in. tall and weighs 45 lb. The recommended IM dosage is 2500 units/m²/dose.

    BSA: _____ m²; Safe dosage: _____ units

26. Oncaspar is reconstituted to 750 units per 1 mL. Calculate one dose for the child in question 25. Give: _____ mL

27. Should the Oncaspar in question 26 be given in one injection? _____

28. Ordered: Vincristine 2 mg direct IV stat for a child who weighs 85 lb and is 50 in. tall. Recommended dosage of vincristine for children: 1.5–2 mg/m², 1 time/week; inject slowly over a period of 1 minute.

    On hand: vincristine 1 mg/mL

    BSA (per formula) of this child: _____ m²

    Recommended dosage range for this child: _____ mg to _____ mg

29. Use the BSA nomogram to calculate the safe oral dosage and amount to give of amoxicillin for a child of normal proportions who weighs 25 lb.

    Recommended dosage: 80 mg/m²/day once daily p.o.

    On hand: amoxicillin 50 mg/mL

    BSA: _____ m²

    Safe dosage: _____ mg

    Give: _____ mL

30. Use the BSA nomogram to calculate the safe IV dosage of sargramostim for a 1-year-old infant who is 25 in. tall and weighs 20 lb.

    Recommended dosage: 250 mcg/m²/day once daily IV

    BSA: _____ m²

    Safe dosage: _____ mcg

31. Sargramostim is available in a solution strength of 500 mcg/10 mL. Calculate one dose for the child in question 30. Give: _____ mL

32. Ordered: D_5 0.45% NaCl IV at 66 mL/hr with Fortaz 620 mg IV q8h to be infused over 40 min

    Use a volume control set and flush with 15 mL.

    On hand: Fortaz 0.5 g/5 mL

    Add _____ mL Fortaz and _____ mL D_5 0.45% NaCl to the chamber.

Critical Thinking

1. A pharmacy technician received an order to dispense Halotex® (antifungal) for topical use for a 4-year-old child. Fortunately, the technician was alerted by the pharmacy computer system that Halotex should not be administered to patients younger than 5 years of age. This patient should not receive Halotex. Whom should the pharmacy technician notify about this?

   _____

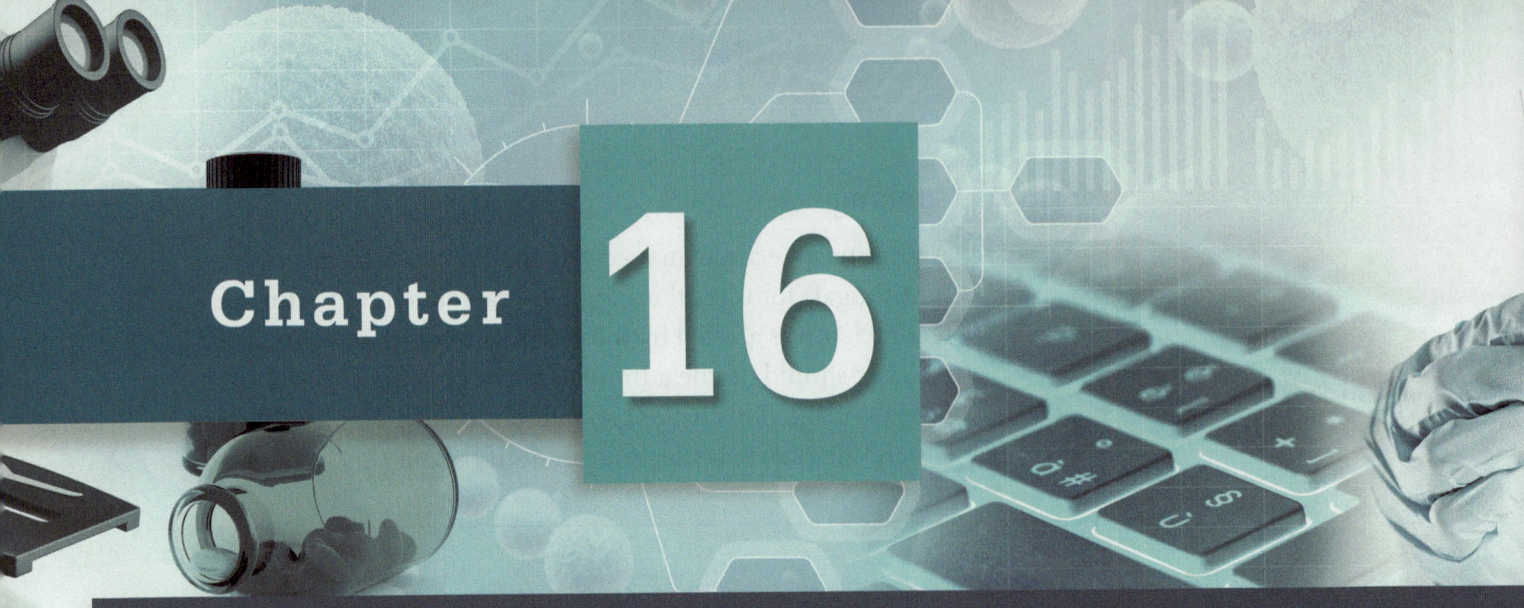

Chapter 16

Business Math for Pharmacy Technicians

Outline

Overview
Markup
    Percent Markup
    Percent Markup Plus a Professional Fee
Gross Profit
Net Profit
Discounts
Depreciation
Inventory Turnover
    Average Wholesale Price
Wholesale Acquisition Cost
Insurance Reimbursements

Objectives

Upon completion of this chapter, you should be able to:

1. Compute gross profit.
2. Explain net profit.
3. Explain inventory turnover.
4. Compute discounts.

Objectives continued

5. Calculate actual product costs when rebates are offered for certain quantities purchased.
6. Calculate credits for expired drug products that are returned to the manufacturer.
7. Compute total pharmacy profit based on total operating cost, and average monthly purchases and sales.
8. Calculate the cost of a 6-month supply of a drug based on its daily cost.
9. Compute a drug's selling price, taking into account its actual cost and the profit added in.
10. Calculate the cost of an entire bottle of medication, taking into account its per-dose price, pharmacy operating costs, and the desired profit.

Key Terms

average wholesale price
capital assets
copayment
expenses
gross margin
gross profit

inventory
inventory control
inventory turnover rate
markup
markup method
net profit

return on investment
sales
tangible
third-party payer
turnover
waste control

Overview

Pharmacy practice has changed dramatically over the last several years. Most pharmacists work for large organizations, such as hospitals, chain pharmacies, and managed care pharmacies, rather than in small, independently owned pharmacies. Pharmacy managers are responsible for planning, organizing, and controlling resources so that their organizations meet desired goals, along with the finances of the pharmacy. Without establishing the pharmacy's ability to make a regular profit, pharmacy managers will not be able to achieve the pharmacy's ultimate goal of serving the community. There has been a dramatic decline in the number of pharmacists who own their businesses, but this has not affected the number of pharmacists who are managers. However, most states require pharmacy managers to actually be pharmacists.

Markup

The term **markup** refers to the difference between the cost of merchandise and its selling price. Markup is sometimes called "margin of profit" or "gross profit." For example, if a pharmacist buys an item for $2.75 and sells it for $3.75, the markup is $1.00. The **markup method** bases price and dollar margin on the ingredient cost of the dispensed product. Consequently, as ingredient cost increases, both price and margin increase proportionally. The markup may be calculated as a percentage, which refers to the markup divided by the selling price. The percent of markup may be somewhat ambiguous because it may be based on either the cost or the selling price of merchandise. As of this writing, the percentage is based on selling price, and the term *markup percent* means a percentage of the selling price.

Calculating the merchandise's selling price to yield a certain percent of gross profit involves the following.

■ **Example 1:**

The cost of 100 antihistamine tablets is $1.98. What should the selling price be for 100 tablets to yield a 66% gross profit on the cost?

$$\text{Cost} \times \text{\% of gross profit} = \text{Gross profit}$$
$$\$1.98 \times 66\% = \$1.30$$
$$\text{Cost} + \text{Gross profit} = \text{Selling price}$$
$$\$1.98 + \$1.30 = \$3.28$$

A markup system automatically adjusts prices to accommodate changes in ingredient costs. You can also calculate the markup rate by using this formula:

$$\text{Markup rate} = \frac{\text{Markup}}{\text{Cost}} \times 100\%$$

■ **Example 2:**

If Zocor® 10 mg in a 30-pack costs the pharmacy $98.64 and the price is $147.96, what is the markup rate?

The markup is $147.96 − $98.64 = $49.32

The markup rate is calculated via the formula given previously:

$$\text{Markup rate} = \frac{49.32}{98.64} \times 100\% = 50\%$$

Percent Markup

In this type of prescription pricing, the cost of the ingredients of a prescription is added to the cost of ingredients multiplied by the desired percentage of markup.

$$\text{Cost of ingredients} + (\text{cost of ingredients} \times \text{\% of markup})$$
$$= \text{Prescription price}$$

Percentages vary but, in general, lower-priced items are marked up with a higher percentage, and higher-priced items are marked up with a lower percentage.

■ **Example 3:**

What would be the prescription price in the following situation?

A package of a certain drug product costs $5. The pharmacist applies a 50% markup on cost.

$$\$5 + (\$5 \times 50\%) = \$5 + \$2.50 = \$7.50$$

Percent Markup Plus a Professional Fee

Utilizing this method, both a percent markup *and* a professional fee are added to the ingredient's cost. In this type of prescription pricing, the percent markup is usually a bit lower than in the preceding *percent markup* example. A minimum professional fee is added to help recover the costs of professional services, labeling, containers, and overhead.

Cost of ingredients + (cost of ingredients × % of markup) + professional fee = Prescription price

■ **Example 4:**

If the package of a quantity of drug product costs $5 and the pharmacist applies a 50% markup on cost plus a professional fee of $3, what would the prescription price be?

$5 + ($5 × 50%) + $3 = $5 + $2.50 + $3 = $10.50

Gross Profit

The pharmacy, like other businesses, must make a profit. It must have more revenue than **expenses** to continue providing customer services. The pharmacy technician is also involved in this effort to help ensure that revenue exceeds expenses. The technician must understand the importance of cost, overhead, markup, discount, and **inventory control** as they relate to profit. The overall cost for the pharmacy may include the cost of drug purchases, salaries, operating expenses, utilities, and insurance (business and liability).

Because **net profit** is usually reported annually or semiannually, the retail pharmacy department may frequently measure the cost of goods as compared to the revenue generated by the sale of those goods. This reported margin of profit is known as **gross profit**. Gross profit is the marginal difference between actual cost and total reimbursement and is also known as "**gross margin**." The insurance reimbursement or private pay customer's service charge most dramatically influences the "gross profit" margin.

■ **Example 1:**

(sales − acquisition cost = gross profit)

If a pharmacy has **sales** totaling $1,000,000 and the cost of the items sold is $750,000, then the *gross profit* is $250,000.

Depending on the nature of the pharmacy, most institutional pharmacies do not operate under the profit-margin system. Hospitals, nursing homes, and other "closed" pharmacies must maintain cost efficiency but are not required, by their nature, to generate a significant profit.

Net Profit

The net profit for each drug sold is calculated as the difference between the overall cost and the selling price. The overall cost is made up of the cost to dispense added to the purchase price. The net profit amount can be calculated by multiplying the overall cost by the desired percent of profit.

■ **Example 1:**

A liquid drug for oral administration costs $20/pint. The pharmacy technician calculates that it costs $5 (including pharmacy supplies, shipping, supply maintenance, pharmacist consultation, and personnel time) to dispense one bottle's entire contents. If a 15% profit is desired, what selling price is required for the pint bottle?

Purchase price	+ dispensing cost	= overall cost
$20	+ $5	= $25
Overall cost	× 0.15	= net profit
$25	× 0.15	= $3.75
Overall cost	+ net profit	= selling price
$25	+ $3.75	= $28.75

Retail pharmacy establishments answer to private, corporate, or public investors, that is, stock shareholders, and must maintain a level of pharmacy profit dictated by the business. The cost of goods along with overhead costs, including professional labor, clerical support, utilities, capital investment, and government fees must be considered in developing the actual margin of profit. The actual profit generated is known as net profit. This is the reported profit a pharmacy generates when all costs of the business are considered.

■ **Example 2:**

Assume that Family Drug Mart has the following annual overhead expenses:

Pharmacist's Salary	$ 70,000
Technician's Salary	$ 23,250
Rent	$ 16,000
Utilities	$ 7300
Liability Insurance	$ 3400
Business Insurance	$ 4000
Supplies and Drug Purchases	$1,691,000
Total Overhead	$1,814,950

When Family Drug Mart has an annual income of $2,087,192.50, it will be making a 15% profit. If a 15% profit is desired, what amount of income has to be received to meet this goal?

$$\text{Overhead} \times 0.15 = \text{Profit}$$

$$\$1,814,950 \times 0.15 = \$272,242.50$$

Because profit is equal to incoming receipts minus overhead:

$$\text{Overhead} + \text{Profit} = \text{Income}$$

$$\$1,814,950 + \$272,242.50 = \$2,087,192.50$$

Discounts

When a manufacturer or a supplier offers an item at a lower price to a pharmacy, this lower price is considered to be "discounted." A discount is, simply put, a deduction from what is normally charged. Discounts provided by suppliers may be based on quantity purchased and/or payment of invoices within a specified time period. These discounts provide the pharmacy with a means of increasing the gross profit on selected merchandise. Discounts are offered as incentives to purchase the products being discounted. They are calculated as follows:

$$\text{DISCOUNT} = \text{Discount rate} \times \text{total purchase price}$$

$$\text{Purchase price} - \text{discount} = \text{DISCOUNTED PRICE}$$

■ **Example 1:**

Ten cases of ointment are purchased at $180 per case. If the account is fully paid within 15 days, the manufacturer offers a discount of 12%. What is the total discounted purchase price?

First, you must calculate the full purchase price: 10 cases × $180 per case = $1800

Next, calculate the discount if paid for within 15 days:

$$(\text{DISCOUNT} = \text{Discount rate} \times \text{total purchase price})$$

$$12\% \times \$1800$$

The DISCOUNT is equal to $216.

Finally, to obtain the discounted price, you would subtract the discount from the original total purchase price.

$$\text{Total purchase price} - \text{discount} = \text{discounted purchase price}$$

$$\$1800 - \$216 = \$1584$$

Prescription pricing is designed so that the pharmacy receives a fair **return on investment** and costs. It gives the pharmacy the ability to provide the services that its community needs in a uniform and consistent manner. The following sections explain the most common methods of prescription pricing.

Depreciation

In the pharmacy, depreciation is a regular part of business. Assets become worth less and less over time, as in any business. Depreciation allows for writing off the expense of pharmacy equipment throughout its useful life, which decreases the tax burden for several years. In order for an item to be depreciated, it must be considered a *capital asset*, which is one that is defined as property, part of the facility, or equipment. Capital assets help generate a profit but are not considered to be inventory. They have a life span of multiple years. Therefore, items such as office supplies cannot be depreciated. **Capital assets** must also be **tangible**, such as the actual pharmacy building, which can be depreciated, while the land it is built on cannot. There are three basic types of information about each item that must be considered for depreciation, as follows:

- *Asset basis*—the total cost of the asset, including shipping, installation fees, and training costs.
- *Useful life (recovery period)*—a predetermined period of time, as listed by the Internal Revenue Service's Publication 946.
- *Salvage value*—the estimated value of the asset after it reaches the end of its useful life. This is estimated by the pharmacy, though quite often, items are depreciated to zero dollars.

Once these three values have been determined, each item's depreciation can be calculated. There are a few ways to calculate depreciation, as follows:

- *Straight-line* (the simplest method)—asset basis minus salvage value equals useful life.
- *Declining balance*—larger amounts of depreciation are recorded at the beginning of each item's life, and less toward the end; this is often done for extremely technical products that become obsolete rather quickly. The depreciation rate is found by taking 100% of the item's value and dividing it by the useful life. If the item depreciated over five years, the depreciation rate would be 20%. Next, the current book value of the item is multiplied by its depreciation rate. The result is the amount of depreciation for the first year. During the next year, the depreciation is calculated from the current book value.
- *Sum of years' digits* (SYD depreciation)—the sum of all the digits in the asset's useful life is determined. For a five-year depreciation, this would be 1 + 2 + 3 + 4 + 5, which equals 15, so the depreciation would be as follows:

    a. Year 1: 5/15 (depreciate by 33%)
    b. Year 2: 4/15 (depreciate by 27%)
    c. Year 3: 3/15 (depreciate by 20%)
    d. Year 4: 2/15 (depreciate by 13%)
    e. Year 5: 1/15 (depreciate by 7%)

- *Units of production*—usually used for depreciation of machinery or production equipment that "wears out over time." Take the asset basis and subtract the salvage value. Divide this by the estimated total production capability. Then divide the number of units produced in the current year. For example, if a pharmacy prescription filling machine cost $20,000; has a salvage value of $2000; could fill 500,000 units over its lifetime; and filled 30,000 prescriptions in a particular year, the depreciation would be calculated as follows:

$$[(\$20{,}000 - \$2000)/500{,}000] \times 30{,}000 = \$1080$$

This means that, based on how much the machine was used, $1080 of depreciation would be expensed.

After depreciation, at the end of an item's useful life, it still may be somewhat useful, but it has been fully depreciated and cannot be expensed any more. The item can continue to be used as long as it is still working, in a situation known as "off the books." The asset's salvage value is still recorded as an asset until a decision is made to sell it or scrap it (take it to a junkyard or landfill).

Inventory Turnover

Inventory may be defined as a list of merchandise itemized by various types and their costs. The goal of sound inventory management in today's environment is a reasonable turnover of products combined with rapid billing and receiving along with minimal waste. The objective is to purchase an adequate supply of often-used pharmaceuticals. Today's highly competitive market demands optimal cost management for the pharmacy to operate efficiently and productively.

A well-managed inventory program will include **waste control**. In institutional settings, the amount and size of injectable pharmaceuticals is often analyzed to reduce costs through minimizing waste. In the retail pharmacy department, timely return for credit of a near-expired product may be considered a controllable cost-effective tool for inventory management. The technician should become familiar with the pharmacy's policies and procedures on inventory management in an effort to prevent product depreciation and improve turnover.

Turnover is a measure of time that the product remains in stock and is not used by the pharmacy. For higher-cost pharmaceuticals, this value may be used to prevent excessive expenditures by the pharmacy. Select drugs that have short expiration dating or limited need would be required to have a very high turnover rate to prevent excessive waste and financial loss. An **inventory turnover rate** is a specific time period over which the total inventory is sold. The more often this occurs, the higher the turnover rate. The turnover rate is calculated by dividing the total purchases by the average inventory.

■ **Example 1:**

During the past year, a pharmacy spent $900,000 on the items in its inventory. The average inventory value during the past year was determined to be $150,000.

What was the *turnover rate* of the inventory?

So, $900,000 divided by $150,000 = 6 times

Average Wholesale Price

The term **average wholesale price** (AWP) is used to describe the national average cost of a drug product to the pharmacy. This price usually represents the highest cost available for pharmaceuticals purchased from the most readily available vendor source. However, in practice, this is simply a "benchmark" price set by manufacturers.

While the drug product (cost of goods) represents the major cost in the business aspect of pharmacy, it is often the cost the pharmacy has least control over. Pharmacies use a variety of contracts and limited purchase agreements to reduce the cost of goods. The "laid-in" or actual cost of a drug product is the product cost after all contract discounts are applied. This often differs from the AWP.

Pharmacies may restrict multiple-source products to a select manufacturer or distributor as a means of reducing the cost of goods. For example, Cefazolin 1 g IV powder for injection is produced by a variety of manufacturers. The pharmacy may choose to contract with a specific manufacturer or distribution group to reduce the cost substantially. When a drug product is available generically, the cost of goods represents an opportunity for the pharmacy to control the cost of the product. For single-source or branded products protected by U.S. patent, the pharmacy has less of an opportunity to control the cost of goods unless the department maintains a pharmacy formulary and restricts therapy choices.

Wholesale Acquisition Cost

The supply of medications (pharmaceuticals) involves a chain of wholesalers that help distribute them to pharmacies. Wholesalers purchase large orders of medications and drug products from manufacturers and sell them to pharmacies at higher prices. The *wholesale acquisition cost (WAC)* is an estimate of the manufacturer's list price for a drug to wholesalers or other direct purchasers. It does not include discounts or rebates. The price is determined by federal law. Without including rebates and other manufacturer-provided incentives, it can be difficult to estimate a drug's actual cost. The WAC represents the manufacturer's published catalog price ("list price") for sales of a brand name or generic drug to wholesalers. It is usually higher than the average wholesale price.

Insurance Reimbursements

Average wholesale price (AWP) is often used by insurance carriers and third-party providers to determine a contract price. Third parties reimburse a pharmacy based on the AWP, less an established percentage, as the cost basis for the drug in reimbursement programs. The AWP is obtained from commercial listings. The reimbursed amount is calculated from a predetermined formula, for example, "AWP less 10% plus $3.50 professional fee." Many third-party programs have a **copayment** provision, which requires the patient to pay a portion of the charge for each prescription filled.

■ **Example 1:**

If a **third-party payer** reimburses a pharmacy "AWP less 15%" plus a professional fee of $3.50, what would the total reimbursement be on a prescription written for 40 capsules having an AWP of $22 per 100 capsules?

AWP for 40 capsules = $5 − 15% = $7.50

$7.50 + $3.50 = $11

If the patient must pay a copayment of $2 for each prescription filled, how much would the third party reimburse the pharmacy in the preceding example?

$11 − $2 = $9

 Test Your Knowledge

Choose the most correct answer from the choices provided.

1. Twice annually, your pharmacy department analyzes and reports the net profit of the business. When calculating net profit, which of the following statements is true?

   a. Net profit is the gross profit (difference between the cost of goods and services and the total reimbursement to the pharmacy for those goods and services) *minus* all overhead costs.

   b. Salaries and bonuses paid to all pharmacy employees must be calculated.

   c. Benefits paid for all pharmacy employees (i.e., health care, retirement account) must be calculated.

   d. All of the above

2. Product turnover is best described as

   a. the average amount of time your pharmacy retains a product before it is sold.

   b. the amount of time before a pharmaceutical expires.

   c. the amount of revenue a product generates by the time it is dispensed and sold.

   d. the interest charge that the pharmacy pays for inventory purchased and not used.

3. Sales minus cost equals gross profit. What is the gross profit for a pharmacy whose sales total $199,991 and whose costs total $19,191?

   a. $108,072

   b. $108,000

   c. $108,080

   d. $180,800

4. The manufacturer's average wholesale price is $1200 per unit of product. If the pharmacy purchases 24 units or more per year, the pharmacy will receive a 15% rebate. If the pharmacy purchases 12 units or more, the rebate is 10%. What is the product's actual cost if 15 units are purchased?

   a. $14,400

   b. $15,000

   c. $1200

   d. $1080

5. Using the actual cost of $1080, what is the gross profit percent of the prescription sold to a patient with an insurance program that pays the pharmacy as follows: average AWP minus 6% plus a $2 dispensing fee?

   a. 4.4%

   b. 1.25%

   c. 6%

   d. 27%

6. Insurance company A will reimburse the pharmacy at AWP minus 8% with a further deduction of a $4.50 dispensing fee. Insurance company B will reimburse the pharmacy at AWP minus 10% plus a $6 dispensing fee. Which insurance company will generate the greatest gross profit?

a. Insurance company B

b. Insurance company A

c. Both insurance companies

d. Neither insurance company

7. The pharmacy manager wants a comparison of gross profit dollars between insurance plan A and insurance B for 2022. Insurance plan A will reimburse the pharmacy at AWP minus 8% with a further deduction of a $4.50 dispensing fee. Insurance plan B will reimburse the pharmacy at AWP minus 10% plus a $6 dispensing fee. You are asked to examine the pharmacy purchase history to find the rebate your pharmacy received in 2022 so you can then calculate the correct actual cost. The purchase history from January 1 to December 31, 2022, shows 28 units purchased. Which insurance plan would reimburse more for the drug described in question 6, and by how many total dollars?

a. Plan A by $22.50

b. Plan A by $630

c. Plan B by $66

d. Plan B by $88.50

8. If a drug product expires and is returned to the vendor, the pharmacy receives 45% of AWP for credit. The pharmacy returned two units in 2022. How much credit did the pharmacy receive?

a. $1300

b. $1080

c. $918

d. $997

9. The pharmacy receives a 10% discount if a case of 12 ammonium lactate lotion, 365 mL, is ordered from the manufacturer. If the invoice is paid within 14 days, the pharmacy receives an additional 2% rebate. If the AWP unit cost of the lotion is $7.25, and the pharmacy pays the invoice in 10 days, what is the "laid-in" or actual acquisition cost of one bottle (365 mL) for the pharmacy?

a. $7.25

b. $6.53

c. $6.38

d. $6.66

10. The total operating cost for the pharmacy department is approximately $172,000 per month. The average monthly invoice total for all goods purchased is $164,000. The average monthly sales amount the pharmacy department generates is $358,000. What is the total profit from the pharmacy?

    a. $186,000
    b. $172,000
    c. $194,000
    d. $22,000

For questions 11 to 14, write each correct calculation on the line provided.

11. A drug prescribed to treat AIDS costs $300 per 60 tablets. Calculate the cost for a 6-month supply if the patient takes one tablet per day.

    _____

12. A treatment for an eye infection is priced at $50 per gallon, minus a limited-time discount of 25%. If the pharmacy purchases the solution and receives this discount, what would the net cost be of 32 ounces (1 quart) of the medication?

    _____

13. Antacid tablets cost $100 per 500 tablets, less a discount of 30%. What would 100 tablets cost if purchased at the discounted price?

    _____

14. Mouthwash sells for $2.50. A 25% profit had been added to its actual cost in order to reach the selling price. What was the actual cost of the mouthwash?

    _____

Critical Thinking

1. Each tablet in a bottle of 30 costs $4.60. The pharmacy's cost (including pharmacy supplies, shipping, pharmacist consult, and personnel time to dispense) is $1.40 per pill. If a 12% profit is desired, how much would the entire bottle cost?

   _____

Answers to Stop and Review Exercises

Appendix A

Chapter 1: Fundamentals of Math

Metric Measures
1. 2.5
2. 0.63
3. 1.6
4. 1.3
5. 0.5
6. 0.15
7. 0.85
8. 0.25
9. 5.5
10. 0.1

Measures in Abbreviations and Notation
1. 5 g
2. 200 mL
3. 0.5 L
4. 0.03 g
5. 400 mcg
6. 0.2 mg
7. 0.4 mg
8. 900 mcg
9. 10.3 mcg
10. 2.7 kg
11. 0.05 g
12. 6.4 kg

Metric Unit Abbreviations
1. mg
2. mm
3. g
4. mcg
5. kg
6. m
7. mL
8. L
9. cm
10. kl

The Apothecary System
1. gr iii
2. dr $\frac{2}{3}$
3. ʒ viii
4. lb iv
5. gr $\frac{1}{200}$
6. dr $\overline{ss}$
7. ʒ iii
8. lb ii
9. lb ii ʒ xi
10. gr $\overline{ss}$

The Household System
1. 1
2. 3
3. 1.5
4. 32
5. 2.67

Chapter 2: Celsius and Fahrenheit Temperature Conversions

Converting Temperatures
1. 98.6°F
2. 33.9°C
3. 16.7°C
4. 40°C
5. 108.9°F
6. 86.7°C
7. 212°F
8. 188.6°F
9. 42.8°C
10. 71.6°F
11. 37°C
12. 31.1°C
13. 39.3°C
14. 42.8°C
15. 101.3°F

Chapter 3: Fractions and Decimals

Common Fractions
1. 80
2. 5
3. 60
4. 25
5. 9
6. 82

Appendix A • Answers to Stop and Review Exercises   327

7. c
8. a
9. 3
10. 1
11. $6\frac{1}{2}$
12. $1\frac{4}{5}$
13. $4\frac{13}{15}$
14. 25
15. 2
16. $10\frac{1}{3}$

17. $\frac{20}{3}$
18. $\frac{370}{19}$
19. $\frac{51}{10}$
20. $\frac{9}{4}$
21. $\frac{35}{9}$
22. $\frac{113}{2}$
23. $\frac{452}{3}$
24. $\frac{578}{3}$

Lowest Common Denominator and Reducing Fractions

1. 12
2. 6
3. 60
4. 20
5. 16
6. 12
7. 24
8. 16
9. 8
10. 4
11. $\frac{1}{2}$
12. $\frac{2}{3}$
13. $\frac{3}{4}$
14. $\frac{1}{9}$
15. $\frac{1}{2}$
16. $\frac{1}{2}$
17. $\frac{1}{3}$
18. $\frac{7}{8}$
19. $\frac{3}{4}$
20. $\frac{7}{9}$

Adding and Subtracting Fractions

1. $\frac{13}{24}$
2. $\frac{71}{72}$
3. $4\frac{3}{5}$
4. $1\frac{17}{24}$
5. $\frac{2}{3}$
6. $\frac{2}{5}$
7. $3\frac{8}{11}$
8. $\frac{13}{42}$
9. $\frac{71}{105}$
10. $\frac{2}{3}$
11. $\frac{47}{60}$
12. $1\frac{11}{18}$
13. $2\frac{7}{10}$
14. $\frac{13}{15}$
15. 6
16. $3\frac{1}{5}$
17. $\frac{1}{5}$
18. $3\frac{1}{3}$
19. $5\frac{1}{2}$
20. $\frac{4}{5}$
21. $6\frac{4}{7}$
22. $\frac{3}{7}$
23. $\frac{7}{12}$
24. $5\frac{1}{8}$
25. $2\frac{1}{8}$
26. $11\frac{2}{5}$
27. $13\frac{4}{7}$
28. $4\frac{5}{6}$
29. $7\frac{2}{9}$
30. $\frac{7}{12}$

Multiplying Fractions

1. $\frac{1}{15}$
2. $\frac{8}{35}$
3. $\frac{3}{10}$
4. $1\frac{1}{3}$
5. $\frac{2}{9}$
6. $4\frac{1}{2}$
7. $\frac{25}{72}$
8. $\frac{1}{6}$
9. $1\frac{1}{3}$
10. $\frac{14}{15}$
11. 2
12. $14\frac{3}{10}$
13. $27\frac{1}{12}$
14. $1\frac{1}{2}$
15. $\frac{21}{128}$
16. $\frac{48}{125}$
17. $\frac{49}{108}$
18. $\frac{5}{6}$
19. $1\frac{17}{88}$
20. $\frac{35}{96}$

Dividing Fractions

1. $\frac{3}{4}$
2. $\frac{20}{33}$
3. $\frac{8}{9}$
4. $\frac{4}{15}$
5. $2\frac{1}{7}$
6. $1\frac{5}{9}$
7. $1\frac{1}{2}$
8. $\frac{90}{161}$
9. $2\frac{1}{7}$
10. $\frac{5}{14}$
11. $2\frac{106}{171}$
12. $4\frac{5}{7}$
13. $\frac{4}{42}$
14. 16
15. $1\frac{1}{8}$
16. $\frac{16}{21}$

Converting Fractions and Decimals

1. 0.5
2. 0.4
3. 0.17 (rounded)
4. 0.625
5. 0.13 (rounded)
6. 0.006 (rounded)
7. 0.015
8. 0.83 (rounded)
9. 0.002
10. 0.0003 (rounded)
11. $\frac{1}{200}$
12. $\frac{9}{1000}$
13. $\frac{33}{10,000}$
14. $\frac{1}{20}$
15. $\frac{1}{4}$
16. $\frac{1}{5000}$
17. $\frac{3}{40}$
18. $\frac{3}{20}$
19. $\frac{21}{25}$
20. $2\frac{3}{4}$

Adding and Subtracting Decimals

1. 14.24
2. 186.09
3. 17.469
4. 77.224
5. 4.86
6. 5.459
7. 0.705
8. 8.033
9. 53.55
10. 17.135
11. 7.8
12. 15.6
13. 4.62
14. 12.023
15. 8.977
16. 16.93

Multiplying Decimals

1. 83.42
2. 3.43
3. 20.724
4. 0.5648
5. 0.539
6. 0.0492
7. 0.00027
8. 0.2125
9. 90.72
10. 1.36
11. 0.0591
12. 0.38535

Dividing Decimals

1. 4.43
2. 61.33
3. 47
4. 2
5. 3
6. 1.55
7. 4
8. 7.3
9. 100
10. 0.1
11. 0.3906
12. 0.004
13. 2222.2
14. 20705
15. 0.06313
16. 18.295
17. 60
18. 23.5454
19. 0.00089
20. 2.7308

Chapter 4: Ratios, Proportions, and Percents

Converting Fractions into Ratios. (Reduced to the lowest terms).

1. 1 : 4
2. 1 : 5
3. 2 : 3
4. 3 : 4
5. 1 : 3
6. 1 : 8
7. 1 : 20
8. 1 : 20
9. 1 : 3
10. 1 : 2
11. 2 : 5
12. 1 : 10
13. 1 : 20
14. 2 : 25
15. 1 : 200
16. 1 : 20
17. 1 : 4
18. 1 : 5
19. 1 : 4
20. 1 : 10

Proportions

1. 75
2. 15
3. 12
4. 50
5. 135
6. 16
7. 45
8. 40
9. 3
10. 640
11. 125
12. 50

Percentages

1. 12
2. 500
3. 0.02
4. 10
5. 250
6. 7.5
7. 8
8. 187.5
9. 3
10. 35
11. 10.8
12. 250
13. 1.25
14. 60
15. 30

Chapter 5:
Percentage of Errors Due to Equipment

1. 6%
2. 1.4%
3. 0.5 g or 500 mg
4. 10%
5. 75 mg

Chapter 6:
Ratio and Proportion Method

Using the Ratio and Proportion Method

1a. 0.16
1b. 38.1
1c. 0.46
1d. 0.625
1e. 1.89
1f. 32,000
1g. 7.28
1h. 32.4
1i. 8.1
1j. 0.25
2a. True
2b. True
2c. True
2d. False
2e. True
3a. 2.9 mL
3b. 1.9 mL
3c. 0.4 mL
3d. 1.3 mL
3e. 0.6 mL
3f. 1.5 mL
3g. 2.4 mL
3h. 2.7 mL
3i. 0.5 mL
3j. 2 mL

Ratio and Proportion Expressed Using Colons

1. True
2. True
3. True
4. False
5. True

Calculations When Dosages Are in Different Units of Measure

1. 0.8 mL
2. 1.1 mL
3. 1.1 mL
4. 2.2 mL
5. 1.3 mL
6. 15 mL
7. 2.7 mL

Chapter 7:
Dimensional Analysis

Basic Dimensional Analysis

1. 0.06 mL
2. 2.7 mL
3. 1.3 mL
4. 15 mL
5. 1.1 mL

Chapter 8:
Formula Method

Basic Formula

1. 1.5 mL
2. 0.9 mL
3. 1.2 mL
4. 0.55 mL

Use with Metric Conversions

1. 0.9 mL
2. 4.5 mL
3. 1.2 mL
4. 1 mL

Use with Units and mEq Calculations

1. 1.9 mL
2. 0.6 mL
3. 5 mL
4. 1.9 mL

Chapter 9:
Concentrations

Concentrations and Volumes of Solutions

1. 180 g
2. 6 g
3. 1800 mL of stock solution and 1200 mL of water

Weight and Weight (w/w)
1. 0.95%

Volume and Volume (v/v)
1. 700 mL
2. 270 mL
3. 240 mL
4. $166\frac{2}{3}$ mL
5. 157 mL

Weight and Volume (w/v)
1. 0.03 mL concentrate; 1.97 mL diluent
2. 5 mL concentrate; 20 mL diluent
3. 500 mg; 18 mL diluent
4. 17.5 mL diluent
5. 4 mL concentrate
6. 0.05 mL concentrate
7. 1 mL concentrate
8. 3.57 mL concentrate
9. 2% w/v concentration
10. 2.25% w/v concentration

Chapter 10: Dilutions and Solutions

Dilutions, Stock Solutions for Solids, and Liquid Dilutions
1. water; saline
2. solvents
3. total
4. stock
5. 1; 7
6. 800
7. 1500
8. 40
9. 3; 7
10. 1; 10

Alligation
1. 129 g of 10% and 321 g of 3%
2. 400 mL of 30% and 100 mL of 20%
3. 231 mL of 23.4% and 5769 mL of water
4. 167 mL of 60% and 83 mL of water
5. 333 mL of NaCl and 667 mL of water
6. 1 L of 31% and 1 L of 27%
7. 1000 mL of 42% and 500 mL of 18%; 86 mL of stock solution and 34 mL of water

Chapter 11: Oral Medication Labels and Dosage Calculation

Calculating Dosages of Tablets and Capsules

1a. 2 tablets   400X = 800
1b. 2 tablets   10X = 20
1c. 1 tablet   60:1::X mg:5 gr
1d. 4 tablets   15X = 60 = 4
1e. 2 tablets   0.4 mg:1 tab::X mg:2 tab X = 0.4 × 2 = 0.8 mg (which, in practice, would be 1 tablet)
1f. 3 tablets = $\frac{600}{200} = 3$
1g. 1.5 tablets = $x = \frac{7.5}{5} = 1.5$
1h. 2 tablets = $x = \frac{250}{125} = 2$
1i. 1 tablet
1j. $2\frac{1}{2}$ tablets
2a. B, 1 caplet
2b. I, 2 tablets
2c. F, 1 tablet
2d. H, 2 tablets
2e. C, 1 tablet
2f. E, 2 tablets
2g. D, 2 tablets
2h. G, 2 tablets
2i. A, 1 tablet
2j. C, 1 tablet

Calculating Liquid Dosages

1a. 10 mL
1b. 7.5 mL
1c. 2.5 mL
1d. 4 mL
1e. 10 mL
1f. 10 mL
1g. 7.5 mL
1h. 3 mL
1i. 6 mL
1j. 5 mL
1k. 2.5 mL
1l. 20 mL
1m. 2.5 mL
1n. 8 mL
1o. 10 mL
1p. 2 mL
1q. 2 mL
1r. 5 mL
1s. 0.75 mL
1t. 10 mL
1u. 3 mL

Chapter 12: Reconstitution of Powdered Drugs

Reconstitution of a Single-Strength Solution

Label 1

1. Sterile water for injection or bacteriostatic water for injection
2. 0.9 mL
3. 1.7 mL
4. 3.4 mL
5. 6.8 mL
6. 250 mg per 1 mL
7. 5 mL
8. Inject slowly over 3 to 5 minutes
9. Rapid administration may result in seizures

Label 2

1. 250,000 units per mL
2. Yes
3. Expires June 8 at 2 p.m.
4. 20 million units
5. Your initials
6. Package insert

Label 3

1. 10 mL
2. 20 mL
3. Sterile water for injection
4. 50 mg per mL
5. 14 days
6. Expires May 18 at 1350 hours
7. Your initials

Label 4

1. 1 g
2. 2.1 mL
3. 350 mg/mL

Label 5

1. 200 mcg; 0.2 mg
2. 5 mL
3. 0.9% sodium chloride
4. Must be used immediately
5. 40 mcg/mL
6. Package insert

Label 6

1. 10 mL
2. Bacteriostatic water for injection with benzyl alcohol
3. 1 gram
4. 25°C (77°F)
5. 100 mg per mL
6. 48 hours
7. Expires February 16 at 0840 hours

Label 7

1. 19 mL
2. Water for injection
3. 10 mg/mL
4. 200 mg

Label 8

1. 29 mL
2. Distilled water
3. Shake the bottle to loosen granules, add half (15 mL) of the distilled water, shake vigorously to dissolve the granules, and then add the balance of the water and shake vigorously
4. 100 mg/5 mL
5. 14 days

Label 9

1. 500 mg
2. Bacteriostatic water with benzyl alcohol
3. 10 mL
4. 50 mg per mL
5. 48 hours

Chapter 13: Parenteral Medication Labels and Dosage Calculation

Calculating Insulin Doses

1a. Humulin R Regular, rapid-acting

1b. Novolin N, intermediate-acting

1c. Humulin U, long-acting

1d. Humalog, rapid-acting

1e. Humulin L, intermediate-acting

1f. Standard, dual-scale 100 unit/mL U-100 syringe;
Lo-dose, 50 unit/0.5 mL U-100 syringe;
Lo-dose, 30 unit/0.3 mL U-100 syringe

1g. Lo-dose, 30 unit U-100 syringe

1h. Lo-dose, 50 unit U-100 syringe

1i. 0.6

1j. 0.25

1k. Standard dual-scale 100 unit U-100 syringe

1l. False

2a. 68

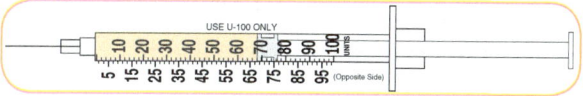

2b. 15

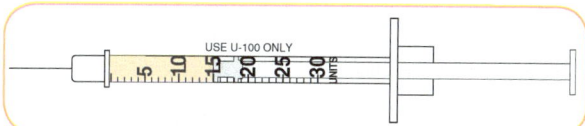

2c. 23

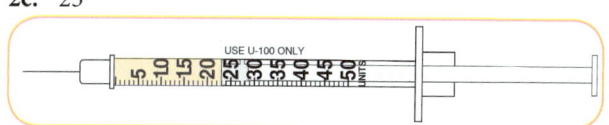

2d. 57

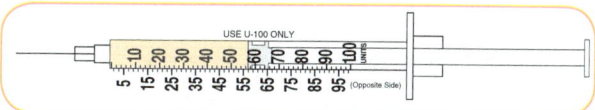

3a. 80 units

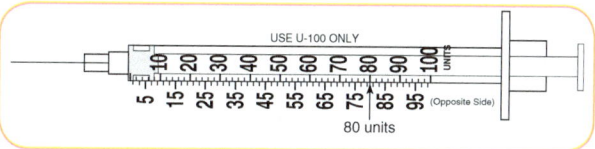

3b. 15 units

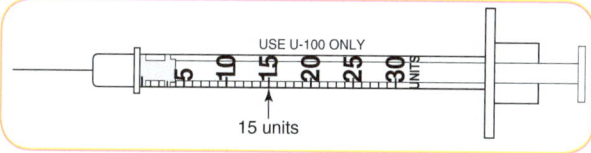

3c. 66 units

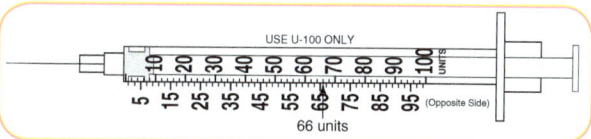

3d. 16 units

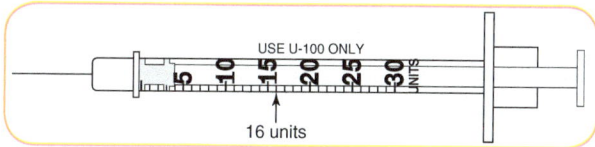

3e. 32 units

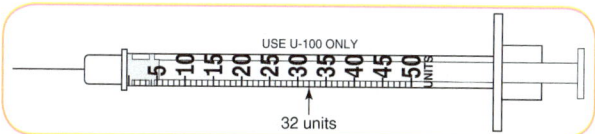

4a. 15 and 21 units

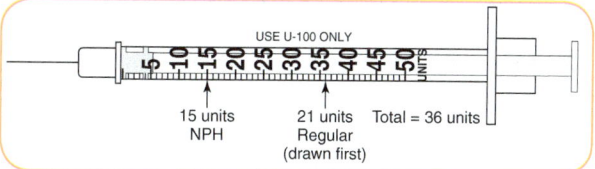

4b. 42 and 16 units

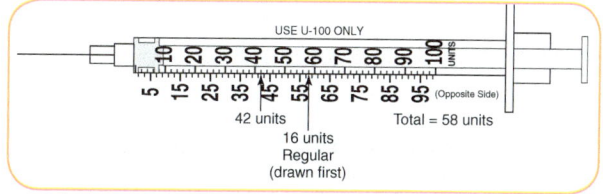

4c. 40 and 32 units

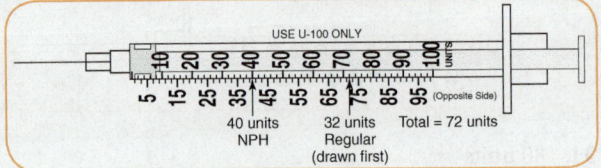

4d. 12 and 8 units

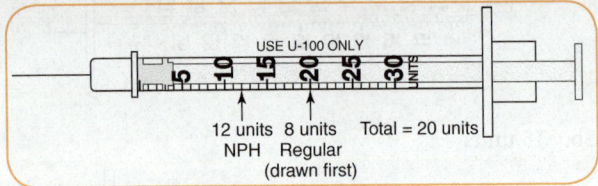

Solutions Measured as Milliequivalents

1. 30 mEq; 15 mL
2. 2 mEq/mL
3. 7.5 mL
4. 2 mEq/mL
5. 20 mL
6. 10 mL
7. 1 mEq/mL
8. 50 mL/50 mEq; 1 mEq/mL
9. 4.2 g/mL
10. 10 mL

Chapter 14: Intravenous Flow Rate Calculations

Calculating IV Push Rates

1. 0.6 mL; 2.4; 144
2. 167
3. 1.5; 0.19
4. 120
5. 50
6. 25
7. 133
8. 200
9. 3; 3
10. 2; 18; 2.5

Intravenous Solutions and Additives

1a. C; sodium chloride 0.9%, 0.9 g/100 mL; 308 mOsm/L

1b. E; dextrose 5%, 5 g/100 mL; 252 mOsm/L

1c. G; dextrose 5%, 5 g/100 mL; sodium chloride 0.9 g/100 mL; 560 mOsm/L

1d. D; dextrose 5%, 5 g/100 mL; sodium chloride 0.45 g/100 mL; 406 mOsm/L

1e. A; dextrose 5%, 5 g/100 mL; sodium chloride 0.225%, 0.225 g/100 mL; 329 mOsm/L

1f. H; dextrose 5%, 5 g/100 mL; sodium lactate 0.31 g/100 mL, NaCl 0.6 g/100 mL; KCl 0.03 g/100 mL; CaCl 0.02 g/100 mL; 525 mOsm/L

1g. B; dextrose 5%, 5 g/100 mL; sodium chloride 0.45%; 0.45 g/100 mL; potassium chloride 20 mEq per liter; 447 mOsm/L

1h. F; sodium chloride 0.45%; 0.45 g/100 mL; 154 mOsm/L

Calculating IVs as Percentages

1a. 2.25
1b. 150; 27
1c. 25; 1.65
1d. 25
1e. 50; 9
1f. 6.75
1g. 3.375
1h. 36; 2.7
1i. 25; 2.25
1j. 50; 1.125

Calculating IV Flow Rates

1a. 15
1b. 10
1c. 60
1d. 60
1e. 10

Calculating gtt/min Flow Rates

1. 28
2. 42
3. 16
4. 42
5. 49
6. 42

Calculating gtt/min Flow Rates Using Dimensional Analysis

1. 26
2. 23
3. 28
4. 31
5. 42
6. 23

Manually Calculating IV Flow Rates Using the Formula Method

1a. 50
1b. 40
1c. 80
1d. 50
1e. 20
1f. 55
1g. 33
1h. 83

Manually Calculating IV Flow Rates Using the Shortcut Method

1a. 11
1b. 28
1c. 31
1d. 8
1e. 25
1f. 50
1g. 60
1h. 28

Adjusting Flow Rates

1a. 31; 1350; 10; 135; 34; 10%; reset to 34 gtt/min (10% increase is acceptable)

1b. 100; 5; 100; 100; 0%; IV is on time, so no adjustment is needed

1c. 21; 4; 188; 31; 48% (48% increase is unacceptable); consult the physician

1d. 33; 3; 83; 28; −15% (−15% slower is acceptable), IV is ahead of schedule; slow rate to 28 gtt/min, and observe the patient's condition

1e. 42; 6; 142; 47; 12%; reset to 47 gtt/min (12% increase is acceptable)

1f. 42; 4; 200; 67; 60%; recalculated rate 67 gtt/min (60% increase is unacceptable); consult the physician

1g. 13; 10; 60; 15; 15%; reset to 15 gtt/min (15% increase is acceptable)

1h. 42; 2; 180; 45; 7%; reset to 45 gtt/min (7% increase is acceptable)

Calculating IV Flow Rates for Electronic Infusions

1a. 42
1b. 75
1c. 200
1d. 150
1e. 125
1f. 120
1g. 125
1h. 83

Calculating IV Flow Rates from Units Per Hour Ordered

1. 38 mL/hr
2. 40 mL/hr
3. 16 mL/hr
4. 80 mL/hr
5. 50 mL/hr

Heparin Intravenous Calculations

1. 1000 units/hr
2. 1200 units/hr
3. 1200 units/hr
4. 600 units/hr
5. 1500 units/hr
6. 1000 units/hr
7. 500 units/hr
8. 875 units/hr
9. 400 units/hr
10. 1400 units/hr

Chapter 15: Pediatric Drug Administration

Calculating Pediatric Dosages by Body Weight

1. 20; 500; 125; 1000; 250; yes
2. 5
3. 2.2; 110; 55; yes
4. 0.55
5. 15; 120; yes
6. 8
7. 5; 7.5; 9.5; yes
8. 0.8
9. 1.8; 4.5; no
10. 17.7; 354; 118; 708; 236; no
11. 120; 60; 7.5; yes
12. 7.5; $1\frac{1}{2}$
13. 25; 375; 125; 625; 208; no

Determining Pediatric Dosages by Body Surface Area

1. $0.57\ m^2$
2. $0.69\ m^2$
3. $0.42\ m^2$
4. $0.52\ m^2$
5. $0.78\ m^2$
6. $1.40\ m^2$
7. $0.69\ m^2$
8. $0.29\ m^2$
9. $0.88\ m^2$
10. $0.64\ m^2$
11. $0.5\ m^2$
12. $1.08\ m^2$
13. $0.34\ m^2$
14. $1.08\ m^2$
15. $0.38\ m^2$

Calculating Pediatric Intravenous Drug Administrations

1. 7.2; 36.8
2. 2; 8
3. 7.5; 88.5
4. 2; 23
5. 120; 3; 22
6. 87; 2; 48
7. 80; 6; 44
8. 75; 3; 57

Calculating Daily Maintenance Fluids for Pediatric Patients

1. 350; 14.6
2. 1150; 48
3. 1800; 75
4. 1600; 67
5. 800; 33
6. 880; 35
7a. 1720
7b. 600
7c. 1100
7d. 1960

Chapter 16: Business Math for Pharmacy Technicians

Due to this chapter's shorter length, Stop & Review questions were not needed, but Test Your Knowledge questions were created, which appear in Appendix B.

Answer Key to Test Your Knowledge Questions

Appendix B

Chapter 1: Fundamentals of Math

Convert Arabic Numbers to Roman Numerals

1. V
2. XVIII
3. IX
4. XVI
5. XIX
6. XXII
7. XXIV
8. XXVII
9. XXIX
10. XXX
11. XLV
12. LXXXIX
13. CXII
14. CLV
15. CXCVIII
16. CCII
17. DVI
18. DXXXIV
19. M
20. MXXV

Convert Roman Numerals to Arabic Numbers

21. 4
22. 7
23. 9
24. 13
25. 14
26. 18
27. 19
28. 24
29. 27
30. 29

Convert Roman Numerals to Arabic Numbers

31. 18
32. 12
33. 11
34. 31
35. 21
36. 6
37. 18
38. 10
39. 9
40. 3

Abbreviations of Units of Measure

41. m
42. pt
43. gr
44. fl oz
45. dr
46. gtt
47. fl dr
48. qt
49. kg
50. L
51. mg
52. g
53. mL
54. mcg
55. m
56. cm
57. T or tbsp
58. c
59. t or tsp
60. gal
61. oz

Metric Measures in Abbreviations and Notation

62. 0.04 g
63. 17.5 kg
64. 3.5 kg
65. 5.3 mL
66. 10.4 mcg
67. 200 mcg
68. 15.2 mcg
69. 0.6 L
70. 8 g
71. 0.4 mL
72. 0.09 mg

Apothecary or Household Amounts

73. gr v
74. $\frac{1}{2}$ t or $\frac{1}{2}$ tsp
75. 9 oz
76. $7\frac{1}{2}$ oz
77. gr xvi
78. gr $\overline{ss}$

79. dr iv
80. 25 mEq
81. 10,000 units
82. $\frac{1}{2}$ T or $\frac{1}{2}$ tbsp
83. $3\frac{1}{2}$ oz
84. $\frac{1}{2}$ oz

Equivalents

85. 15
86. 6
87. 32
88. 40
89. 76 (rounded)
90. 3
91. 1.2 (rounded)
92. 2

Interpreting Symbols

93. meter
94. dram
95. minim
96. grain
97. quart
98. ounce
99. ounce
100. $\frac{1}{2}$
101. millimeter
102. gram

Writing Symbols

103. gtt
104. gr
105. t or tsp
106. ɱ
107. T or tbsp
108. dr
109. mEq
110. pt
111. oz

Completion

112. length
113. volume
114. weight

Equivalents

115. 1000
116. 1
117. 10
118. 1000
119. 10
120. 1000
121. 0.1

Metric Notation

122. 10 mg
123. 4.5 mL
124. 7 kg
125. 2.5 mm
126. 8.5 mcg

Critical Thinking

1a. The patient should use a tablespoon to administer the medication.

1b. The patient should take one tablespoon three times a day.

1c. 45 mL per day × 10 days equals 450 mL total. Because 450 mL is equivalent to 0.95 of a pint, the patient needs 2 half-pint bottles to contain enough medication for the 10-day period.

2. The pharmacy technician should ask the pharmacist or check a website to understand what the "L" stands for in the Roman numeral system.

3. 2 tablets

4. 240

5. 7.438915 kg, which is rounded to 7.4 kg

Chapter 2: Celsius and Fahrenheit Temperature Conversions

1. 17.44°C
2. 37.5°C
3. 30.7°C
4. 81.1°C
5. 55.6°C
6. 0°C
7. 44.4°C
8. 100°C
9. 6.7°C
10. 36.6°C
11. 73.3°C
12. 8.9°C
13. 32°F
14. 44.2°F
15. 36.3°F
16. 99.3°F
17. 212°F
18. 110.5°F
19. 89.6°F
20. 47.1°F
21. 131°F
22. 62.6°F
23. 32.2°F
24. 80.6°F

Critical Thinking

1. 38.33°C
2. 46.4°F
3. 68°F
4. The pharmacy technician must document the incorrect temperature and make the pharmacist aware of the situation.
5. The Pfizer and Moderna vaccines must be frozen during transport.
6. The liquid form of amoxicillin should be refrigerated at temperatures as low as 52°F (11°C).
7. Lipitor and Toprol should be stored at room temperature.
8. All medications become degraded at 86°F (30°C) or higher.

Chapter 3: Fractions and Decimals

Calculating Fractions

1. $2\frac{1}{3}$
2. 2
3. $\frac{13}{25}$
4. $9\frac{3}{8}$
5. $1\frac{1}{3}$
6. $\frac{1}{20}$
7. $3\frac{5}{8}$
8. $2\frac{5}{7}$
9. $\frac{2}{3}$
10. $\frac{3}{14}$
11. 12
12. $8\frac{1}{4}$
13. $\frac{3}{8}$
14. $24\frac{16}{39}$
15. $8\frac{5}{8}$
16. $\frac{1}{5}$

Converting Mixed Numbers to Improper Fractions

17. $\frac{9}{7}$
18. $\frac{171}{8}$
19. $\frac{43}{5}$
20. $\frac{13}{2}$
21. $\frac{9}{2}$
22. $\frac{34}{3}$

Reducing Fractions

23. $\frac{1}{4}$
24. $\frac{33}{46}$
25. 6
26. $11\frac{1}{2}$
27. $1\frac{25}{31}$
28. 2

Least Common Denominators

29. The least common denominator is 10; the fraction is 1 and $\frac{1}{10}$.
30. The least common denominator is 18; the fraction is $\frac{17}{18}$.
31. The least common denominator is 60; the fraction is 1 and $\frac{37}{60}$.
32. The least common denominator is 30; the fraction is 2 and $\frac{4}{15}$.

Round to Nearest Tenth

33. 4.6
34. 7.8
35. 9
36. 0.1

Round to Nearest Hundredth

37. 8.09
38. 0.44
39. 64
40. 9.88

Round to Nearest Whole Number

41. 20
42. 7
43. 1
44. 13

Calculating Decimals

45. 0.901
46. 21.56
47. 5.39
48. 17.308
49. 5.08
50. 2.95
51. −0.206
52. 18.373
53. 41.87
54. 0.00268
55. 8.928
56. 12.19881
57. 23.1524 (rounded)
58. 2.0464 (rounded)
59. 40
60. 20

Circle the Correct Answer

61. 0.15
62. 0.073
63. False
64. False
65. True

Critical Thinking

1. The instruments should be arranged as follows (smallest to largest):

$$\frac{1}{16}, \frac{3}{16}, \frac{1}{4}, \frac{5}{16}, \frac{7}{16}, \frac{1}{2}$$

2. The missing instrument sizes in sequence are the following:

$$\frac{1}{8} \text{ and } \frac{3}{8}$$

3. 212.75 mg
4. 287.25 mg
5. 787.25 mg

Chapter 4:
Ratios, Proportions, and Percent

Percentages to Decimals

1. 0.06
2. 0.35
3. 0.003
4. 0.0001
5. 0.00004

Decimals to Percentages

6. 16%
7. 9%
8. 140%
9. 1280%
10. 260%

Percentages to Fractions, Reduced to Lowest Terms

11. $\frac{1}{20}$
12. $\frac{1}{5}$
13. $\frac{3}{1000}$
14. $\frac{1}{400}$
15. $\frac{1}{2000}$

Fractions to Percentages

16. 12%
17. 80%
18. 75%
19. 30%
20. 35%

Fractions to Ratios

21. 1:3
22. 1:500
23. 8:9
24. 1:75
25. 2:1

Percentages to Ratios

26. 1:100
27. 1:2
28. 1:8
29. 1:400
30. 1:300

Solve for "X" in Proportions

31. 4
32. 1
33. 2
34. $\frac{1}{3}$
35. 500
36. 4
37. 0.375
38. 0.5
39. 9
40. $\frac{2}{3}$

True or False

41. T
42. T
43. F
44. T
45. F
46. F
47. F
48. F
49. T
50. F

Critical Thinking

1. No, the technician made a mistake during calculation.

2. The pharmacy technician should use the ratio formula as follows:

$$\frac{250 \text{ mcg}}{1 \text{ tablet}} = \frac{125 \text{ mcg}}{X \text{ tablets}}$$

By cross-multiplying, the answer reveals that one-half of a tablet contains 125 micrograms of medication. Therefore, the patient must take only one-half of a tablet per dose.

3. 0.8
4. 125
5. 1 : 125

Chapter 5:
Percentage of Errors Due to Equipment

1. 6.67%
2. 1%
3. 69%
4. 6.5%
5. 5.19%
6. 7.14%
7. 247.5 mg would have actually been weighed because of the 10% overage.
8. 1.25%
9. The smallest weight would be 0.12 g, and an aliquot could be made to get the desired amount of weight.
10. The smallest weight would be 0.08 g, and an aliquot could be made to get the desired amount of weight.

Critical Thinking

1. This spoon is not calibrated identically to a conventional teaspoon.
2. The child is still sick because she is not receiving enough medication per spoonful because the spoon being used is not equivalent to a full teaspoon.
3. 0.5%
4. 10%
5. A conical graduate must be used, because it is calibrated in apothecary as well as metric units, while a cylindrical graduate is only calibrated in metric units.

Chapter 6:
Ratio and Proportion Method

mL Required of Dosage Ordered

1. 0.8 mL
2. 1.5 mL
3. 0.4 mL
4. 5 mL
5. 0.9 mL
6. 1.5 mL
7. 0.38 mL
8. 0.8 mL
9. 2.4 mL
10. 0.8 mL
11. 8 mL
12. 2 mL
13. 1.5 mL
14. 0.45 mL
15. 2 mL
16. 1.8 mL
17. 15 mL
18. 0.8 mL
19. 1.7 mL
20. 2.5 mL
21. 8 mL
22. 1.6 mL
23. 1.5 mL
24. 1.6 mL
25. 1.5 mL
26. 0.8 mL
27. 1.3 mL
28. 2.4 mL
29. 0.9 mL
30. 0.7 mL

Critical Thinking

1. The ratio should be written as follows:

   $$\frac{20 \text{ mg}}{1 \text{ mL}} = \frac{30 \text{ mg}}{X \text{ mL}}$$

2. The correct steps to make the calculation are to cross-multiply:

   20 mg multiplied by X mL = 20. Place this as a denominator.

   30 mg multiplied by 1 mL = 30. Place this as a numerator.

   Divide 30 by 20 to solve for X, which is equal to 1.5 mL.

Chapter 7: Dimensional Analysis

Calculate Dosage Using Dimensional Analysis

1. $2\frac{1}{2}$ tablets
2. 1.3 mL
3. 0.5 mL
4. 2.5 mL
5. 2.3 mL
6. 2.6 mL
7. 3 mL
8. 1.5 mL
9. 7 mL
10. 3 mL

Calculate Using Medicine Labels and Syringes

1. 0.8 mL
2. 1.4 mL
3. 3 mL
4. 0.9 mL
5. 1.5 mL
6. 0.38 mL
7. 0.8 mL
8. 1.2 mL
9. 1.5 mL
10. 0.45 mL
11. 1.6 mL
12. 2 mL
13. 2.3 mL
14. 2.4 mL
15. 15 mL
16. 1.5 mL
17. 0.8 mL
18. 1.6 mL
19. 2.5 mL
20. 3 mL
21. 8 mL
22. 1.2 mL
23. 1.6 mL
24. 0.6 mL
25. 1.5 mL
26. 1.6 mL
27. 1.3 mL
28. 1.5 mL
29. 1.5 mL
30. 2.5 mL
31. 1.7 mL
32. 2 mL
33. 0.9 mL
34. 1.4 mL
35. 10 mL
36. 1.8 mL
37. 0.8 mL
38. 2 mL
39. 0.8 mL

Critical Thinking

1. Using dimensional analysis,

   $$\text{mL} = \frac{5 \text{ mL}}{125} \times \frac{100}{1} = \frac{500}{125} = 4 \text{ mL}$$

2. If the same 100 mg was ordered, but the pharmacy had the medication available as 125 mg in 2 mL, the answer would be as follows:

   $$\text{mL} = \frac{2 \text{ mL}}{125} \times \frac{100}{1} = \frac{200}{125} = 1.6 \text{ mL}$$

3. Using dimensional analysis,

   $$\frac{0.25}{0.125} \times \frac{0.25}{1} = 0.5 \text{ tablet}$$

Chapter 8: Formula Method

Calculating Dosages and Expressing Them as Decimal Fractions

1. 1.3 mL
2. 0.8 mL
3. 1.5 mL
4. 1.6 mL
5. 1.4 mL
6. 1.2 mL
7. 1.2 mL
8. 2.4 mL
9. 0.7 mL
10. 0.8 mL

11. 2 mL
12. 12 mL
13. 3 mL
14. 4 mL
15. 2.6 mL
16. 4 mL
17. 1.4 mL
18. 20 mL
19. 1.6 mL
20. 0.8 mL
21. 1.5 mL
22. 30 mL
23. 1.5 mL
24. 0.8 mL
25. 2.5 mL
26. 1.6 mL
27. 0.8 mL
28. 1.6 mL
29. 2.5 mL
30. 20 mL
31. 0.7 mL
32. 0.8 mL
33. 1.3 mL
34. 25 mL
35. 1.2 mL
36. 0.8 mL
37. 30 mL
38. 1.3 mL
39. 2.5 mL
40. 35 mL

Critical Thinking

1. The first step that the pharmacy technician needs to take is to convert mg to mcg, to eliminate the decimal point, as follows: 0.4 mg = 400 mcg

2. The amount of mL to be administered is calculated as follows:

$$\frac{200 \text{ mcg}}{400 \text{ mcg}} \times 1.5 \text{ mL} = 0.75 \text{ mL}$$

3. The amount of mL to be administered is calculated as follows:

$$\frac{40 \text{ mEq}}{70 \text{ mEq}} \times 5 = \frac{200}{70} = 2.85 \text{ mL}$$

4. If a dosage of 80 mEq was ordered, the amount of mL to be administered is calculated as follows:

$$\frac{80 \text{ mEq}}{70 \text{ mEq}} \times 5 = 5.71 \text{ mL}$$

Chapter 9: Concentrations

Calculating Concentrations

1. 1.5%
2. 0.8%
3. 5%
4. 25%
5. 1.5%
6. $\frac{1}{5}$
7. $\frac{1}{2}$
8. $\frac{1}{4}$
9. $\frac{1}{3}$
10. 0.2%
11. 1%
12. 10%

Concentrations and Volumes

1. 4.8%
2. 7.5%
3. 90 mL
4. 87.5 mL
5. 125 mL
6. 96 mL
7. 1.25%
8. 0.5%
9. 1.75%
10. 0.75%
11. 0.4%
12. 400 mL
13. Approx 171 mL
14. Approx 233 mL
15. 700 mL

w/w, v/v, and w/v Equations

1. Need 22.5 g
2. Need 37.5 g
3. Need 6.75 g
4. 90 g
5. Add 45 mL isopropyl alcohol to 205 mL water
6. Add 40 mL isopropyl alcohol to 160 mL water
7. Add 22.5 mL isopropyl alcohol to 202.5 mL water

8. Add 49 mL isopropyl alcohol to 21 mL water
9. Dissolve 37.5 g NaCl in 150 mL diluent
10. Dissolve 12 g ampicillin in 200 mL diluent
11. Dissolve 1 g NaCl in 50 mL diluent
12. Dissolve 15 g cephapirin in 125 mL diluent
13. Dissolve 21 g cephapirin in 150 mL diluent
14. 150 g
15. 1350 g
16. 2 g
17. 20 g
18. 600 mL
19. 1000 mL = 1 L
20. Approx 583 mL
21. 250 mL
22. 3%
23. 8%
24. 6%
25. Approx 8.3%
26. 20%
27. 18.75%

Critical Thinking

1. By using the formula of $V_1 \times C_1 = V_2 \times C_2$,

    $C_1 = 5\%$, $C_2 = 2\%$, and $V_2 = 100$ mL

    Therefore, $V_1 = 40$ mL, so 40 mL of the 5% solution were poured into the container.

2. By using the same formula,

    $C_1 = 20\%$, $C_2 = 2\%$, and $V_2 = 100$ mL

    Therefore, $V_1 = 20$ mL, so 20 mL of the 20% solution were poured into the container.

Chapter 10: Dilutions and Solutions

1. $3\frac{1}{3}$ mg
2. 15 mg
3. $6\frac{2}{3}$ mg
4. 100 g
5. $\frac{2}{5}$; $\frac{2}{7}$
6. $\frac{3}{7}$; $\frac{3}{10}$
7. $\frac{4}{11}$; $\frac{11}{15}$
8. $\frac{5}{7}$; $\frac{7}{12}$
9. $\frac{1}{7}$; $\frac{1}{7}$
10. $\frac{3}{14}$; 3; 14
11. $\frac{2}{17}$; $\frac{2}{17}$
12. $\frac{5}{23}$; $\frac{5}{23}$
13. $\frac{2}{5}$
14. $\frac{5}{13}$
15. $\frac{1}{11}$
16. $\frac{3}{13}$
17. Take 162 mL urine and add it to 108 mL water
18. Take 40 mL urine and add it to 60 mL water
19. Take 50 mL urine and add it to 30 mL water
20. $\frac{3}{12} = \frac{1}{4}$
21. $\frac{2}{14}$ or $\frac{1}{7}$

22. $\frac{2}{7}$

23. 15 microliters serum and 105 microliters diluent are needed.

24. 18 mL total solution; 14 mL diluent are needed.

25. 10 microliters serum and 140 microliters diluent are needed.

26. 12 mL total solution; 9 mL diluent are needed.

27. Take 300 mL concentrate and add it to 200 mL diluent

28. Take 160 mL concentrate and add it to 240 mL diluent

29. 12.5 microliters

30. Take 125 mL concentrate and add it to 125 mL diluent.

31. 2 microliters

32. 12.5 mL

33. 20 g of 20% ichthammol ointment and 40 g of 15% ichthammol ointment

34. 20 g of 20% zinc oxide ointment and 40 g of 5% zinc oxide ointment

35. 60 g of 10% coal tar and 100 g of 2% coal tar

36. 45 g of benzocaine 10% ointment and 75 g of benzocaine 2% ointment

37. 19 g of 10% hydrocortisone cream and 71 g of 2.5% hydrocortisone cream

38. 250 mL of 90% alcohol and 1750 mL of 10% alcohol

39. 9 bottles

40. Combine 750 mL of D10W and 250 mL of SWFI

41. 15 g of petrolatum

42. 180 mL of 1:10 solution and 300 mL of 1:50 solution

Critical Thinking

1. 400 mL ÷ 8 = 50 mL

2. 350 mL of sterile water must be added to the solution.

Chapter 11: Oral Medication Labels and Dosage Calculation

Calculating Oral Medication Dosages

1. 2 capsules
2. 2 tablets
3. 1 tablet
4. 1 tablet
5. $\frac{1}{2}$ tablet
6. 2 capsules
7. 4 tablets
8. 4 tablets
9. 1 capsule
10. 1 tablet
11. 2 tablets
12. 2 tablets
13. 1 tablet
14. 2 tablets
15. 2 tablets
16. 2 tablets
17. 4 tablets
18. 2 tablets
19. 4 tablets
20. 1 tablet
21. 10 mL
22. 1.5 mL at bedtime
23. 5 mL
24. 12.5 mL
25. 7.5 mL
26. 1.9 mL
27. 0.5 mL
28. 1 oz per dose
29. 6 mL
30. 5 mL
31. 2.5 mL
32. 2.5 mL
33. 5 mL
34. 20 mL
35. 5.5 mL
36. 3.3 mL
37. 3 oz per dose
38. 3.3 mL
39. 2.5 mL
40. 20 mL

Critical Thinking

1. 480 mg would have been administered to the patient; no, the correct dosage is 120 mg per day, or six 20 mg tablets.

Chapter 12: Reconstitution of Powdered Drugs

Label 1

1. Sterile water for injection
2. 10 mL
3. 500 mg
4. Within 12 hours

Label 2

1. 2 g
2. 20 mL
3. Bacteriostatic water for injection USP with benzyl alcohol
4. 100 mg/mL
5. 48 hours

Label 3

1. One million units
2. 10 mL
3. 1.8 mL
4. 20 mL
5. Package insert
6. Refrigerate
7. Expires at 1:10 a.m. on Dec. 25
8. Your initials
9. Space considerations; handwriting is difficult to read

Label 4

1. azithromycin
2. 500 mg
3. Sterile water for injection
4. 4.8 mL
5. 100 mg per mL

Critical Thinking

1. No, they do not have enough vials on hand to prepare this order.
2. To fulfill this order, 4 vials are needed.
3. If the dose ordered was for 1600 mg of Unasyn® instead, 4.266666 mL must be dispensed. This rounds up to 4.27 mL, which actually provides 1601.25 mg.

Chapter 13: Parenteral Medication Labels and Dosage Calculation

1. 0.3

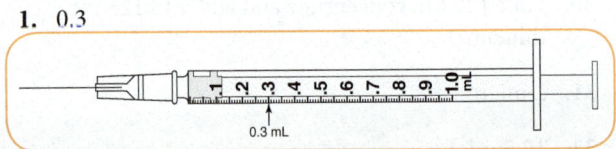

2. 1.6

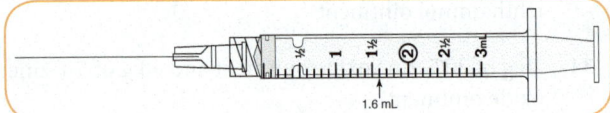

3. 0.4

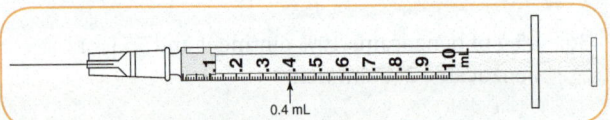

4. 2.5

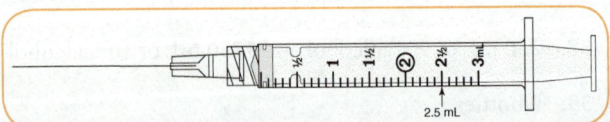

5. 1.2

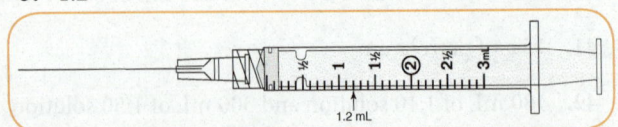

6. 22

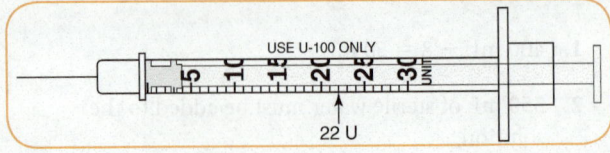

7. 0.8

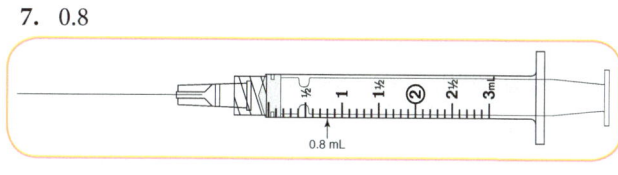

8. 0.6

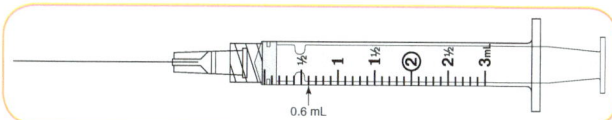

9. 1.4

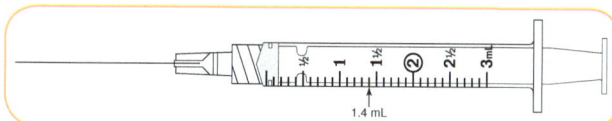

10. 0.75

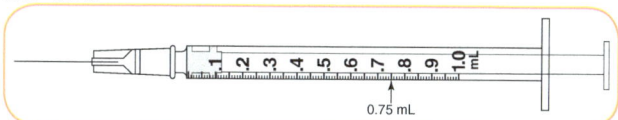

11. 86

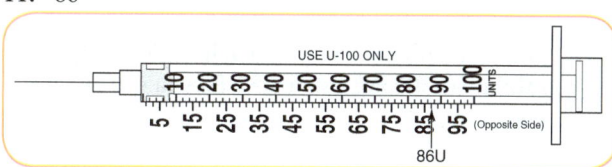

12. 46

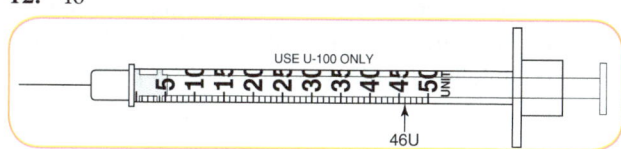

13. 0.7; 1 mL or 3 mL, with 1 mL being best
14. 0.8; 1 mL or 3 mL
15. 1; 1 mL or 3 mL
16. 0.7; 1 mL or 3 mL
17. 6; 10 mL
18. 0.7; 1 mL or 3 mL, with 1 mL being best
19. 0.75; 1 mL or 3 mL, with 1 mL being best
20. 2.5; 3 mL
21. 1.5; 3 mL
22. 2; 3 mL
23. 0.5; 1 mL or 3 mL
24. 0.6; 1 mL or 3 mL, with 1 mL being best
25. 1; 1 mL or 3 mL
26. 0.4; 1 mL
27. 0.7; 1 mL or 3 mL, with 1 mL being best
28. 0.4; 1 mL
29. 0.25; 1 mL
30. 2.5; 3 mL
31. 0.24; 1 mL
32. 0.75; 1 mL

Critical Thinking

1. Compazine would be injected intramuscularly (IM). Therefore, it would be absorbed through the blood capillaries around the muscle injected.

2. There is a possibility of infection and nerve damage due to the patient's lack of knowledge of properly self-injecting.

3. The smallest capacity insulin syringe that can be used is the Standard U-100 insulin syringe.

4. Regular insulin must always be withdrawn from the vial into the syringe first. This prevents contaminating the vial of regular (clear) insulin with the NPH (cloudy) insulin since if contaminated, it can affect the action of the insulin.

Chapter 14: Intravenous Flow Rate Calculations

1. 33
2. 50
3. 67
4. 8
5. 11
6. 15
7. 45
8. 83
9. 21
10. 14
11. 28
12. 33
13. 100
14. 17
15. 25
16. 125
17. 42
18. Assess the patient. If stable, recalculate and reset to 50 gtt/min; observe the patient closely.
19. 42
20. 42

21. 3000 mL
22. Abbott Laboratories
23. 15 gtt/mL
24. 4
25. $$\text{mL/hr} = \frac{500 \text{ mL}}{4 \text{ hrs}} = 125 \text{ mL/hr}$$

$$\frac{\text{mL/hr}}{\text{Drop factor constant}} = \text{gtt/min}$$

$$\frac{125 \text{ mL/hr}}{4} = 31.2 \text{ gtt/min} = 31 \text{ gtt/min}$$

26. $$\frac{V}{T} \times C = \frac{125 \text{ mL}}{60 \text{ min}} \times 15 \text{ gtt/mL}$$

$$= \frac{125 \text{ gtt}}{4 \text{ min}} = 31.3 \text{ gtt/min or } 31 \text{ gtt/min}$$

27. 1930 (or 7:30 p.m.)
28. 250
29. Recalculate 210 mL to infuse over the remaining 2 hours. Reset the IV to 26 gtt/min and observe the patient closely.
30. 125
31. 200 mL/hour
32. 160 mL/hour
33. 14 gtt/min
34. 233 gtt/min
35. 75 gtt/min
36. 35 gtt/min
37. 60 minutes
38. 70.8 or 71 gtt/min
39. 30 gtt/min over 300 minutes (5 hours)
40. 125 mL/hour
41. 66.6 or 67 mL/hour
42. 41.6 or 42 gtt/min
43. 160 gtt/min
44. 30 gtt/min over 1200 minutes (20 hours)
45. 0.5 mL
46. 750 mL/hour
47. 25 gtt/min
48. 55.5 gtt/min
49. 300 mL/hour
50. 25 gtt/min
51. 1125 units/hr
52. 750 units/hr
53. 1575 units/hr
54. 800 units/hr
55. 750 units/hr
56. 1500 units/hr
57. 50 mL/hr
58. 34 mL/hr
59. Total mL ordered (500) ÷ total hr ordered (3) = mL/hr. So, 500 mL ÷ 3 hr = a flow rate of 167 mL per hour.
60. Units per hour is calculated by dividing 25,000 units of heparin by 250 mL, then multiplying the result by 18 mL per hour. So, 25,000 ÷ 250 = 100, which is multiplied by 18. The correct answer is 1800 units per hour.

Critical Thinking

1. 25 gtt/min
2. 10 hours

Chapter 15: Pediatric Drug Administration

1. 1500–1875; 250–312.5; yes; 2.8
2. 35; 2.8; 32.2
3. 25; 2,500,000–6,250,000; 416,667–1,041,667
4. Yes
5. 20; 2.6; 17.4
6. 330–495; 110–165
7. 25; 3.3; 21.7
8. 1.11
9. 1.69
10. 1.92

11. 1.68
12. 1.63
13. 0.69
14. 0.32
15. 0.52
16. 10.8; 5.4
17. 14; 7
18. 3.8; 1.9
19. 1809; 75
20. 1520; 63
21. 240; 10
22. 1250; 52
23. 1.3; 26
24. 13
25. 0.8; 2000
26. 2.7
27. No
28. 1.17; 1.8–2.3
29. 0.52; 42; 0.84
30. 0.43; 108
31. 2.2
32. 6.2; 37.8

Critical Thinking

1. The pharmacy technician should alert the pharmacist.

Chapter 16: Business Math for Pharmacy Technicians

1. d
2. a
3. d
4. d
5. a
6. b
7. b
8. b
9. c
10. d
11. $900
12. $9.38
13. $14.00
14. $2.00

Critical Thinking

1. $4.60 + ($4.60 × 12%) + $1.40 = $6.55

    $6.55 × 30 = $196.50

Appendix C

Case Studies with Answers

1. The physician prescribes dopamine 400 mg in 250 mL D_5W to start at 5 mcg/kg/min in a 55-year-old man weighing 178 lb. The nurse would set the infusion pump to how many milliliters per hour?

   A. 12.8
   B. 15.1
   C. 17.5
   D. 21.1

2. A 60-year-old woman is brought to the hospital because of her hypertensive condition. Her weight is 165 pounds, and her physician prescribed Nipride 3 mcg/kg/min. IV. Nipride 50 mg is added to a 250 mL solution of D_5W. What would be the concentration of Nipride in this solution?

   A. 120 mcg/mL
   B. 150 mcg/mL
   C. 200 mcg/mL
   D. 250 mcg/mL

3. In question 2, by using an infusion pump, the nurse would set the flow rate at how many milliliters per hour?

   A. 47–48
   B. 57–58
   C. 67–68
   D. 97–98

4. A pediatrician ordered Benadryl® for a 9-year-old to relieve itching from chickenpox. Benadryl® comes in an elixir of 12.5 mg/5 mL. The normal adult dose is 25 mg every 12 hours as needed. Which of the following doses would you give?

   A. 5 mg in 2 mL
   B. 5 mg in 4 mL
   C. 7.5 mg in 2 mL
   D. 10 mg in 4 mL

5. A family practitioner prescribed 1.0 mg IM of leucovorin calcium to be administered once a day for the treatment of megaloblastic anemia. The medication is available as a powder in a 50 mg vial. The nurse reconstitutes it with 5.0 mL of sterile water for injection and shakes it well. Solution concentration will yield 10 mg/mL and fluid volume will equal 5.0 mL. How much would the nurse give once a day?

   A. 0.1 mL
   B. 0.3 mL
   C. 0.5 mL
   D. 0.9 mL

6. A pediatrician ordered 100 mg of Augmentin every 8 hours for a 4-year-old. These antibiotics come in a powder for an oral suspension with a concentration of 200 mg/5 mL. The nurse would administer ___ mL for each dose. The child would receive ___ mg and ___ mL in 24 hours.

7. The physician prescribed 0.4 mg of atropine sulfate to be administered intramuscularly. The medication was labeled in grains/mL. The pharmacy technician knew to look for an ampule labeled ___ grains/mL.

8. The physician ordered 120 mg of furosemide to administer intramuscularly every 8 hours for 2 days. The medication is available for injection as 10 mg/mL. How much should the nurse give every 8 hours?

   A. 2 mL
   B. 4 mL
   C. 6 mL
   D. 10 mL

9. A cardiologist prescribes a continuous labetalol infusion to control hypertension. The label indicates that you should remove 90 mL from a 250 mL NSS bag, and add 200 mg of labetalol. The labetalol vial has 5 mg/mL. You would add ___ mL of labetalol to the IV bag. The concentration of labetalol would be ___ mg/mL (remember to include the volume of labetalol in the calculation of the total volume). In order to administer 1 mg/min, you would set the infusion pump at ___ mL/hr.

10. A child was prescribed 1 fluidram of cough syrup, four times a day, as needed. The child's mother wants to know how many teaspoon(s) should be given.

    A. 1
    B. $1\frac{1}{2}$
    C. 2
    D. $2\frac{1}{2}$

11. A physician prescribed 300 mg of Tagamet four times a day. The nurse would administer ___ tablet(s) for each dose. The patient would receive ___ mg of Tagamet in 24 hours.

12. A patient is to receive Nitrostat 20 mcg/min IV. Nitrostat is available in a 10 mL vial labeled 5 mg/mL. To prepare a 200 mcg/mL solution with a concentration of 50 mg in 250 mL, the nurse would add ___ mL of Nitrostat to 250 mL of D_5W, and set the infusion pump flow rate at ___ mL/hr to deliver 20 mcg/min.

13. The usual adult dose for Celebrex is 100 mg twice daily for a total dose of 200 mg/day. How much should a child weighing 52 lb receive per dose?

    A. 49.34 mg
    B. 59.34 mg
    C. 69.34 mg
    D. 82.26 mg

14. A 4-year-old child is to receive 250 mg of Ceclor three times daily. The medicine is available in oral suspension, 250 mg per 5 mL. The nurse would give how many teaspoons?

    A. $\frac{1}{2}$
    B. 1
    C. $1\frac{1}{2}$
    D. 2

15. The physician prescribed an IV of Ringer's lactate at 75 mL/hr. There is a drop factor of 15. How much would the nurse administer to the patient?

    A. 13 gtt/min
    B. 19 gtt/min
    C. 22 gtt/min
    D. 27 gtt/min

16. The nurse increases a lidocaine infusion of 2 g in 250 mL D_5W to 30 mL/hr to control the patient's dysrhythmia. She should document that the patient is now receiving how many milligrams per minute?

    A. 2   C. 4
    B. 3   D. 5

17. Mrs. Brown goes to her participating HMO provider for a checkup and a flu shot. The allowed charge for a checkup is $65, and the physician's usual fee is $70. The allowed charge for the flu shot is $40, and the physician's usual fee is $25. How much is Mrs. Brown charged for the visit?

    A. $7   C. $18
    B. $12   D. Nothing

18. A pharmacy technician has been given 100 mL of a 10% acetic acid solution. The pharmacist asks the technician to dilute the solution to 500 mL with sterile water and to label the solution. What percentage should appear on the label?

    A. 1.5%
    B. 2.0%
    C. 2.5%
    D. 3.0%

19. A drug is available in the following strengths and dosage forms: 125 mg tablets, 250 mg capsules, and 125 mg/5 mL liquid. A child weighs 55 lb and the recommended dose is 10 mg/kg/24 hr (to be given in 6- or 12-hour intervals). Determine which of the following would not be an appropriate dosage regimen using the information provided.

    A. One-half of a 125 mg tablet every 6 hours
    B. 5 mL of 125 mg/5 mL liquid every 12 hours
    C. One 250 mg capsule every 12 hours
    D. One 125 mg tablet every 12 hours

20. The cost of 250 tablets of furosemide 80 mg is $246.84. If your pharmacy marks up the cost by 13% and adds a $2.35 dispensing fee, what would be the retail charge for 60 tablets?

    A. $54.51
    B. $62.43
    C. $69.29
    D. $76.64

21. The pediatrician ordered ampicillin 75 mg/kg/24 hr to be given in divided doses every 8 hours for days. The child weighs 44 lb. The pharmacy has a 150 mL bottle that contains 250 mg/5 mL. What is the patient's weight in kg?

    A. 10 kg
    B. 20 kg
    C. 25 kg
    D. 32 kg

22. A nurse received an order to administer 5 mEq of potassium acetate per hour. The bag of IV fluid contains 30 mEq/L. How many drops per minute would be needed to provide the prescribed dose using a set that delivers 15 gtt/mL?

    A. 26
    B. 42
    C. 51
    D. 64

23. The recommended dose of Demerol® is 6 mg/kg/24 hr for pain. It is given in divided doses every 4 to 6 hours. How many milliliters of Demerol® injection (50 mg/mL) should be administered to a 33 lb child as a single dose every 6 hours?

    A. 0.45 mL
    B. 0.65 mL
    C. 0.85 mL
    D. 1.25 mL

24. A pharmacy technician receives a prescription that orders 12.5% dextrose solution. There are 20% dextrose and 5% dextrose solutions available in stock. If the technician wants to mix these stock solutions, which of the following ratios would be correct?

    A. 1 : 1
    B. 1 : 2
    C. 1 : 3
    D. 2 : 1

25. A patient is to receive cefamandole (Mandol®) 500 mg IM by injection. The vial of powdered medication on hand is labeled Mandol® 1 gram. The directions state: For IM solution, add 3 mL of sterile diluent to provide an approximate volume of 3.5 mL = 1 gram. How many milliliters should the nurse inject?

    A. 1.25
    B. 1.50
    C. 1.75
    D. 2.25

26. The physician prescribed Aldomet 125 mg IV stat for Mrs. Johnston to be added into 100 mL NSS and hung as an intermittent infusion. The medication is available as 250 mg/5 mL. The nurse should prepare how many milliliters?

    A. 1.5
    B. 2.5
    C. 3.5
    D. 4.5

27. A pediatrician ordered Benadryl® 25 mg orally every 8 hours for a 2-year-old child who weighs 16 kg. Pediatric dosage range is 5 mg/kg/day. If this drug is available as 12.5 mg/5 mL, how many milliliters would you give?

    A. 2.5 mL
    B. 5.0 mL
    C. 7.5 mL
    D. 10 mL

28. The physician has prescribed tobramycin sulfate injection (Nebcin®) 70 mg in 100 mL of D_5W via IVPB to be infused in 75 minutes. Nebcin® 80 mg in 2 mL is available. The drop factor of the infusion set is 60. How much Nebcin® should be added to the 100 mL bag of D_5W? ___ mL

    How many drops per minute should be infused to deliver Nebcin® 70 mg in 75 minutes? ___ gtt/min

    If an electronic infusion device is used, the nurse should set the hourly rate at ___ mL/hr.

29. A child is brought to the emergency department with an asthma attack. His weight is 64 lb, and he requires aminophylline IV at 1 mg/kg/hr. The solution is prepared using premixed aminophylline 400 mg in 500 cc D_5W. Which of the following will be the correct rate?

    A. 22.32 mL/hr
    B. 32.46 mL/hr
    C. 64.64 mL/hr
    D. 94.94 mL/hr

30. A pregnant woman was prescribed 60 mg of Fergon® daily. Her cumulative monthly dose (30 days) would be approximately how many grams?

    A. 0.8 g
    B. 1.8 g
    C. 2.8 g
    D. 4.8 g

Answer Key

1. B
2. C
3. C
4. D
5. A
6. 2.5; 300; 7.5
7. $\dfrac{1}{150}$
8. B
9. 40; 1; 60
10. C
11. 1; 1200
12. 10; 6
13. C
14. B
15. B
16. C
17. D
18. B
19. C
20. C
21. B
22. B
23. A
24. A
25. C
26. B
27. D
28. 1.75 or 1.8; 82; 82
29. C
30. B

Glossary

A

alligation A mathematical process that allows for calculation of amounts of substances based on their different percentage strengths. (Ch. 10)

apothecary system A system of measurement that was used in pharmacies until the early twentieth century. It has been replaced by the metric system. (Ch. 1)

Arabic numbers The numerical system commonly used; based on the digits 0, 1, 2, 3, 4, 5, 6, 7, 8, and 9. (Ch. 1)

average wholesale price The national average cost of a drug product for a pharmacy. In practice, however, this is simply a "benchmark" price set by manufacturers. (Ch. 16)

B

body surface area (BSA) Calculated by using a graph called a nomogram that consists of weight and height variables. It is expressed as meters squared (m^2). (Ch. 15)

C

capital assets An asset defined as property, part of a facility, or equipment. They help generate a profit but are not considered to be inventory. (Ch. 16)

capsules Solid oral dosage forms in which a medication is enclosed in a hard or soft soluble container, usually made of gelatin. (Ch. 11)

Celsius scale A temperature measurement scale wherein water freezes at 0 degrees and boils at 100 degrees. Celsius was the last name of the scale's inventor. (Ch. 2)

centigrade Identical to the Celsius scale. The terms are used interchangeably. (Ch. 2)

class A prescription balances One- or two-pan balances that are commonly used by pharmacists. They may be electronic or torsion balances. (Ch. 5)

clinical ratios Common fractions used in dimensional analysis calculations. (Ch. 7)

common fraction A fraction in which both the numerator and denominator are whole numbers as opposed to fractions themselves. (Ch. 3, 6)

complex fraction A fraction in which the numerator or the denominator, or both, may be a whole number, proper fraction, or mixed number. (Ch. 3, 6)

concentrate A highly condensed drug product that is diluted prior to administration. (Ch. 9)

concentration The amount of a particular substance in a given volume. (Ch. 9)

conical graduates Cone-shaped containers with graduated markings for measuring liquids. Their slanted sides may make estimations of quantity difficult. (Ch. 5)

continuous IV infusion Replaces or maintains fluids and electrolytes and serves as a vehicle for medication administration. (Ch. 14)

controllers Devices that are often referred to as electronic flow clamps because they control the infusion rate by either drop counting or volumetric delivery, using gravity to maintain desired flow rates. (Ch. 14)

copayment A specific amount required to be paid by a patient for a prescription. (Ch. 16)

cylindrical graduates Cylinder-shaped containers with graduated markings for measuring liquids. (Ch. 5)

D

D_5W (dextrose 5% in water) In this mixture, the solute is dextrose, and the solvent is water. (Ch. 14)

decimal fraction A fraction with a denominator of 10, 100, 1000, or any multiple or power of 10; also known as a decimal. (Ch. 3)

denominator The number the whole is divided into. (Ch. 3)

desired dosage The amount of a medication that is needed for administration. (Ch. 8)

diluent A liquid such as saline or sterile water mixed with a powder to convert medications into a liquid form. (Ch. 12)

diluents Substances used to dilute another substance, such as solvents used to prepare solutions. When added, they decrease concentrations. (Ch. 10)

dilutions Parts of concentrate in total volume. They make a mixture weaker in concentration. (Ch. 10)

dimensional analysis The process of mathematically changing or converting units of measure; also referred to as unit conversion or units conversion. (Ch. 7)

dividend The number that is being divided. (Ch. 3)

divisor The number performing the division. (Ch. 3)

dosage ordered The amount of a medication in milligrams, grams, and so forth specified by a prescriber for a patient. (Ch. 8)

dosage strength available The amount of medication on hand in milligrams, grams, and so forth. (Ch. 8)

E

electronic balances   Scales that use electronic components and digital readouts to calibrate the weighing of different substances. (Ch. 5)

expenses   Costs associated with the operation of a pharmacy, which are often called overhead. Expenses include salaries, wages, rent, utilities, telephone, insurance, legal and accounting fees, advertising, and depreciation. (Ch. 16)

exponent   A method of expressing a number that is multiplied by itself. (Ch. 1)

extremes   The two outside terms in a ratio. (Ch. 4)

F

Fahrenheit scale   A temperature measurement scale wherein water freezes at 32 degrees and boils at 212 degrees. Fahrenheit was the last name of the scale's inventor. (Ch. 2)

fraction   An expression of division with a number that is the portion or part of a whole. (Ch. 3)

G

gram   The basic unit of weight in the metric system. (Ch. 1)

gross margin   Also called gross profit; the marginal difference between actual cost and total reimbursement. (Ch. 16)

gross profit   The marginal difference between actual cost and total reimbursement. It is also known as gross margin. (Ch. 16)

H

heparin lock   A device attached to the hub of the IV catheter that allows access to the vein for IV push medications; also known as a saline lock or an intermittent peripheral infusion device. (Ch. 14)

household system   A system of measurement primarily used by patients at home. It is less accurate than the metric system. Its most common units of measure include drops, teaspoons, and tablespoons. (Ch. 1)

hypertonic solution   Used to maintain daily fluid needs; is generally a combination of saline, glucose, and potassium chloride. (Ch. 15)

I

improper fraction   A fraction with the numerator larger than or equal to the denominator. (Ch. 3)

infusion pump   A device that maintains flow by displacing fluid at an ordered rate, rather than relying on gravity. (Ch. 14)

intermittent intravenous infusion   Medication administration as a single dose into a vein that has been kept open with an IV catheter. (Ch. 14)

intermittent peripheral infusion device   A device attached to the hub of the IV catheter that allows access to the vein for IV push medications; also known as a heparin lock or a saline lock. (Ch. 14)

international unit   A measurement used to describe potency of vitamins and chemicals. The quantity that measures biological activity, or effect, of substances, developed from the French Système Internationale. (Ch. 1, 13)

inventory   A list of merchandise, itemized by various types, and their cost. (Ch. 16)

inventory control   The process of managing inventory in order to meet customer demand at the lowest possible cost, with a minimum of investment in inventory. Average inventory is calculated by adding beginning and ending inventory, and dividing by two. (Ch. 16)

inventory turnover rate   A specific time period over which the total inventory is sold. The more often this occurs, the higher the turnover rate. (Ch. 16)

IV bolus   A quantity of IV fluid that can be run over a specified period of time through an IV setup attached to the lock. (Ch. 14)

IV push   Drugs that are administered by the direct IV injection route. (Ch. 14)

L

liter   The basic unit of volume in the metric system. (Ch. 1)

M

markup   The difference between the purchase price and the selling price of an item, often expressed as a percentage; markup percentage is calculated by subtracting the purchase price from the selling price, and then dividing by the purchase price. (Ch. 16)

markup method   The cost of a medication based on price and dollar margin on the ingredient cost of the dispensed product. (Ch. 16)

means   The two inside terms in a ratio. (Ch. 4)

meniscus   The bottom portion of the concave surface of a liquid; used to measure the volume of a liquid in a container such as a graduate. (Ch. 5)

meter   The basic unit of length in the metric system. (Ch. 1)

metric conversion   A process of converting between different metric values, such as from milligrams to grams. (Ch. 7)

metric system   The most commonly used system of measurement. It is simple to use because it is based on parts and multiples of 10. (Ch. 1)

milliequivalent   One-thousandth of an equivalent; the mass of a chemical ion that will combine with 1 gram of hydrogen or 8 grams of oxygen. (Ch. 1)

milliunit   One-thousandth of a unit. (Ch. 1)

mixed fraction   A fraction consisting of a whole number and a proper fraction combined. (Ch. 3)

multiplicand A number to be multiplied by another. (Ch. 3)

multiplier A number by which another is multiplied. (Ch. 3)

N

National Formulary A part of the United States Pharmacopeia that contains public pharmacopeia standards. (Ch. 11)

net profit The net amount of money left after all operating or overhead expenses have been subtracted from the gross margin. This amount may be a profit or a loss. (Ch. 16)

nomogram A quick reference graph for calculating pediatric doses. (Ch. 15)

normal saline A general term referring to a sterile solution of sodium chloride in water. (Ch. 9)

numerator The portion of the whole being considered. (Ch. 3)

P

parenteral Injectable. This term indicates medications that are administered other than by the oral (enteral) route. (Ch. 13)

percentages Ratios of numbers to 100; preferred to be used in reference to any lesser amount in relation to a whole amount. (Ch. 4)

percentage solutions Liquid mixtures that may be calculated with percentages pertaining to mass/mass, mass/volume, or volume/volume. (Ch. 13)

pipets Graduated tubes used to transfer small volumes of liquids; also spelled *pipettes*. (Ch. 5)

proper fraction A fraction with the numerator smaller than the denominator. (Ch. 3)

proportion A statement of two equal ratios. (Ch. 4, 6)

Q

quotient The answer to a division problem. (Ch. 3)

R

ratio A statement of the relation of one quantity to another. (Ch. 6)

ratio strength A numerator expressing an active ingredient and a denominator expressing the number of parts of a whole preparation. (Ch. 9)

reconstitution The return of a substance to its original liquid state. (Ch. 12)

return on investment A measure of the percentage of net profit as related to net worth. Net profit divided by net worth, multiplied by 100, gives this percentage. (Ch. 16)

Roman numerals The numerical system in which symbols (letters) are used to represent Arabic numbers. (Ch. 1)

S

safe-dosage range Varying amounts of a drug that can be taken in a single dose and still have therapeutic value. (Ch. 15)

sales The revenue generated by the sale of the pharmacy's inventory (or goods) and services. (Ch. 16)

saline lock A device attached to the hub of the IV catheter that allows access to the vein for IV push medications; also known as a heparin lock or an intermittent peripheral infusion device. (Ch. 14)

scientific notation A shorthand method of expressing numbers that are a product of a number between 1 and 10 and a power of 10. (Ch. 1)

scored Manufactured with a groove or indentation so that it may be easily broken; scored tablets are designed to be broken into one or more pieces so that lower dosages can be administered. (Ch. 11)

solute The substance being dissolved in a solvent to form a solution. (Ch. 9, 12)

solution A liquid preparation of several soluble chemical substances, often dissolved in water. (Ch. 12)

solvents Materials (usually fluids) that can dissolve other substances. Common solvents include water, alcohol, and acetone; often referred to as diluents. (Ch. 10)

syringe pump A kind of electronic infusion pump used to infuse fluids or medications directly from a syringe. (Ch. 14)

Système International (SI) A complete metric system of measurement for scientists. It includes measurements for length, weight, electric current, temperature, matter, and luminous intensity. (Ch. 1)

T

tablets Solid oral dosage forms containing a medication with or without a diluent. (Ch. 11)

tangible An asset that has physical substance, such as inventory, buildings, rolling stock, manufacturing equipment or machinery, and office furniture. (Ch. 16)

temperature The measure of heat associated with metabolism of the body, or from any heat source. (Ch. 2)

third-party payer A company that pays part of the cost of an invoice between a health-care provider and a patient. (Ch. 16)

true proportion A proportion in which the ratios have been proven to be equal by multiplying the means and extremes. (Ch. 6)

turnover A measure of time that a product remains in stock and is not used by a pharmacy. (Ch. 16)

U

unit A standard of measurement based on the biological activity of a drug rather than its weight; used to express measurement quantities of vitamins, some antibiotics, and certain biologics such as vaccines. (Ch. 1, 13)

unit conversion Dimensional analysis; also known as units conversion. This is the process of mathematically changing or converting units of measure. (Ch. 7)

United States Pharmacopeia (USP) An organization that sets official public standards for all prescription and OTC medications, dietary supplements, and other health care products. (Ch. 11)

W

waste control A system used by an organization to dispose of, reduce, reuse, and prevent waste; includes recycling, incineration, landfills, bioremediation, and waste minimization. (Ch. 16)

Index

A

abbreviations
   apothecary system, 14
   household system, 15
   IV, 243–44
   metric system, 9–10
action, timing of, 213
addition
   decimals, 54
   fractions, 42–43
adjusting IV flow rates, 263–64
alligation, 155, 158–62
alligation alternate, 158
ampules, 156
apothecary system, 13–14
Arabic numbers, 4
   conversion between Roman numerals and, 6–7
asset basis, 320
average wholesale price (AWP), 322–23

B

balances, 77
body surface area (BSA), 286
   dosage calculations, 295–98

C

capital asset, 320
capsules, 171–82
Celsius scale, 25
centi-, 9
centigrade, 25
centimeter, 10
children. *See* pediatric drug administration
Clark's rule, 300
Class A prescription balances, 77
clinical ratios, 110
common fractions, 33, 89
complex fractions, 35
components, calculating, 249–51
concentration, 139–42
conical graduates, 79
continuous IV infusions, 243–46
controllers, 268
conversion, 6–7
converting/conversions
   decimals/percentages, 70
   fractions/percentages, 71
   percentages/decimals, 70
   percentages/fractions, 70
   Roman numeral/Arabic systems, 6–7
   temperature, 25–26
copayment, 323
cylindrical graduates, 79

D

daily maintenance fluid needs, 307–8
deci-, 9
deciliter, 9
decimal fraction, 33

decimals, 51–63
  adding, 54
  converting to/from fractions, 52–54
  converting to/from percentages, 70
  dividing, 57–59
  multiplying, 56–57
  rounding, 59
  subtracting, 54–56
declining balance, 320
deka-, 9
denominator, 33
depreciation, 320–21
desired dosage, 129
diluents, 155
dilutions, 155
  liquid, 156–58
dimensional analysis
  basic, 110–12
  calculating IV flow rates using, 258–59
  dosage calculations using, 116–27
discount, 319
division
  decimals, 57–59
  fractions, 45–47
dosage calculations
  ration and proportion expressed using colons, 96
  ration and proportion expressed using common fractions, 91–93
  using dimensional analysis, 116–27
dosage ordered, 129
dosage strength available, 129
drugs, 301–5

E

electronic balances, 77
electronic regulation, 268–71

error, percentage of, 81
expenses, 317
exponents, 11
extremes, 67

F

Fahrenheit scale, 25
formula method, 129–31
  calculating IV flow rates using, 259–61
  use with metric conversions, 131–32
  use with units and milliequivalent calculations, 132–33
fractions, 25–51
  adding, 42–43
  changing percentages to, 70
  changing to percentages, 71
  common, 33
  comparing, 35–36
  complex, 35
  decimal, 33
  definition, 33
  distinguishing types of, 33–35
  dividing, 45–47
  improper, 34–35
  mixed, 35
  multiplying, 44–45
  proper, 33–34
  reducing to lowest terms, 41
  subtracting, 43–44
Fried's rule, 300–301

G

giga-, 9
gram, 8, 9
gross margin, 317
gross profit, 317

H

hecto-, 9
heparin IV calculations, 271–76
heparin lock, 276
household system, 15–16
hyperalimentation, 249
hypertonic solutions, 307

I

improper fractions, 34–35
    converting to/from mixed or whole numbers, 37
infusion pumps, 260
insulin
    dosage combination, 216–23
    injections, 212
    labels, 213–14
    measuring, insulin syringe, 215–16
    mixing, 214
    timing of action, 213
    types of, 212–13
insulin dosage, combination, 216–23
insurance reimbursement, 323
intermittent intravenous infusions, 276–84
intermittent peripheral infusion device, 276
international units (IU), 16, 210
    solutions measured in, 212–23
intramuscular drugs, 301
intravenous drugs, 302–5
inventory, 321
inventory control, 317
inventory turnover, 321–22
inventory turnover rate, 321
IV bolus, 277
IV flow rates, 251–55
    adjusting, 263–68
    calculating units per hour infusing from, 274–76
    calculations
        from units per hour ordered, 273–74
        using dimensional analysis, 258–59
        using formula method, 259–61
        using ratio and proportion, 255–57
        using shortcut method, 262–63
    for electronic regulation, 268–71
IV fluids, percentage in, 248–49
IV piggyback (IVPB), 276–77
IV push, 240–43

K

kilo-, 9
kilogram, 9
kiloliter, 10
kilometer, 10

L

labels
    insulins, 213–14
    oral solutions, 183–89
    tablets/capsules, 171–82
least common denominator (LCD), 39–41
liquid dilutions, 156–58
liter, 8, 10
lo-dose U-100 insulin syringe, 215–16

M

markup, 315–16
markup method, 315
means, 67
measure, unit of, 8
measurements
    volume, 78–81
    weight, 77–78
mega-, 9

meniscus, 79
meter, 8, 10
metric conversions
    equations requiring, 113–15
    use of formula method with, 131–32
metric notation, 10–12
    definition, 10–11
    exponents, 11
    Scientific notation, 11
metric solution labels, 210–11
metric system, 7–12
    abbreviations, 9–10
    definition, 7–8
    metric notation, 10–12
    terminology, 9–10
    unit of measure, 8
micro-, 9
microgram, 9
milli-, 9
milliequivalents, 16–17
    solutions measured as, 223–25
milligram, 9
milliliter, 9
millimeter, 10
milliunit, 16
mixed fractions, 35
mixed numbers, 37
multiple-strength solutions, 205–8
multiplication
    decimals, 56–57
    fractions, 44–45

N

nano-, 9
nanogram, 9
National Bureau of Standards Handbook, 80
National Formulary, 171
net profit, 317–19
nomogram, 295, 297

number systems, 4–6
    Arabic numbers, 4
    Roman numerals, 4–6
numerator, 33

O

oral drug dosages, tablets/capsules, 171–82. *See also* oral solutions
oral solutions
    labels, 183–89
    measurement of, 184
oral syringe, 81

P

parenteral, 210
parenteral drug dosages, calculating, 225–30
parenteral nutrition, 249
partial parenteral nutrition (PPN), 249
pediatric drug administration
    body weight dosage calculations, 287–88
    BSA dosage calculations, 295–98
    calculating pediatric dosages, 286–87
    Clark's rule, 300
    daily maintenance fluid needs, 307–8
    Fried's rule, 300–301
    intramuscular drugs, 301
    intravenous drugs, 302–5
    single-dosage ranges, 288–89
    Young's rule, 300
percent markup, 316
    plus professional fee, 317
percentage in IV fluids, 248–49
percentage of error, 81
    calculating, 81–83
percentage solutions, 211

percentages, 69–75
   converting from/to, 70–71
   determining, 71
pharmacy, common medication temperatures in, 27
pipets, 79
proper fractions, 33–34
proportions, 67–69

Q

quotient, 57

R

ratio and proportion. *See also* proportion
   calculating IV flow rates using, 255–57
   expressed using colons, 95–96
   expressed using common fractions, 89–95
ratio and proportion method
   calculations using different units of measure, 97–98
ratio strength, 148–49
ratios, 65–66, 89
   clinical, 111
   complete, 91
reconstitution, 196
   of multiple-strength solutions, 205–8
   of single-strength solution, 196–205
Roman numerals, 4
   conversion between Arabic numbers and, 6–7
   reading, 4–5
   use of, 6
rounding, 59

S

safe-dosage range, 288–89
sales, 317
saline lock, 276
salvage value, 320
Scientific notation, 11
scored, 171
sensitivity requirement, 78
shortcut method, calculating IV flow rates using, 262–63
single-strength solution, 196–205
solute, 142, 196
solution, 196
solution additives, 246–48
solution labels
   metric, 210–11
   percent and ratio, 211–12
solutions
   measured in international units, 212–23
   measured in milliequivalents, 223–25
solutions, concentrations and volumes of, 139–42
solvents, 155
straight-line, 320
standard U-100 insulin syringe, 215
stock solutions for solids, 156
stock vials, 156
subtraction
   decimals, 54–56
   fractions, 43–44
sum of years' digits (SYD depreciation), 320
syringe pump, 269
syringe, insulin, 215–16
Système International (SI), 8

T

tablets, 171–82
tangibility, 320
temperature
    converting between Celsius and Fahrenheit scales, 25–26
    definition, 25
    in medication, 27
terminology, metric system, 9–10
third-party payer, 323
total parenteral nutrition (TPN), 249
true proportion, 89
turnover, 321

U

unit, 16–17
unit conversion, 110
unit of measure, 8
United States Pharmacopeia, 80
United States Pharmacopeia (USP), 171
units, 210
units of production, 321
useful life, 320

V

volume
    measurements of, 78–81
    per unit volume, 143–45
    and percentage of error, 81–83
volume control set, 303–5

W

waste control, 321
weight
    measurements of, 77–78
    per unit volume, 145–48
    per unit weight, 142–43
    and percentage of error, 81–83
whole numbers, 37
wholesale acquisition cost (WAC), 322

Y

Young's rule, 300